OVARIAN CANCER - A CLINICAL AND TRANSLATIONAL UPDATE

Edited by **Iván Díaz-Padilla**

Ovarian Cancer - A Clinical and Translational Update
http://dx.doi.org/10.5772/56234
Edited by Iván Díaz-Padilla

Contributors

Malgorzata Banys, Natalia Krawczyk, Tanja Fehm, Andreas Hartkopf, Junzo Kigawa, Laurie Elit, Clare J. Reade, Laura Cortesi, Vania Gonçalves, Janica C. Wong, Ronald Fiscus, Sherif Abou Elela, Jean-Philippe Brosseau, Sherri Stewart, Ana Fernández Montes, Maddalena Falagario, Gennaro Cormio, Vera Loizzi, Doriana Scardigno, Luigi E. Selvaggi, Annekathryn Goodman, Jeanine Staples, Constantine Gennatas, Alexandra Leary, Alain Piché, Nadzeya Gocharenko Khaider, Isabelle Matte, Denis Lane, Claudine Rancourt, Gregory Edward Rice, Jorge Tapia, Sebastián Illanes, Mercedes De Alvarado, Lucas Minig, Guadalupe Patrono, Iván Diaz Padilla, Rafael Alvarez Gallego, Javier Valero De Bernabe, Gonzalo Tapia Rico, Ivan Diaz-Padilla

Published by InTech

Janeza Trdine 9, 51000 Rijeka, Croatia

Publishing Process Manager Danijela Duric
Technical Editor InTech DTP team
Cover InTech Design team

Additional hard copies can be obtained from orders@intechopen.com

Ovarian Cancer - A Clinical and Translational Update, Edited by Iván Díaz-Padilla
p. cm.
ISBN 978-953-51-1030-9

For EU product safety concerns:
IN TECH d.o.o., Prolaz Marije Krucifikse Kozulić 3, 51000 Rijeka, Croatia,
info@intechopen.com or visit our website at intechopen.com.

Meet the editor

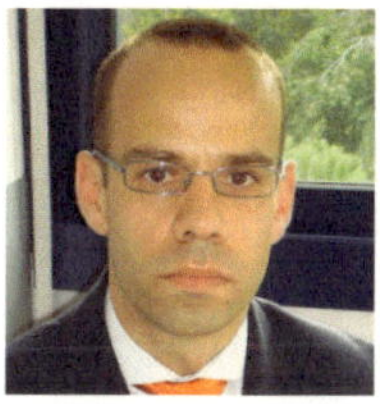

Dr. Ivan Diaz Padilla received his Doctor of Medicine (M.D.) in 2000 from Autonoma University, in Madrid, Spain. He completed his medical oncology training in 2005 at University Hospital La Princesa, Madrid. After a few years serving as staff general medical oncologist in Madrid, Dr. Diaz-Padilla completed a two-year clinical research fellowship in Drug Development and Gynecologic Oncology at the Princess Margaret Hospital in Toronto, Canada. Dr. Diaz-Padilla's main research interest is directed towards an efficient implementation of new molecularly targeted agents into the gynecological cancers. He currently serves as a Consultant Medical Oncologist at the Centro Integral Oncologico Clara Campal in Madrid, Spain. His clinical activity is focused on gynecological cancer and early-phase clinical trials.

Contents

Preface

Ovarian cancer can no longer be considered one disease entity, but a heterogeneous group of diseases. Our understanding of its clinical and molecular complexity is improving notably over the last decade. This is of utmost importance when it comes to determine the most adequate treatment strategy for each individual patient. Despite not being the most frequent tumor, ovarian cancer has the highest mortality rate amongst gynecological cancers. The absence of specific symptoms and the lack of a universally and validated screening strategy leads to a delayed diagnosis, when the tumor has spread beyond the ovaries. Despite most patients are diagnosed at advanced stages, aggressive cytoreductive surgery and combination chemotherapy is recommended. This therapeutic approach may control the disease for some time, but a great majority of patients experience relapses within the first two years of primary treatment. Relapsed ovarian cancer is no longer a curable disease and chemotherapy is the mainstay of treatment in that scenario. Ovarian cancer has been traditionally considered a chemosensitive tumor. However, the development of resistance to cytotoxics is a major problem. New molecularly targeted agents are actively being investigated in an attempt to improve the outcome of this patient population.

Stemmed from the complexity of ovarian cancer, high-scale medical specialization is therefore needed. Ideally, ovarian cancer patients should be treated in tertiary institutions, where higher volumes of complex cytoreductive procedures are performed. It is likely that a strong link with a clinical research facility may also derive in benefit for patients, having immediate access to the latest treatment opportunities within clinical trials. Considerable efforts are also underway in early diagnosis and identification of new biomarkers that may help in predicting response to treatment.

The present book encompasses most of the key aspects pertaining the current of diagnosis and treatment of ovarian cancer. It is intended to cover topics from clinical epidemiology to the latest advances in biomarker development and new drugs. The present publication has counted with the valuable contribution of renowned international experts in the field of ovarian cancer, to whom I want to express my most sincere gratitude. We hope that our target readership (general gynecologists, medical oncologists, gynecologic oncologists) will find this book as a useful and valuable reference in their daily practice.

Ivan Diaz-Padilla, M.D.
Consultant Medical Oncologist
Head, Gynecologic Cancer Program
Centro Integral Oncologico Clara Campal
Hospital Universitario HM Sanchinarro

Section 1

Clinical Epidemiology of Ovarian Cancer

Chapter 1

In what Setting Should Women with Ovarian Cancer Receive Care?

Laurie Elit and Clare Reade

Additional information is available at the end of the chapter

http://dx.doi.org/10.5772/52936

1. Introduction

In Canada, ovarian cancer affects 2600 women and 1750 women die annually from this disease.[1] The case fatality rate for ovarian cancer is quite high at 0.67 because women usually present with wide-spread disease. Symptoms of ovarian cancer are non-specific, and there is no effective screening test which identifies ovarian cancer early, when the cure rate is highest.[2] When patients present with advanced disease, long term survival is elusive and the goals of care focus on increasing duration of survival and improving quality of life by managing symptoms of disease.

Ovarian cancer is usually managed with a combination of surgery and chemotherapy. The role of surgery is to make a histologic diagnosis, determine the extent of disease spread (staging) and remove as much disease as possible (debulking). The role of chemotherapy is to reverse the vascular permeability of tumour capillaries, thereby decreasing the presence of ascites and pleural effusions, and to cause cellular apoptosis of tumour cells, resulting in disease regression.

Evaluation of the patterns of care provided to patients with ovarian cancer in Ontario, Canada demonstrated a variety of specialists are involved in the delivery of surgery including gynaecologists, general surgeons and gynaecologic oncologists.[3] The delivery of chemotherapy can be provided by medical or gynaecologic oncologists. Surgery and/or chemotherapy can be delivered in low, medium or high volume centres in rural or urban settings and by teaching or non-teaching faculty.[3] This paper addresses the question of whether the context in which a woman receives care for her ovarian cancer affects her outcome.

2. Quality of care

The focus of this chapter falls within the rubric of quality of care. The Institute of Medicine has defined quality of care as "the degree to which health services for individuals and populations increase the likelihood of desired health outcomes and are consistent with current professional knowledge".[4] Good quality means providing patients with appropriate services in a technically competent manner, with good communication, shared decision making and cultural sensitivity.[4] Quality assurance can be defined as all those planned and systematic actions necessary to provide adequate confidence that a product or service will satisfy given requirements for quality.[5]

Donabedian originally coined the phrase quality of care.[6,7] He assessed quality of care by looking at the triad of *structures, processes and outcomes*.

Structure attributes describe the physical and organizational settings in which care is provided and evaluate whether these characteristics are conducive to the kind of care that can be expected to improve health and to be acceptable to patients and the community. Evaluation of the adequacy of facilities, qualifications of medical staff, availability of equipment, and organizational structure and operations of programs within the institution providing care fall under the category of structure of care. Often-evaluated structural variables include the demographic characteristics, training and experience of care providers and the environment in which they work. Other structural variables of interest include access to specific technologies, access to intensive care facilities and nurse-to-patient ratios. The most commonly cited variable used as a surrogate for assessing surgical quality is hospital or physician case volume.

Process of care describes the care the patient actually receives and evaluates the degree to which interventions provided to patients correspond to what is known or believed to be most effective in improving health. This includes: 1) the patient's activity in seeking care and carrying it out, and 2) the practitioner's activities in making a diagnosis and recommending and implementing therapy. Whether care is effective can be judged according to the evidence from good studies demonstrating a link between a particular process (ie., debulking surgery) and better outcomes (ie., prolonged survival). Process indicators are easily measured in a timely fashion and can provide actionable feedback for quality improvement initiatives. Other examples of process variables include guidelines for surgery and use of care pathways. These variables are usually used in the context of quality assessment audits.

Outcomes are the actual changes in health and wellbeing obtained by patients and communities, and the degree to which the care provided is acceptable. In other words, outcome is the effect of care on the health status of patients and populations. This may be improvement in patient knowledge, behaviour and satisfaction. Endpoints of interest in ovarian cancer could include 30-day peri-operative mortality, overall survival, and quality of life. Overall survival data takes a long time to mature and it reflects a culmination of many processes and structures that have contributed to care. There is currently a strong focus on outcomes for patients with ovarian cancer, especially in the context of health care payers obtaining high quality care for the health care dollars spent.[8]

http://dx.doi.org/10.5772/52936

To demonstrate the concepts of structure, process and outcomes as ways to measure quality of care in ovarian cancer, we will review population-based studies published over the last 10 years. We have restricted our scope to population-based studies because they provide outcomes for the whole population in a region and avoid biases inherent with single institution studies (ie., related to socioeconomic status, race or comorbidities). As well, population-based studies allow us the opportunity to identify where variations in care may lead to superior outcomes for the population. If these processes and/or structures are incorporated into practice, they may lead to improved health outcomes.

3. Methods

A systematic search of the published English language literature from Jan 1, 2000 to Jun 29, 2012 was undertaken in order to present an unbiased view of the current population-based literature in the field of quality of care. Several key articles were identified[9-11] and MeSH terms from these references were used to create a search strategy for PubMed (Figure 1).

```
http://www.ncbi.nlm.nih.gov/entrez/query.fcgi?CMD=search&term=(genital
neoplasms,
female[mh]+AND+(th[sh]+OR+su[sh]+OR+rt[sh]+OR+dt[sh]+OR+surgery[tiab]+OR+surgi
cal* [tiab]))+AND+(health planning[mh]+OR+"health care quality, access, and
evaluation"[mh]+OR+"outcome and process assessment (health
care)"[mh])+AND+(outcome* [ti]+OR+population* [ti]+OR+treatment
outcome[majr])+AND+2000:2012[dp]+AND+english[la]&db=PubMed
```

Figure 1. PubMed search strategy

The search yielded 1178 articles of which 172 were identified as potentially relevant by title and abstract. To be included the article had to include population-based data collection related to primary management of ovarian cancer. The article needed to report on structure or processes of care in relation to outcomes. Articles were excluded if they were reporting on screening for ovarian cancer, pre-cancerous or benign conditions; if they were focused solely on quality of life, biologic therapies, biomarkers and personalized medicine, survivorship or palliative care. We identified two systematic reviews of quality of care indicators.[12,13] However, in both cases the authors did not restrict their study inclusion to population-based reports, therefore these studies are not included in our analysis.

4. Results

The 30 population-based studies in this review represent findings from many high-income countries, including Australia (1), Canada (3), USA (12), Austria (2), Finland (2), Germany

(1), Netherlands (3), Norway (1), Switzerland (1), UK (3), and Japan (1). Twenty-five unique studies report the impact of structure on outcomes, and 13 studies report the impact of various processes on outcomes. Included are 91,866 patients.

4.1. Outcomes

The 5-year overall survival rate is the indicator of most interest to clinicians caring for patients with ovarian cancer. Other outcomes of interest include quality of life, patient satisfaction, and cost. However, when 5-year survival rates are so poor, surrogate outcomes, including progression-free survival (PFS), can be used to reflect small changes in outcomes that are important to patients and society. Changes in processes or structures that result in improved surrogate outcomes should eventually be reflected in improved 5-year survival rates. Surrogate outcomes in ovarian cancer include PFS and 30 or 60-day mortality.

4.2. Structure

In 25 unique population-based studies of quality of care in ovarian cancer, structural variables evaluated include a hospital's annual ovarian cancer surgical volume, physician annual ovarian cancer surgical volume, hospital type (university affiliated vs community hospital), and physician type (gynaecologic oncologist, general gynaecologist, or general surgeon). These studies are listed in Table 1.

Studies evaluating hospital volume demonstrate hospitals with higher volumes of ovarian cancer surgery per year are often associated with better long-term survival (Table 2). The improvement in overall survival did not appear to be a reflection of peri-operative deaths, because the 30 and 60-day mortality was not affected by hospital volume in the studies evaluating those outcomes. The long-term survival advantage produced by high-volume hospitals is due to other differences in structures and processes of care in these institutions.

Studies evaluating physician volume did not demonstrate a uniform improvement in survival when high-volume physicians operated on patients with ovarian cancer (Table 3). Findings were inconclusive for both shorter and longer-term survival.

In just over half of the studies identified, hospitals classified as teaching facilities or university hospitals were associated with better short and long-term survival outcomes (Table 4). Usually these specialized facilities provide access to physicians with expertise in complicated gynaecologic oncology surgical procedures necessary for appropriate surgical management of ovarian cancer patients.

Studies evaluating physician specialization usually compare outcomes for patients operated by gynaecologic oncologists versus general gynaecologists versus general surgeons. Operation by a gynaecologic oncologist was associated in most studies with better outcomes in terms of long-term survival (Table 5). It is likely that general surgeons are more likely to perform emergency surgeries in advanced situations like bowel obstruction. However, the difference in outcomes persisted even after adjusting for prognostic factors like the Charlson comorbidity score.

Study	Country	Data Source	Number of patients	Did structure impact survival?
Stockton 2000[14]	UK	Retrospective database	989	Yes
Olaitan 2001[15]	UK	Prospective cohort	595	n/a
Carney 2002[16]	USA	Retrospective database	734	Yes
Elit 2002[17]	Canada	Retrospective database	3,815	Yes
Grossi 2002[18]	Australia	Retrospective database + chart review	434	No
Kumpulainen 2002[19]	Finland	Retrospective database	3,851	Yes
Cress 2003[20]	USA	Retrospective database	1,088	n/a
Harlan 2003[21]	USA	Retrospective database	1,167	n/a
Ioka 2004[22]	Japan	Retrospective database	2,450	Yes
Diaz-Montez 2005[23]	USA	Retrospective database	2,417	n/a
Bailey 2006[24]	UK	Prospective cohort	361	No*
Earle 2006[25]	USA	Retrospective database	3,067	Yes
Elit 2006[11]	Canada	Retrospective database	2,502	No
Engelen 2006[26]	Netherlands	Retrospective database + chart review	632	Yes
Goff 2006 and 2007[27,28]	USA	Retrospective database	10,432	n/a
Kumpulainen 2006 and 2009[29,30]	Finland	Prospective cohort	275	Yes
Oberaigner 2006[31]	Austria	Retrospective database	911	Yes
Paulsen 2006[32]	Norway	Prospective registry	198	Yes
Schrag 2006[33]	USA	Retrospective database	2,952	Yes
Elit 2008[34]	Canada	Retrospective database	1,341	No
Bristow 2009[35]	USA	Retrospective database	1,894	Yes
Marth 2009[36]	Austria	Prospective cohort	1,948	Yes
Vernooij 2009[37]	Netherlands	Retrospective cohort	1,077	Yes
Mercado 2010[38]	USA	Retrospective cohort	31,897	Yes
Rochon 2011[39]	Germany	Prospective cohort	476	No

n/a: not applicable—these studies used surrogate outcomes, *the authors of this study reported it was underpowed to find an association between structure and survival

Table 1. Studies reporting on structural variables in relation to outcomes for ovarian cancer

Outcomes	Number of studies finding an association between higher volume and improved outcomes	Number of studies finding no association between volume and outcomes	Total
Overall survival	7	3	10
DFS	1	0	1
30-day mortality	0	2	2
60-day mortality	0	1	1

DFS: disease-free survival

Table 2. Relationship between hospital volume and patient outcomes

Outcome	Number of studies finding an association between higher volume and improved outcomes	Number of studies finding no association between volume and outcomes	Total
Survival	1	2	3
30-day mortality	1	2	3
60-day mortality	0	1	1

Table 3. Relationship between physician volume and patient outcomes

Outcomes	Number of studies finding an association between specialized hospitals and improved outcomes	Number of studies finding no association between hospital type and outcomes	Total
Overall survival	4	3	7
30-day mortality	1	1	2

Table 4. Relationship between hospital type and patient outcomes

Outcomes	Number of studies finding an association between increased physician specialization and improved outcomes	Number of studies finding no association between physician specialization and outcomes	Total
Overall survival	6	3	9
30-day mortality	1	1	2

Table 5. Relationship between physician specialization and patient outcomes

Several studies have reported a link between structural variables (hospital volume, physician volume, hospital type and physician specialization) and outcomes. Population-based studies published over the past ten years identify more consistent evidence linking increased hospital volume and increased physician specialization with long-term outcomes than for other structural variables. Surgery by a gynecologic oncologist appears to provide superior outcomes in terms of long term survival. These studies pertain to the surgical management of patients with ovarian cancer. The single study looking at chemotherapy for ovarian cancer patients found no association between oncologist volume of chemotherapy and outcomes.[11] Of note, no study demonstrated worse outcomes with higher volumes or specialization of hospitals or physicians. Some jurisdictions have used these findings to implement a strategy of centralization of surgery for ovarian cancer in an effort to improve quality of surgical care and outcomes.[40,41]

There are important limitations in this data. Not all studies were able to obtain individual data to allow adjustment for every important confounding variable which can impact survival. The majority of these studies were retrospective or dependant on accurate data-entry into databases. It is possible some of the advantages observed for type or volume of provider may be due to more diligent data-entry and documentation of patient demographics, stage and treatment received. For example, teaching hospitals may have more accurate and detailed documentation of the surgical procedures provided to patients which may lead to an assumption that they provided more complete surgical care when in fact the differences were in documentation only. The use of re-operation as a surrogate outcome is questionable when discussing physician type, since more specialized physicians are typically the ones making the decision to perform a second operation and this decision is more likely to occur if the primary surgery was performed by a less specialized surgeon.

4.3. Process

Evidence-based guidelines on the surgical care of women with ovarian cancer generally recommend hysterectomy, bilateral salpingo-oophorectomy, and omentectomy. In early-stage disease, staging should be performed, including cytology, peritoneal biopsies, and pelvic and para-aortic lymphadenectomy. In late-stage disease, debulking should be performed, including the removal of all macroscopic tumour. This sometimes requires the use of bowel resection, splenectomy, diaphragmatic and peritoneal stripping.[42-44] Adjuvant or neoadjuvant chemotherapy with a combination of a platinum and a taxane agent has been the standard of care for epithelial ovarian cancers over the past ten years.[45] Appropriate surgery and chemotherapy have a demonstrated impact on outcomes for ovarian cancer patients and represent processes of care indicating quality.

Next we look at whether the processes evaluated in the literature are related to the four structural variables reported, and whether these impact on survival.

	Number of studies finding an association between higher volume and improved processes	Number of studies finding no association between volume and processes	Total
Adequate surgery	1	1	2
Optimal debulking	5	1	6
LND	3	0	3
Re-operation	2	0	2
Length of Stay	2	0	2
Complications	0	1	1
Adjuvant chemotherapy	1	0	1

LND: lymph node dissection

Table 6. Relationship between hospital volume and evidence-based processes

Higher hospital volumes of ovarian cancer surgery were associated with better compliance to process steps in the optimal care of women with ovarian cancer (Table 6). These processes included: surgery according to guidelines (optimal debulking, lymph node dissection) and use of adjuvant chemotherapy.

	Number of studies finding an association between higher volume and improved processes	Number of studies finding no association between volume and processes	Total
LND	2	0	2
Optimal debulking	1	0	1
Length of stay	1	0	1
Re-operation	2	0	2
Adjuvant chemotherapy	1	0	1
Complications	0	1	1
Length of Stay	1	0	1

LND: lymph node dissection

Table 7. Relationship between physician volume and evidence-based processes

Surgery by physicians with higher volumes of ovarian cancer surgeries was also associated with better compliance to process steps such as surgery according to guidelines and use of adjuvant chemotherapy (Table 7).

	Number of studies finding an association between specialized hospitals and improved processes	Number of studies finding no association between hospital type and processes	Total
Optimal debulking	3	0	3
LND	6	0	6
Re-operation	1	0	1
Adjuvant chemotherapy	5	0	5
LND: lymph node dissection			

Table 8. Relationship between hospital type and evidence-based processes

Type of hospital (ie. teaching versus non-teaching, academic versus community) where surgery for ovarian cancer is performed was clearly associated with more appropriate surgery and adjuvant chemotherapy in accordance with guidelines (Table 8).

Processes	Number of studies finding an association between increased physician specialization and improved outcomes	Number of studies finding no association between physician specialization and outcomes	Total
Optimal debulking	6	0	6
LND	5	0	5
Re-operation	3	0	3
Adjuvant chemotherapy	4	0	4
LND: lymph node dissection			

Table 9. Relationship between physician specialization and evidence-based processes

Physician specialization (ie., gynaecologic oncologist vs general gynaecologist vs general surgeon) was also associated with appropriate surgery and adjuvant chemotherapy in accordance with guidelines (Table 9).

In summary, 13 population-based studies involving 22,255 patients across 3 continents linked processes of care to improved survival. The relationship of important processes of care with survival is so clear that this work that has led to defining quality indicators for the treatment of ovarian cancer care. In Ontario, Canada, Gagliardi and colleagues[40] used the Delphi technique to define quality indicators. More recently, Verleye and the EORTC has defined and set surgical benchmarks for quality care in ovarian cancer (Table 11., Appendix).[46]

Study	Country	Data Source	Number of patients	Which process variables affected survival?	
				Surgery	Chemo
Bailey 2006[24]	UK	Prospective cohort	361	X	
Chan 2008[47]	USA	Retrospective database	8,372	X	
Elit 2006[11]	Canada	Retrospective database	2,502	X	X
Elit 2008[34]	Canada	Retrospective database	1,341	X	X
Engelen 2006[26]	Netherlands	Retrospective database + chart review	632	X	
Fairfield 2010[48]	USA	Retrospective database	4,589	X	
Grossi 2002[18]	Australia	Retrospective database + chart review	434	X	
Hershman 2004[49]	USA	Retrospective database	236		X
Maas 2005[50]	Netherlands	Retrospective database	1,116	X	X
Marth 2009[36]	Austria	Prospective cohort	1,948	X	
Paulsen 2006[32]	Norway	Prospective registry	198	X	X
Petignat 2007[51]	Switzerland	Retrospective database	50	X	
Rochon 2011[39,52]	Germany	Retrospective database	476	X	X

Table 10. Studies reporting on process variables in relation to outcomes in ovarian cancer

5. Processes or structures of care that require further evaluation

There are many processes considered by experts to be important in the care of women with ovarian cancer. These process variables have face validity but have not yet been clearly evaluated for their impact on outcomes in ovarian cancer. Additionally, the organizational structure for care provision is a complex construct; it is unclear what components contribute most positively to outcomes. We wish to focus on three variables that may or may not be related to survival but may impact treatment and decision making.

5.1. Pathology assessment

When making a diagnosis of ovarian cancer, the histology may be assessed by a pathologist, a pathologist with interest and experience in gynaecologic malignancies, or a subspecialist gynaecologic pathologist. Heatley[53] defines a pathologist as someone who has completed training and passed the appropriate examinations. A pathologist with a special interest (PSI) is a general pathologist who takes the lead in a subspecialty area within their department such as gynaecological pathology, attending meetings of specialist societies, participating in the appropriate subspecialist external quality assurance scheme, providing specialist opinions for colleagues in the department, and on occasion, neighbouring departments. A subspecialist pathologist is a pathologist with a special interest but who now, possibly after a period working as a general pathologist, devotes all or the vast majority of their time to one area of practice.[53] Subspecialisation leads to standardisation of pathology reports and improved communication of findings, participation in multidisciplinary tumour board meetings, enhanced knowledge and standards, decreased turnaround times, quality assurance of diagnoses, improved quality of resident training, ability to distinguish appropriate variation from the standard of care, and advancement of academic knowledge through participation in research.[54]

In gynaecologic oncology, there are several studies reporting up to a 16.9% discrepancy with the referral diagnosis when a PSI or a subspecialist gynaecologic pathologist provides a review of the original pathology.[55] In 4.7% -12% of cases there is a change in diagnosis which has a major therapeutic or prognostic implication.[55-58] Although these findings were from studies including all gynaecologic malignancies rather than ovarian cancer specifically, they demonstrate subspecialist pathology review has an important role to play in the care of patients with ovarian cancer. Verleye and colleagues[59] found that pathology reports for ovarian cancer surgery originating from high-volume centres and academic hospitals are of higher quality than those originating from lower volume or non-academic centres. The availability of subspecialist gynaecologic pathologists may be one structural aspect of care in these centres leading to better outcomes. The impact of expert pathology review in ovarian cancer needs to be evaluated as a process step that could impact survival.

5.2. Multidisciplinary care

Multidisciplinary care is an integrated team-based approach to cancer care where medical and allied health care professionals consider all relevant treatment options and collaboratively develop an individual treatment and care plan for each patient. Evidence in oncology suggests that multidisciplinary care leads to improved survival and quality of life, satisfaction with treatment, and mental well-being of clinicians.[60] An important component of multidisciplinary care is availability of regularly scheduled tumour board meetings[61] with participation of gynaecologic oncologists, pathologists, radiologists, radiation and medical oncologists, and allied health professionals with a special interest in care of gynaecologic oncology patients. Tumour board conferencing in Auckland City Hospital from 2005-2006 led to a 5.9% rate of major changes in patient management.[62] This resulted from radiologic review (major discrepancy rate 1.4%) and pathology review (major discrepancy rate of 4.5%) which led to identification of major diagnostic discrepancies. However, they could not quantify how the changes in diagnosis and management might impact patient outcomes. Santoso did a comparison of the initial gynecologic cancer diagnosis and management plan to the diagnosis and management plan after discussion at a multidisciplinary tumor board meeting. They showed that 6.9% of cases discussed at tumor board had changes made to the diagnosis or plan, and in 5% there were major changes in treatment.[63] The most convincing research suggesting care by a multidisciplinary team is a process that improves outcomes was published by Junor and colleagues using population-based data from Scotland. In a retrospective analysis of all 533 cases of ovarian cancer diagnosed in Scotland in 1987, referral to a multidisciplinary team was one of five factors significantly associated with improved 5 yr survival after adjusting for patient and disease characteristics (hazard ratio 0.60, $p<0.001$).[64]

5.3. Institutional participation in clinical trials

Several studies have identified clinical trial participation as an institutional marker of quality care. In 1994, Stiller published a review of several cancer disease sites and found that across disease sites, patients treated as part of a clinical trial had better outcomes.[65] du Bois and colleagues evaluated outcomes in a population-based cohort of patients diagnosed with ovarian cancer in Germany in 2001.[52] After adjusting for disease stage, patients treated in an institution participating in multi-centre clinical trials had improved overall survival (35 months vs 25 months for patients with stage III-IV ovarian cancer treated at participating vs non-participating hospitals).[39,52] Notably, patients treated in participating hospitals had better outcomes even if they were not themselves participating in a trial. Patients treated in hospitals participating in trials were more likely to receive care in accordance with clinical practice guidelines including staging, debulking and combination chemotherapy where appropriate.[39] Trial participation at an individual patient level may indicate good performance status that can, in and of itself, lead to better outcomes. However, it appears all patients treated at hospitals participating in trials may benefit from improved outcomes. This is likely due to differences in processes of care at these institutions.

6. What does all this mean?

When geographic variation in outcomes exist at a population level, there are opportunities to assess whether changes in structures or processes of care could improve outcomes. There have been several strategies to improve outcome. One is to standardize care using evidence-based guidelines and techniques to optimize processes like a structured care path, whether in a paper chart or as part of an electronic medical record. Another approach to try to improve outcomes at a population level has been to centralize care. In some situations where care requires an experienced surgical team and highly developed perio-operative care, such as for the surgical management of pancreatic cancer, there is evidence that centralization of care to high-volume centres decreases 30-mortality.[66] However, not all reports are consistent with this finding.[67] Another strategy to improve outcomes is to focus on improving processes by the involvement of highly regarded opinion leaders providing education. More consistent improvement in processes of care has been noted using the audit and feedback system.[68] These approaches have been variously referred to as quality assessment, quality management quality improvement and knowledge translation. In this paper, we refer to quality assessment as the audit process whereby performance is measured and compared with a reference standard. Quality improvement includes the steps taken to actively change practice to improve adherence to processes and to improve outcomes.

7. Quality assurance and monitoring

Quality assurance and monitoring of outcomes is essential to allow for quality improvement initiatives. Regions, hospitals, and care providers must understand which outcomes are not reaching a targeted standard in order to identify structures and processes which may improve outcomes. Initiatives such as the International Cancer Benchmarking Partnership[69] have used population-based registry data to identify significant discrepancies in survival for women with ovarian cancer based on geographic location. Striking differences were observed, with women in Australia and Canada having significantly longer survival than women in the UK and Denmark after adjusting for stage.[70]

Measuring the quality of surgical procedures has lagged behind quality-assurance initiatives in other areas because of the difficulty in identifying parameters to evaluate.[71] Early studies suggested operative morbidity and mortality, adequacy of resection, local recurrence and survival as parameters to measure surgical quality.[71] However several of these factors are also highly influenced by the use of appropriate adjuvant therapy. Several programs have now begun systematically tracking outcomes for surgical oncology patients in an effort to identify areas where quality improvement measures should be implemented.

One such program is the American College of Surgeons (ACS) National Surgical Quality Improvement Program (NSQIP).[72] This is a nationally validated, multi-specialty, risk-adjusted 30-day outcomes measurement program which originated in the Veterans Health Administration in 1991. Since 2004, NSQIP has been expanding and now includes more than 400 hospitals in the US, Canada, Lebanon and the UAE. The aim of the program is to provide institutions and surgeons with 30-day outcomes which can be used to compare performance to other institutions. Risk adjustment incorporates pre-operative comorbidities and intra-operative risk factors using hierarchical modelling. Twice per year, institutions are given a report with their risk-adjusted outcomes in the form of odds ratios, which can be used for bench-marking. After implementation of NSQIP in 10 Tennessee hospitals, significantly fewer surgical site infections, failed grafts and flaps, episodes of acute renal failure, and prolonged ventilation of more than 48 hours was achieved.[73] The ACS evaluated outcomes across all participating institutions from 2005 to 2007 and found 66% of hospitals showed improvement in 30-day mortality and 82% of hospitals achieved a reduction in complications after enrollment in the NSQIP program.[74] These improvements also led to significant cost savings. The remarkable success of this program will likely lead to further expansion.

8. Quality improvement

Quality improvement naturally follows from quality assessment. Review of performance in terms of adherence to best-practices (processes of care) in a methodologically rigorous and transparent manner (quality assessment) can lead to improvement in outcomes if interventions are undertaken to improve areas of weakness in performance. Interventions based on quality assurance data attempt to improve processes of care in order to improve outcomes. A framework for quality improvement could include the following steps:[75]

1. Debate and select values and goals that will inform the effort
2. Select a clinical area requiring improvement
3. Select team members
4. Select relevant quality markers for improvement
5. Collect data for selected markers
6. Select and operationalize interventions to achieve improvements in markers
7. Re-evaluate, modify and repeat the steps

The American Society of Clinical Oncology (ASCO) initiated the Quality Oncology Practice Initiative (QOPI)[76] for US-based Hematology-Oncology practices in order to improve quality of cancer care by using measurement and feedback and by providing improvement tools. Processes of care indicative of quality were identified by a group of oncologists using consensus and clinical practice guidelines.[77] QOPI provides individual care providers with quality of care benchmarking information twice per year, allowing clinicians to make improvements within their own practices. Implementation of QOPI and sharing results with physicians at one academic oncology centre in the US led to significant improvements in several areas of quality.[78] Although this program is only available to medical oncology practices in the US, it serves as a good example of how measurement and feedback can lead to improvement in quality of care.

A quality management program was implemented in one German academic oncology centre in 2001 with the aim of improving the quality of surgery provided to patients with ovarian cancer.[79] The components of the quality management system included establishment of a prospective tumour registry, creation and training of dedicated surgical teams operating on patients with advanced ovarian cancer, inter-disciplinary surgical care, intra-operative second opinion by another gynecologic oncologist if the first surgeon did not believe debulking to microscopic residual disease was attainable, interdisciplinary management of complications, and quality conferences including assessment and benchmarking of morbidity and survival outcomes. This effort, along with a significant increase in the volume of ovarian cancer surgery performed at this centre over time, led to a significant improvement in processes and outcomes. Debulking to microscopic residual disease increased from 33% in 1997-2000, and 47% in 2001-2003, to 62% in 2004-2008. This led to median survival of 26 months for patients treated in 1997-2000, 37 months in 2000-2003 and to 45 months in

2004-2008 and 5-year survival in 24%, 34% and 36% of patients in the three time periods. Changes in both structures and processes of care were achieved using this quality management system, leading to improved survival for patients.[79]

A quality improvement program for the surgical care of patients with advanced ovarian cancer was implemented at the Mayo Clinic using an audit and feedback approach, with the aim of increasing the proportion of patients debulked to microscopic residual disease.[44] A surgical complexity score was developed to categorize the aggressiveness of the surgical approach.[80] The quality improvement program consisted of weekly conferences where patient outcomes and treatment approaches were discussed, confidential benchmarking allowing individual surgeons to see their rates of complete surgical debulking in comparison to peers, teaching fellows and staff how to perform techniques needed for complete debulking, and intra-operative mentoring of staff and fellows by surgeons experienced in advanced procedures. After the quality improvement program was implemented, rates of debulking to microscopic disease increased from 31% to 43%.

9. Knowledge translation

Knowledge translation is the science of moving knowledge into action.[81] Several studies across various disciplines in medicine have demonstrated many patients do not receive care known to improve outcomes.[81,82] One of the first groups to show this in ovarian cancer was Munstedt and colleagues who found a large proportion of patients treated in Hesse, Germany between 1997 and 2001 did not receive care recommended in national guidelines.[83] Knowledge translation aims to bridge the gap between what is known from research, and implementation of this knowledge in an effort to improve outcomes for patients and efficiency for the health care system.[81]

Knowledge translation has been described as a cycle, where a clinical problem is identified (possibly by quality assurance or monitoring efforts), processes of care are identified from research to address the problem, these processes are adapted to the local context and any barriers to implementation are identified and addressed, and the new processes are implemented. After implementation, adherence to the process is monitored, and final patient outcomes are evaluated.[81] Evaluation of outcomes and monitoring of processes may then identify additional clinical problems. If no evidence-based solution to the problem is identified, this leads to a need for additional research. In this way, new research informs clinical practice, and problems from clinical practice help to identify research priorities.[82]

A major focus of knowledge translation research is finding ways to change clinician and patient behaviour given the results of research. Simply publishing new findings in peer-reviewed journals, a method termed 'diffusion', is not adequate for wide-spread adoption of new processes.[84] Other methods that have been investigated include audit and feedback,[85] educational outreach by local opinion leaders,[86] and clinical decision support and reminder systems which can be integrated into computer-based patient-care platforms.[87] Audit and feedback, such as the ACS NSQIP or ASCO QOPI programs, are one of the most effective methods for behaviour change in clinicians.[68,88] An excellent overview of these methods has been published by Brouwers and colleagues, who performed a review of systematic reviews on knowledge translation interventions used in cancer control.[68] The science of knowledge translation is relatively new. As research methods continue to improve, strategies are expected to be refined.

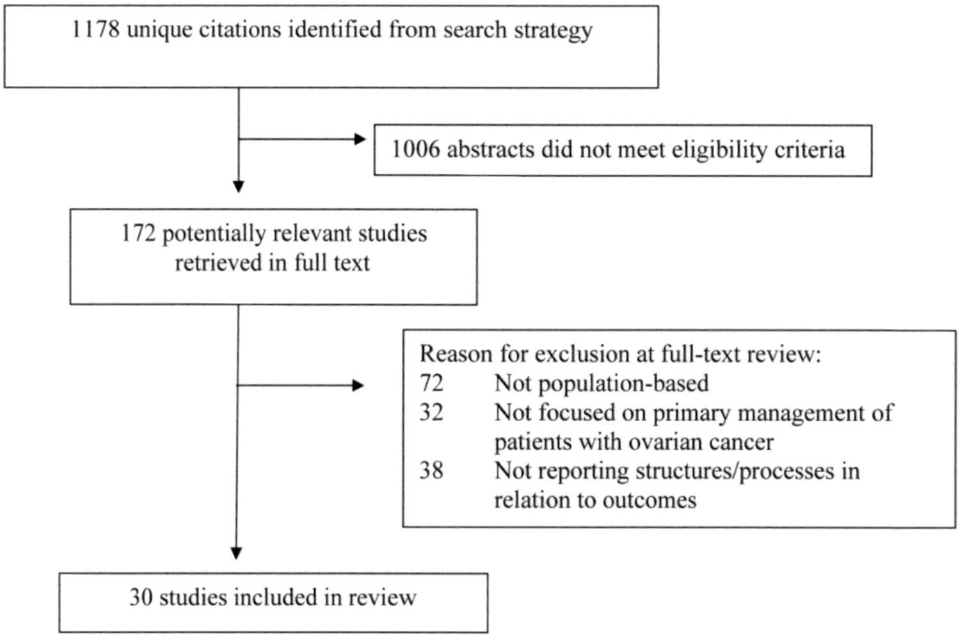

Figure 2. Flow diagram for study selection

10. Conclusion

Women with ovarian cancer should be treated in institutions providing high quality care. Quality of care can be evaluated by examining the processes and structures of care leading to improved outcomes such as survival and quality of life.

In the US, there is a trend to link reimbursement for hospitals and care providers to clinical outcomes in an effort to improve quality of care.[72] Because of financial pressures in the health care system, this trend is expected to continue, since improvement in several metrics used to identify quality surgical care (such as decreased surgical site infections) can save a significant amount of money. Whether health systems are achieving value for money can only be assessed if performance is measured in a systematic way. Tracking outcomes with the use of population-based registries is an essential component of quality assurance, which allows for comparison of outcomes across jurisdictions.[71] Identifying variations in outcomes can then trigger specific quality improvement initiatives. Knowledge translation is

http://dx.doi.org/10.5772/52936

the science of moving knowledge into action, and encompasses both quality assurance and quality improvement. The concepts underlying quality of care are essential information for health care providers caring for women with ovarian cancer given the current global focus on outcomes and value for money in health care systems.

Appendix

Early-stage epithelial ovarian cancer	-Percent of patients with a suspicious ovarian mass undergoing staging laparotomy within 1 month after decision to treat or documented clinical or patient-related reason for delay -Percent of performed staging laparotomies for an ovarian mass suspected to be malignant performed through a vertical incision
	Percent of performed staging laparotomies in which all of the following procedures are included: total hysterectomy, bilateral salpingo-oophorectomy, cytology of the peritoneal cavity, infracolic omentectomy, random peritoneal biopsies and systematic pelvic and para-aortic lymphadenectomy if medium or high risk features
	Percent of surgery reports with documented presence or absence of cyst rupture before or during surgery
	Percent of surgery reports with documented presence or absence of dense adhesions, percent of dense adhesions biopsied
Primary debulking surgery in advanced-stage epithelial ovarian cancer	Percent of patients with advanced-stage ovarian cancer undergoing debulking laparotomy within 31 days after decision to treat or documented clinical or patient-related reason for delay
	Percent of patients undergoing debulking surgery with the spread of disease fully assessed for operability at the start of study and initial findings documented in the operation notes
	Percent of debulking operations including a hysterectomy, bilateral salpingo-oophorectomy and infracolic omentectomy when the surgeon considers optimal debulking feasible
	Percent of debulking operations for advanced ovarian cancer at the end of which complete cytoreduction, defined as no macroscopic residual disease at the end of the operation, was achieved
	Percent of debulking operations including a pelvic and para-aortic lymphadenectomy when otherwise complete debulking has been achieved
	percent of debulking operations for which the size and location of residual disease at the end of the operation is documented in the operation notes

Table 11. EORTC benchmarks for quality surgical care in ovarian cancer[46]

Author details

Laurie Elit[1,2] and Clare Reade[2,3]

1 Dept of Obstetrics and Gynecology, Division of Gynecologic Oncology, McMaster University, Hamilton, Canada

2 Department of Clinical Epidemiology and Biostatistics, Health Research Methodology Program, McMaster University, Hamilton, Canada

3 Division of Gynecologic Oncology, University of Toronto, Toronto, Canada

References

[1] Canadian Cancer Society's Steering Committee on Cancer Statistics. Canadian Cancer Statistics 2012. Toronto, ON: Canadian Cancer Society; May 2012. 0835-2976.

[2] Buys SS, Partridge E, Black A, et al. Effect of screening on ovarian cancer mortality: the Prostate, Lung, Colorectal and Ovarian (PLCO) Cancer Screening Randomized Controlled Trial. JAMA. Jun 8 2011;305(22):2295-2303.

[3] Elit L, Schultz S, Prysbysz R, et al. Chapter 7: Surgery for Ovarian Cancer. In: Urbach D, Simunovic M, Schultz S, eds. Cancer Surgery in Ontario: ICES Atlas. Toronto: Institute for Clinical Evaluative Sciences; 2008.

[4] National Cancer Policy Board, Institute of Medicine, National Research Council. Ensuring Quality Cancer Care: The National Academies Press; 1999.

[5] Hoyle D. ISO 9000 Quality Systems Handbook. 5th ed. Burlington, MA: Butterworth-Heinemann; 2006.

[6] Donabedian A. Evaluating the quality of medical care. Milbank Mem Fund Q. Jul 1966;44(3):Suppl:166-206.

[7] Donabedian A. Contributions of epidemiology to quality assessment and monitoring. Infect Control Hosp Epidemiol. Mar 1990;11(3):117-121.

[8] Hacker NF. Quality control in ovarian cancer surgery. Ann Oncol. Dec 2011;22 Suppl 8:viii19-viii22.

[9] Hillner BE, Smith TJ, Desch CE. Hospital and physician volume or specialization and outcomes in cancer treatment: importance in quality of cancer care. J Clin Oncol. Jun 2000;18(11):2327-2340.

[10] Elit L, Schultz S, Prysbysz R, et al. Patterns of care in the initial management of women with ovarian cancer in Ontario. Eur J Gynaecol Oncol. 2009;30(4):361-364.

[11] Elit L, Chartier C, Oza A, Hirte H, Levine M, Paszat L. Outcomes for systemic therapy in women with ovarian cancer. Gynecol Oncol. Nov 2006;103(2):554-558.

[12] du Bois A, Rochon J, Pfisterer J, Hoskins WJ. Variations in institutional infrastructure, physician specialization and experience, and outcome in ovarian cancer: a systematic review. Gynecol Oncol. Feb 2009;112(2):422-436.

[13] Giede KC, Kieser K, Dodge J, Rosen B. Who should operate on patients with ovarian cancer? An evidence-based review. Gynecol Oncol. Nov 2005;99(2):447-461.

[14] Stockton D, Davies T. Multiple cancer site comparison of adjusted survival by hospital of treatment: an East Anglian study. Br J Cancer. Jan 2000;82(1):208-212.

[15] Olaitan A, Weeks J, Mocroft A, Smith J, Howe K, Murdoch J. The surgical management of women with ovarian cancer in the south west of England. Br J Cancer. Dec 14 2001;85(12):1824-1830.

[16] Carney ME, Lancaster JM, Ford C, Tsodikov A, Wiggins CL. A population-based study of patterns of care for ovarian cancer: who is seen by a gynecologic oncologist and who is not? Gynecol Oncol. Jan 2002;84(1):36-42.

[17] Elit L, Bondy SJ, Paszat L, Przybysz R, Levine M. Outcomes in surgery for ovarian cancer. Gynecol Oncol. Dec 2002;87(3):260-267.

[18] Grossi M, Quinn MA, Thursfield VJ, et al. Ovarian cancer: patterns of care in Victoria during 1993-1995. Med J Aust. Jul 1 2002;177(1):11-16.

[19] Kumpulainen S, Grenman S, Kyyronen P, Pukkala E, Sankila R. Evidence of benefit from centralised treatment of ovarian cancer: a nationwide population-based survival analysis in Finland. Int J Cancer. Dec 10 2002;102(5):541-544.

[20] Cress RD, O'Malley CD, Leiserowitz GS, Campleman SL. Patterns of chemotherapy use for women with ovarian cancer: a population-based study. J Clin Oncol. Apr 15 2003;21(8):1530-1535.

[21] Harlan LC, Clegg LX, Trimble EL. Trends in surgery and chemotherapy for women diagnosed with ovarian cancer in the United States. J Clin Oncol. Sep 15 2003;21(18): 3488-3494.

[22] Ioka A, Tsukuma H, Ajiki W, Oshima A. Influence of hospital procedure volume on ovarian cancer survival in Japan, a country with low incidence of ovarian cancer. Cancer Sci. Mar 2004;95(3):233-237.

[23] Diaz-Montes TP, Zahurak ML, Giuntoli RL, 2nd, et al. Surgical care of elderly women with ovarian cancer: a population-based perspective. Gynecol Oncol. Nov 2005;99(2):352-357.

[24] Bailey J, Murdoch J, Anderson R, Weeks J, Foy C. Stage III and IV ovarian cancer in the South West of England: five-year outcome analysis for cases treated in 1998. Int J Gynecol Cancer. Jan-Feb 2006;16 Suppl 1:25-29.

[25] Earle CC, Schrag D, Neville BA, et al. Effect of surgeon specialty on processes of care and outcomes for ovarian cancer patients. J Natl Cancer Inst. Feb 1 2006;98(3): 172-180.

[26] Engelen MJ, Kos HE, Willemse PH, et al. Surgery by consultant gynecologic oncologists improves survival in patients with ovarian carcinoma. Cancer. Feb 1 2006;106(3):589-598.

[27] Goff BA, Matthews BJ, Wynn M, Muntz HG, Lishner DM, Baldwin L-M. Ovarian cancer: Patterns of surgical care across the United States. Gynecologic Oncology. 2006;103(2):383-390.

[28] Goff BA, Matthews BJ, Larson EH, et al. Predictors of comprehensive surgical treatment in patients with ovarian cancer. Cancer. 2007;109(10):2031-2042.

[29] Kumpulainen S, Kuoppala T, Leminen A, et al. Surgical treatment of ovarian cancer in different hospital categories--a prospective nation-wide study in Finland. Eur J Cancer. Feb 2006;42(3):388-395.

[30] Kumpulainen S, Sankila R, Leminen A, et al. The effect of hospital operative volume, residual tumor and first-line chemotherapy on survival of ovarian cancer - a prospective nation-wide study in Finland. Gynecol Oncol. Nov 2009;115(2):199-203.

[31] Oberaigner W, Stuhlinger W. Influence of department volume on cancer survival for gynaecological cancers--a population-based study in Tyrol, Austria. Gynecol Oncol. Nov 2006;103(2):527-534.

[32] Paulsen T, Kjaerheim K, Kaern J, Tretli S, Trope C. Improved short-term survival for advanced ovarian, tubal, and peritoneal cancer patients operated at teaching hospitals. Int J Gynecol Cancer. Jan-Feb 2006;16 Suppl 1:11-17.

[33] Schrag D, Earle C, Xu F, et al. Associations between hospital and surgeon procedure volumes and patient outcomes after ovarian cancer resection. J Natl Cancer Inst. Feb 1 2006;98(3):163-171.

[34] Elit LM, Bondy SJ, Paszat LP, et al. Surgical outcomes in women with ovarian cancer. Can J Surg. Oct 2008;51(5):346-354.

[35] Bristow RE, Zahurak ML, Diaz-Montes TP, Giuntoli RL, Armstrong DK. Impact of surgeon and hospital ovarian cancer surgical case volume on in-hospital mortality and related short-term outcomes. Gynecol Oncol. Dec 2009;115(3):334-338.

[36] Marth C, Hiebl S, Oberaigner W, Winter R, Leodolter S, Sevelda P. Influence of department volume on survival for ovarian cancer: results from a prospective quality assurance program of the Austrian Association for Gynecologic Oncology. Int J Gynecol Cancer. Jan 2009;19(1):94-102.

[37] Vernooij F, Heintz AP, Coebergh JW, Massuger LF, Witteveen PO, van der Graaf Y. Specialized and high-volume care leads to better outcomes of ovarian cancer treatment in the Netherlands. Gynecol Oncol. Mar 2009;112(3):455-461.

[38] Mercado C, Zingmond D, Karlan BY, et al. Quality of care in advanced ovarian cancer: the importance of provider specialty. Gynecol Oncol. Apr 2010;117(1):18-22.

[39] Rochon J, du Bois A. Clinical research in epithelial ovarian cancer and patients' outcome. Ann Oncol. Nov 2011;22 Suppl 7:vii16-vii19.

[40] Gagliardi AR, Fung MF, Langer B, Stern H, Brown AD. Development of ovarian cancer surgery quality indicators using a modified Delphi approach. Gynecol Oncol. May 2005;97(2):446-456.

[41] Munstedt K, von Georgi R, Misselwitz B, Zygmunt M, Stillger R, Kunzel W. Centralizing surgery for gynecologic oncology--a strategy assuring better quality treatment? Gynecol Oncol. Apr 2003;89(1):4-8.

[42] Bristow RE, Tomacruz RS, Armstrong DK, Trimble EL, Montz FJ. Survival effect of maximal cytoreductive surgery for advanced ovarian carcinoma during the platinum era: a meta-analysis. J Clin Oncol. Mar 1 2002;20(5):1248-1259.

[43] Chi DS, Eisenhauer EL, Zivanovic O, et al. Improved progression-free and overall survival in advanced ovarian cancer as a result of a change in surgical paradigm. Gynecol Oncol. Jul 2009;114(1):26-31.

[44] Aletti GD, Dowdy SC, Gostout BS, et al. Quality improvement in the surgical approach to advanced ovarian cancer: the Mayo Clinic experience. J Am Coll Surg. Apr 2009;208(4):614-620.

[45] Ozols RF, Bundy BN, Greer BE, et al. Phase III trial of carboplatin and paclitaxel compared with cisplatin and paclitaxel in patients with optimally resected stage III ovarian cancer: a Gynecologic Oncology Group study. J Clin Oncol. Sep 1 2003;21(17): 3194-3200.

[46] Verleye L, Ottevanger PB, van der Graaf W, Reed NS, Vergote I. EORTC-GCG process quality indicators for ovarian cancer surgery. Eur J Cancer. Mar 2009;45(4): 517-526.

[47] Chan J, Fuh K, Shin J, et al. The treatment and outcomes of early-stage epithelial ovarian cancer: have we made any progress? Br J Cancer. Apr 8 2008;98(7):1191-1196.

[48] Fairfield KM, Lucas FL, Earle CC, Small L, Trimble EL, Warren JL. Regional variation in cancer-directed surgery and mortality among women with epithelial ovarian cancer in the Medicare population. Cancer. Oct 15 2010;116(20):4840-4848.

[49] Hershman D, Fleischauer AT, Jacobson JS, Grann VR, Sundararajan V, Neugut AI. Patterns and outcomes of chemotherapy for elderly patients with stage II ovarian cancer: a population-based study. Gynecol Oncol. Jan 2004;92(1):293-299.

[50] Maas HA, Kruitwagen RF, Lemmens VE, Goey SH, Janssen-Heijnen ML. The influence of age and co-morbidity on treatment and prognosis of ovarian cancer: a population-based study. Gynecol Oncol. Apr 2005;97(1):104-109.

[51] Petignat P, de Weck D, Goffin F, Vlastos G, Obrist R, Luthi JC. Long-term survival of patients with apparent early-stage (FIGO I-II) epithelial ovarian cancer: a population-based study. Gynecol Obstet Invest. 2007;63(3):132-136.

[52] Du Bois A, Rochon J, Lamparter C, Pfisterer J. Pattern of care and impact of participation in clinical studies on the outcome in ovarian cancer. Int J Gynecol Cancer. Mar-Apr 2005;15(2):183-191.

[53] Heatley MK. Subspecialisation and despecialisation in anatomical pathology. J Clin Pathol. Sep 2010;63(9):761-767.

[54] Chafe S, Honore L, Pearcey R, Capstick V. An analysis of the impact of pathology review in gynecologic cancer. Int J Radiat Oncol Biol Phys. Dec 1 2000;48(5):1433-1438.

[55] Selman AE, Niemann TH, Fowler JM, Copeland LJ. Quality assurance of second opinion pathology in gynecologic oncology. Obstet Gynecol. Aug 1999;94(2):302-306.

[56] Khalifa MA, Dodge J, Covens A, Osborne R, Ackerman I. Slide review in gynecologic oncology ensures completeness of reporting and diagnostic accuracy. Gynecol Oncol. Aug 2003;90(2):425-430.

[57] Santoso JT, Coleman RL, Voet RL, Bernstein SG, Lifshitz S, Miller D. Pathology slide review in gynecologic oncology. Obstet Gynecol. May 1998;91(5 Pt 1):730-734.

[58] Chan YM, Cheung AN, Cheng DK, Ng TY, Ngan HY, Wong LC. Pathology slide review in gynecologic oncology: routine or selective? Gynecol Oncol. Nov 1999;75(2): 267-271.

[59] Verleye L, Ottevanger PB, Kristensen GB, et al. Quality of pathology reports for advanced ovarian cancer: are we missing essential information? An audit of 479 pathology reports from the EORTC-GCG 55971/NCIC-CTG OV13 neoadjuvant trial. Eur J Cancer. Jan 2011;47(1):57-64.

[60] Wilcoxon H, Luxford K, Saunders C, Peterson J, Zorbas H. Multidisciplinary cancer care in Australia: a national audit highlights gaps in care and medico-legal risk for clinicians. Asia Pac J Clin Oncol. Mar 2011;7(1):34-40.

[61] Wright F, De Vito C, Langer B, Hunter A, the Expert Panel on the Multidisciplinary Cancer Conference Standards. Multidisciplinary Cancer Conference Standards. Program in Evidence Based Care. 2006. https://www.cancercare.on.ca/common/pages/UserFile.aspx?fileId=14318. Accessed August 10, 2012.

[62] Cohen P, Tan AL, Penman A. The multidisciplinary tumor conference in gynecologic oncology--does it alter management? Int J Gynecol Cancer. Dec 2009;19(9):1470-1472.

[63] Santoso JT, Schwertner B, Coleman RL, Hannigan EV. Tumor board in gynecologic oncology. Int J Gynecol Cancer. Mar-Apr 2004;14(2):206-209.

[64] Junor EJ, Hole DJ, Gillis CR. Management of ovarian cancer: referral to a multidisciplinary team matters. Br J Cancer. Aug 1994;70(2):363-370.

[65] Stiller CA. Centralised treatment, entry to trials and survival. Br J Cancer. Aug 1994;70(2):352-362.

[66] Simunovic M, Urbach D, Major D, et al. Assessing the volume-outcome hypothesis and region-level quality improvement interventions: pancreas cancer surgery in two Canadian Provinces. Ann Surg Oncol. Oct 2010;17(10):2537-2544.

[67] Massarweh NN, Flum DR, Symons RG, Varghese TK, Pellegrini CA. A critical evaluation of the impact of Leapfrog's evidence-based hospital referral. J Am Coll Surg. Feb 2011;212(2):150-159 e151.

[68] Brouwers MC, Garcia K, Makarski J, Daraz L. The landscape of knowledge translation interventions in cancer control: what do we know and where to next? A review of systematic reviews. Implement Sci. 2011;6:130.

[69] Cancer Research UK. International Cancer Benchmarking Partnership. 2010; http://info.cancerresearchuk.org/spotcancerearly/ICBP/. Accessed August 9, 2012.

[70] Coleman MP, Forman D, Bryant H, et al. Cancer survival in Australia, Canada, Denmark, Norway, Sweden, and the UK, 1995-2007 (the International Cancer Benchmarking Partnership): an analysis of population-based cancer registry data. Lancet. Jan 8 2011;377(9760):127-138.

[71] Landheer ML, Therasse P, van de Velde CJ. The importance of quality assurance in surgical oncology. Eur J Surg Oncol. Sep 2002;28(6):571-602.

[72] American College of Surgeons. ACS NSQIP. 2012; http://site.acsnsqip.org/. Accessed August 9, 2012.

[73] Guillamondegui OD, Gunter OL, Hines L, et al. Using the National Surgical Quality Improvement Program and the Tennessee Surgical Quality Collaborative to improve surgical outcomes. J Am Coll Surg. Apr 2012;214(4):709-714; discussion 714-706.

[74] Hall BL, Hamilton BH, Richards K, Bilimoria KY, Cohen ME, Ko CY. Does surgical quality improve in the American College of Surgeons National Surgical Quality Improvement Program: an evaluation of all participating hospitals. Ann Surg. Sep 2009;250(3):363-376.

[75] Simunovic M, Baxter N. Quality improvement in surgical oncology - measuring and improving clinical outcomes. Surg Oncol. Sep 2011;20(3):179-183.

[76] ASCO. QOPI: The Quality Oncology Practice Initiative. 2012; http://qopi.asco.org/. Accessed August 9, 2012.

[77] Neuss MN, Desch CE, McNiff KK, et al. A process for measuring the quality of cancer care: the Quality Oncology Practice Initiative. J Clin Oncol. Sep 1 2005;23(25): 6233-6239.

[78] Blayney DW, McNiff K, Hanauer D, Miela G, Markstrom D, Neuss M. Implementation of the Quality Oncology Practice Initiative at a university comprehensive cancer center. J Clin Oncol. Aug 10 2009;27(23):3802-3807.

[79] Harter P, Muallem ZM, Buhrmann C, et al. Impact of a structured quality management program on surgical outcome in primary advanced ovarian cancer. Gynecol Oncol. Jun 1 2011;121(3):615-619.

[80] Aletti GD, Santillan A, Eisenhauer EL, et al. A new frontier for quality of care in gynecologic oncology surgery: multi-institutional assessment of short-term outcomes for ovarian cancer using a risk-adjusted model. Gynecol Oncol. Oct 2007;107(1): 99-106.

[81] Graham ID, Logan J, Harrison MB, et al. Lost in knowledge translation: time for a map? J Contin Educ Health Prof. Winter 2006;26(1):13-24.

[82] MacDermid JC, Graham ID. Knowledge translation: putting the "practice" in evidence-based practice. Hand Clin. Feb 2009;25(1):125-143, viii.

[83] Munstedt K, von Georgi R, Zygmunt M, Misselwitz B, Stillger R, Kunzel W. Shortcomings and deficits in surgical treatment of gynecological cancers: a German problem only? Gynecol Oncol. Sep 2002;86(3):337-343.

[84] Farmer AP, Légaré F, Turcot L, et al. Printed educational materials: effects on professional practice and health care outcomes. Cochrane Database of Systematic Reviews. 2008(3). http://www.mrw.interscience.wiley.com/cochrane/clsysrev/articles/CD004398/frame.html.

[85] Ivers N, Jamtvedt G, Flottorp S, et al. Audit and feedback: effects on professional practice and healthcare outcomes. Cochrane Database of Systematic Reviews. 2012(6). http://www.mrw.interscience.wiley.com/cochrane/clsysrev/articles/CD000259/frame.html.

[86] Flodgren G, Parmelli E, Doumit G, et al. Local opinion leaders: effects on professional practice and health care outcomes. Cochrane Database of Systematic Reviews. 2011(8). http://www.mrw.interscience.wiley.com/cochrane/clsysrev/articles/CD000125/frame.html.

[87] Shojania KG, Jennings A, Mayhew A, Ramsay CR, Eccles MP, Grimshaw J. The effects of on-screen, point of care computer reminders on processes and outcomes of care. Cochrane Database of Systematic Reviews. 2009(3). http://www.mrw.interscience.wiley.com/cochrane/clsysrev/articles/CD001096/frame.html.

[88] Grimshaw JM, Thomas RE, MacLennan G, et al. Effectiveness and efficiency of guideline dissemination and implementation strategies. Health Technol Assess. Feb 2004;8(6):iii-iv, 1-72.

Chapter 2

Quality of Life in Ovarian Cancer Treatment and Survivorship

Vânia Gonçalves

Additional information is available at the end of the chapter

http://dx.doi.org/10.5772/54542

1. Introduction

The past two decades have witnessed an unprecedented level of attention devoted to the assessment of Quality of Life (QOL) in cancer patients. This is a result of a major change that occurred in the way cancer management and its impact has been understood and practiced. Contrary to earlier views, which focused primarily on prolonging the quantity of life of the patient, cancer management recognizes now the potential effects of the diagnosis and treatment on the overall functioning and well-being of the patient. QOL issues and its measurement became particularly important in oncology throughout the different phases of the cancer trajectory. In this context, the National Cancer Institute (NCI) has recommended that cancer research focus on both survival and QOL [1]. Many instruments have been developed and used in clinical and research settings. It is noteworthy the inclusion of QOL as one of the main endpoints in important randomized clinical trials [2]. The benefits of studying QOL outcomes are evident. Primarily, QOL measurement has the potential to provide information to guide clinical decision making [3]. The knowledge about the impact of the illness and its treatment on cancer patients can help clinicians and patients to make decisions regarding treatment options and choose appropriate supportive therapy adjusted to the patient's needs. The toxicity and tolerability of a given treatment can be as important as its efficacy, as is the ability to help decrease or prevent associated toxicities that have a negative impact on QOL [4]. Furthermore, QOL data can foster patient-clinician interactions in routine practice, identify problems that have a significant impact on QOL, prioritize problems, develop interventions to deal with these problems and evaluate the impact of palliative and rehabilitative efforts [5]. Additionally, it can help to shape public policy and health care decisions made by governmental and private institutions [6] and allow the economic evaluation of healthcare provision [7].

When considering ovarian cancer in particular, researchers follow the general trend by regarding QOL as one of the most important outcomes. Several reasons make the study of QOL in ovarian cancer patients especially worthy and relevant. First, ovarian cancer is an aggressive illness which is associated with very poor survival and high recurrence rates. It is the most fatal malignancy of the female genital tract and the fourth most common cause of female cancer death [8]. Generally, it is detected at an advance stage, with a 5-year survival rate of 46% for all the stages and 31% for advanced stages [8]. The management of ovarian cancer normally includes radical pelvic surgery and multiple aggressive courses of chemotherapy. The stress of receiving the diagnosis of such an aggressive and life threatening illness, which can be unexpected for many women, may be associated with uncertainty and anxiety about the future. This may be regarded as an immediate threat to a woman's life and an associated fear of death. Additionally, women may suffer disease-related symptoms, which may be very difficult to cope with. These include weight loss, bloating and ascites, fatigue and pain. Women may also experience a wide range of sequalae related to their treatment that do not dissipate with time and may persist for a long-term period [9, 10]. Examples include neutropenia, body distortion, hair loss, bowel and bladder incontinence, loss of taste and appetite, premature menopause, infertility, decrease physical functioning, poor sleep, edema and sexual problems [9, 10]. Another burden involves the amount of time spend in treatments that is lost from family and work [11]. Second, research carried out, specifically, with ovarian cancer patients has shown that a substantial proportion of women experience psychological disorders. Anxiety, depression [9, 12-16] and Post-Traumatic Stress Disorder (PTSD) [17] have been found among different studies. Reports have also highlighted the occurrence of impairments in physical, vocational, social, familial and sexual functioning. Those are not confined to the diagnosis and treatment periods, but have been also observed in short and long-term ovarian cancer survivors. Lastly, advances in Medicine fuelled the development of new treatments for ovarian cancer. However, these treatments have associated side-effects and toxicities that may impact on the QOL of the women. Therefore, when considering a treatment plan, risks and benefits must be balanced in order to achieve an optimal QOL [11]. Improvements in survival in ovarian cancer have been relatively reduced [18]. The ability of chemotherapeutic regimens in slowing the progression of disease to prolong life with active disease has been responsible for those improvements in survival [19]. Undoubtedly, QOL is a fundamental consideration for patients with ovarian cancer.

This chapter addresses the most recent knowledge regarding the impact of the treatment on QOL of ovarian cancer patients. Additionally, QOL in ovarian cancer survivors is also discussed.

2. Quality of life: Brief overview

Central to this particular subject, is the question: What is QOL? Although, it is somehow consensual by the clinical and research communities the importance of studying QOL, it is much less consensual what exactly QOL means. This lack of consensus fuels the appearance of different definitions and, inevitably, means of measurement. This makes difficult the comparison of findings among studies and to establish more definite conclusions. Issues of definition and measurement continue to be, in fact, the subject of ongoing debate. Despite lack of consensus in its definition, it is widely accepted that QOL is a multidimensional construct that includes several important dimensions (any area of behavior or experience) [4, 7, 20, 21]. These encompass physical functioning (physical well-being, mobility, ability to perform self-care activities, physical activities, role activities such as work or housework, appetite, comorbidities, fatigue/sleep, symptoms, side-effects), cognitive and psychological functioning (emotional well-being, anxiety, depression, coping, perceptions, prior experience, enjoyment, optimism), social functioning (family interactions, time with friends, leisure activities), disease and treatment related symptoms (such as pain and fatigue), spiritual or existential concerns, sexual functioning, body image, patient's satisfaction with health care, control of the disease [7, 21]. According to the WHO [22], QOL is defined as 'an individual's perception of their position in life in the context of the culture and value systems in which they live and in relation to their goals, expectations, standards and concerns. It is a broad ranging concept affected in a complex way by the person's physical health, psychological state, level of independence, social relationships, and their relationships to salient features of their environment". Following these lines, QOL includes all aspects of the individual well-being and must be evaluated from the individual's perspective.

When QOL is considered in the context of health, it is often referred to as health-related QOL (HRQOL). HRQOL is a more specific concept, which reflects the effect of the illness and illness treatment on general well-being. Bowling defined HRQOL as 'optimum levels of mental, physical, role (e.g. work, parent, career, etc) and social functioning, including relationships, and perceptions of health, fitness, life satisfaction and well-being. It should also include some assessment of patient´s level of satisfaction with treatment, outcome and health status and with future prospects. It is distinct from QOL as a whole, which would also include adequacy of housing, income and perceptions of immediate environment' [23]. HRQOL is a dynamic concept, as health status deteriorates, experiences, roles and relationships change [24]. Furthermore, It may be modified by impairments, functional status, perceptions, and social opportunities and may be influenced by disease, treatment, and policy [25].

Particularly in ovarian cancer literature, the term QOL is much more extensively used instead of HRQOL. In general, QOL assessment in ovarian cancer patients has been focusing more on the acute phase of the treatment. Of interest is the evaluation of QOL under treatment conditions in randomized clinical trials, focusing on different treatment options. The measurement of QOL in screening and early diagnosis of ovarian cancer is very scarce. It of note that, in fact, screening and early detection of ovarian cancer are very limited in clinical practice, existing narrow useful technologies to assist in early diagnosis. The majority of the QOL measurement in ovarian cancer screening evaluates populations at high risk, such as women with genetic mutations undergoing risk-reducing salpingo-oophorectomy [26]. However, for individuals undergoing risk-reducing salpingo-oophorectomy, screening is more a process of early detection or diagnosis rather than a true screening test [26]. Regarding survivorship, recently, there is a growing interest in the study of QOL in ovarian cancer survivors. The following section focuses on the instruments designed to capture QOL that are more commonly used in this specific population.

3. Measurement of QOL in patients with ovarian cancer

Many instruments have been developed and validated to capture important QOL issues in cancer patients. These instruments comprise four main groups: generic measures of QOL (used to assess non-cancer medical patients), cancer condition-specific (used in general cancer populations), cancer site and treatment-specific instruments. QOL measures are often supplemented by questionnaires designed to evaluate specific dimensions of QOL, for example depression. The use of generic questionnaires allows comparisons of QOL among conditions [7]; however, they lack specificity necessary to understand particular problems inherent to a specific condition, such as cancer. This specificity can be found when disease – and site-specific instruments are used. These are more likely to be responsive to change but are not comprehensive [7]. The Medical Outcome Study (Short Form) MOS SF-36 [27] is an example of a QOL generic instrument used in oncology. The European Organization for Research and Treatment of Cancer QOL Core Questionnaire (EORTC QOL-C30) [28] and the Functional Assessment of Cancer Therapy – General (FACT-G) [20] are examples of condition (cancer) specific instruments. All are self-administered questionnaires, multidimensional, relatively brief, acceptable to patients and have good psychometric properties [7]. The EORTC QOL-C30 and the FACT-G comprise ovarian cancer modules that constitute examples of site specific QOL instruments.

Particularly in ovarian cancer, the most commonly used measures are the EORTC QOL-C30 and the FACT-G [18]. The EORTC QOL-C30 and the FACT-G have a similar format: a core QOL questionnaire applicable to cancer patients in general and specific modules, applicable to specific cancer sites. These instruments have been developed primarily from research environments; however, they will be extremely helpful if they assist physicians in detecting clinically significant differences or changes in a patient condition.

3.1. EORTC QOL-C30

This cancer-specific questionnaire was developed by the Study Group on Quality of Life from the European Organization for Research on Treatment of Cancer comprising a core set of questions applicable to all cancer patients and modules to be used to specific cancer sides, such as ovarian cancer [28, 29]. This instrument was designed to be used in international randomized clinical trials. It is based on a multidimensional model of QOL, covering cancer-specific symptoms of the disease, psychological distress, treatment side-effects, social interaction, physical functioning, body image, sexuality, global health and QOL, and satisfaction with medical care. The core QOL instrument is composed by 30 items, comprising nine scales of QOL: one global QOL scale (2 items), five functional scales (physical functioning, role functioning, cognitive functioning, emotional functioning, social functioning) (15 iems), three symptom scales (fatigue, pain, nausea and vomiting) (7 items), and six single items, assessing additional symptoms commonly reported by cancer patients (breathlessness, difficulty sleeping, appetite loss, constipation, diarrhea, and financial difficulties). Each scale is scored separately. Seven questions have a dichotomous yes/no response. For the two global QOL items, respondents have to answer by using a 7-point scale, where '1 = very poor' and '7 = excellent'. The remaining questions have a four-point Likert scale, ranging from '1 = Not at all' to '4 = Very much'. No timeframe is specified in the seven dichotomous questions. In the remaining questions, the patient has to answer according to the past week. Each dimension score for each patient is the sum of that patient's item responses for that dimension, transformed, so that the minimum possible value is zero and the maximum possible value is 100. Each scale has a limited set of possible values, determined by the number of items and the range of response options for each item. For the functional scales and the global QOL scale, a higher score corresponds to a better QOL. For the symptom scales and the single items, a higher score indicates more frequent and/or intense symptom experience and thus a lower QOL. Finally, there are two items that ask respondents to rate their overall physical condition. The EORTC QOL-C30 has established reliability and validity [28]. This scale is easy to complete, acceptable to patients and has been translated into several languages. The EORTC QOL-OV28 is the ovarian cancer module designed to supplement the EORTC QOL-C30, for the assessment of QOL in ovarian cancer patients in clinical trials and related studies. It consists of 7 subscales and a total of 28 items, which assess abdominal symptoms (abdominal pain, feeling bloated, clothes too tight, changed bowel habit, flatulence, fullness when eating, indigestion), peripheral neuropathy (tingling, numbness, and weakness), other chemotherapy related side effects (hair loss and upset by hair loss, taste change, muscle pain, hearing problem, urinary frequency, and skin problem), hormonal/menopausal symptoms (hot flushes and night sweat), body image (less attractive, dissatisfied with body), attitude to disease and treatment (disease burden, treatment burden, and worry about future) and sexual functioning (interest in sex, sexual activity, enjoyment of sex and dry vagina) [29, 30]. Each scale is scored separately. For symptom scales, a higher score means a lower QOL, while for function scales, such as body image and sexual function, a higher score means a better QOL. The EORTC QOL-OV28 is a valid and reliable measure to be used in ovarian cancer populations [30].

3.2. FACT-G

The FACT-G was developed by Cella et al to evaluate QOL in oncology settings [20]. This is the core scale of the instrument system and consists of four dimensions, comprising a total of 27 items. The dimensions include functional well-being (7 questions), emotional well-being (6 questions), social/family well-being (7 questions) and physical well-being (7 questions). These four dimensions can be analyzed separately or aggregated to produce a total QOL score. Response categories for all items range from 0 (not at all) to 4 (very much). Higher scores are associated with increased satisfaction with QOL. The timeframe for this instrument is the past 7 days. FACT-G is tested and validated in large international samples, showing reliability, validity and responsiveness to change over time [20]. This instrument is commonly used in ovarian cancer clinical trials and it is available in many languages. The supplement of the FACT-G with a set of twelve items specific to ovarian cancer is referred as the Functional Assessment of Cancer Therapy – Ovarian (FACT-O). Items include stomach swelling, losing weight, bowels control, vomiting, hair loss, appetite, appearance, getting around, feeling like a woman, stomach cramping, interest in sex and concerns about ability to have children. The ovarian cancer specific subscale assesses severity of problems that can be targeted by proper disease management. The FACT-O is a valid instrument to be used in ovarian cancer patients [31]. This questionnaire has been commonly used in clinical trials and other descriptive studies. The FACT-O can be used alone or in combination with other scales or subscales of the FACT, such as the FACT/GOG neurotoxicity subscale, or the Anemia (FACT-An) or Fatigue (FACT-F) subscale, if the research interest is these specific issues. The physical well-being and the functional well-being scales of the FACT-G plus the ovarian cancer subscale can be combined to represent the Trial Outcome Index (TOI). This index has excellent psychometric properties [31].

4. Quality of life in ovarian cancer patients

How is the QOL of ovarian cancer patients? Do patients with ovarian cancer experience a good QOL? These are questions that researchers have been attempting to answer in the many studies available dedicated to this subject. The number of studies carried out increased significantly in recent years [18], and collectively, these studies captured ongoing issues and concerns resulting from the ovarian cancer diagnosis and treatment [9]. However, there is a difficulty in drawing definite conclusions to answer the above questions. This is due to the lack of consistency in the types and format of QOL data collected in ovarian cancer patients [18]. The accumulated knowledge about QOL issues in patients undergoing treatment and in survivors of ovarian cancer is presented below.

4.1. QOL during ovarian cancer treatment

The management of ovarian cancer generally requires a multimodal approach. Surgery has always been the cornerstone, which plays an essential role in both diagnosis and treatment. The aim of which is to leave no residual deposits greater than 1–2 cm in diameter. In cases of apparent early stage disease, proper surgical management involves comprehensive surgical staging. Advanced-stage disease frequently requires aggressive surgical debulking [32]. The standard approach is to follow surgery by either intravenous or intraperitoneal chemotherapy. Two classes of cytotoxic components, the plantinums and the taxanes are key components of chemotherapeutic regimens for advanced disease [33]. Both treatment modalities can impact negatively on the QOL of patients [34]. In recurrent disease, a variety of treatment regimens are used, including re-treatment with a platinum and/or taxane agent, and second line agents such as liposomal doxorubicin, topotecan, and gemcitabine. Chemotherapy side effects may be temporary (e.g. hair loss, nausea and vomiting) or cumulative and/or permanent (e.g. fatigue, neurotoxicity) [34].

It is paramount to understand how ovarian cancer and its treatment may disrupt the overall well-being and QOL of patients. A recent systematic review and meta-analysis, carried out to assess and summarize QOL data before, during and after chemotherapy among ovarian cancer patients, found that baseline QOL may significantly improve, particularly after completion of chemotherapy treatment [18]. Authors identified a total of 139 studies; of those, 48 were randomized clinical trials. However, it was only possible to synthesize data from a subset of studies, due to inconsistencies in the way the data was reported across studies. Pooled data showed that QOL as measured by the EORTC QOL C-30 was found to improve during the treatment period and ovarian cancer specific concerns as measured by the FACT-O subscale, were improved during the treatment period [18]. The EORTC QOL C-30, FACT-G and FACT-O found significant improvements in QOL after completion of primary therapy, despite the lack of measurable improvements during treatment as measured by the FACT-G [18]. Following these lines, a recent longitudinal study evaluated the course of QOL, depressive symptoms, anxiety symptoms and fatigue over the course of chemotherapy until 6 months follow-up [35]. Results demonstrated a significant improvement of QOL, as measured by the EORTC QOL C-30 and EORTC QOL OV-28, from the start of chemotherapy and post-surgery period (QOL was severely impaired and high levels of anxiety symptoms, depressive symptoms and fatigue were found), until after care (symptoms reach nearly general population symptom levels). Although, this was a small study of 23 patients, it highlighted the importance of understanding QOL over the course of treatment [35]. Similar results were obtained by other investigators, reporting improvements of QOL in ovarian cancer during chemotherapy until one year follow-up. Von Gruenigen et al [36] in a sample of 42 ovarian cancer patients found that QOL, as measured by the FACT-G and SF-36, markedly decreased after surgery with a slow improvement during adjuvant chemotherapy, mainly in the physical, functional and fatigue domains. Physical functioning decreased during chemotherapy but increased to perioperative levels following treatment. Functional well-being increased following chemotherapy, while emotional and social scores did not change over time [36]. Collectively, these findings highlight that, in addition to chemotherapeutic treatments, surgery may have a negative impact on QOL. Although several factors may influence this impact, tumour stage, and therefore, the extent of the surgical intervention and the existence of intra – or postoperative complications may be crucial [35]. Minig et al [37] found in a study of 181 women with gynaecological cancers, of which 116 had ovarian cancer, that postoperative complications, surgical complexity, advanced stage were associated with lower levels of postsurgical QOL specifically in ovarian cancer patients. The strongest predictor of postsurgical QOL was preoperative QOL, closely followed by surgical complications. Investigators stressed that postoperative complications may be difficult to avoid due to the aggressiveness of the surgery performed in order to achieve maximum cytoreduction in ovarian cancer; however, attention needs to be paid intraoperatively and postoperatively to the early detection of complications to optimize QOL whenever possible in this group of patients [37]. Consequences of surgery are well documented, including loss of fertility, sexual dysfunction, surgical menopause and bowel obstruction. For women at reproductive age, premature menopause and loss of fertility may be devastating [34].

Several clinical trials evaluating ovarian cancer treatments have been carried out, in which QOL is one of the outcomes evaluated. Table 1 describes recent clinical trials that have included QOL as an outcome. QOL measurement in clinical trials has been useful to argue in favor or against novel therapies. Furthermore, there is some evidence demonstrating that QOL is a prognostic indicator for treatment outcomes [26] and future survival [38-41].

Study	Comparison Group	QOL measures	QOL findings
GOG-172[42]	Intraperitoneal (IP) versus intravenous (IV) therapy for first line therapy	FACT-TOI Neurotoxicity and abdominal discomfort subscales	During active treatment, patients on IP had more QOL disruptions when compared to IV therapy
SCOTROC[43]	Carboplatin docetaxel compared with carboplatin paclitaxel for first line therapy	EORTC QOL-C30 EORTC QOL-OV28	Global QOL scores did not differ between treatment arms. Less neurotoxicity was found in the docetaxel group
Vergote (2010)[44] a Gynecologic Cancer Intergroup Collaboration Trial	Neoadjuvant chemotherapy versus primary surgery in stages IIIC or IV	EORTC QOL-C30 EORTC QOL-OV28	No differences in global health scores
OVAR 3[45]	Cisplatin/paclitaxel versus carboplatin/paclitaxel for first line therapy	EORTC QOL-C30	Higher QOL with carboplatin/paclitaxel
Ferrandina (2008)[46] Multicenter Italian Trials in ovarian Cancer group	Pegylated doxorubicin versus gemcitabine for progressive or recurrent disease	EORTC QOL-C30	Higher QOL in the pegylated doxorubicin arm
OV-05[47]	Early versus delayed treatment for recurrent disease	EORTC QOL-C30	QOL decreased shorter in the early treatment arm; significant disadvantages in role, emotional, social and fatigue subscales

Table 1. Some recent clinical trials that have included QOL as an outcome

The aggressiveness of treatments in advanced ovarian cancer patients place more attention upon their QOL than patients diagnosed at an early stage. Several randomized clinical trials have been conducted in the first-line treatment of ovarian cancer. Clinical trials focus in important issues concerning the combination of surgery and chemotherapy, the identification of new targeted therapeutics and the route and timing of chemotherapy administration [48]. Paclitaxel in combination with a platinum compound is considered a standard care as first-line chemotherapy for advanced ovarian cancer. However, paclitaxel is associated with several toxicities (e.g. anemia, thrombocytopenia) that overlap the toxicities of the plantinums, and the co-administration of paclitaxel and a platinum compound can potentially increase the frequency and/or severity of shared toxicities. By itself, paclitaxel is associated with peripheral neuropathy that can add to the disease burden of the patient [4]. Therefore, studies have been conducted to find the least toxic combination of medications used in chemotherapy in order to improve treatment tolerability and QOL [49]. For example, a Phase III Trial conducted by the Scotish Gynaecological Cancer Trials Group (SCOTROC Trial), which included 1077 patients, compared carboplatin docetaxel with carboplatin paclitaxel for first line therapy. Results demonstrated a clear advantage for docetaxel in terms of neurotoxicity [43]. Concurrent with the developments in intravenous treatment, intraperitoneal treatment has also been shown a valuable strategy. The Gynecologic Oncology Group published data from the GOG randomized phase III trial (GOG 172) pertaining QOL outcomes associated with the use of intravenous paclitaxel plus intraperitoneal cisplatin plus paclitaxel, versus intravenous paclitaxel plus cisplatin, for advanced stage cancer [42]. This was the first Phase III GOG ovarian cancer that proposed a change in route for the administration of front-line chemotherapy. In the intraperitoneal arm, overall survival was improved by approximately 16 months; however, during active treatment, patients reported more QOL disruptions, abdominal discomfort and neurotoxicity compared to those patients receiving conventional intravenous chemotherapy. However, only neurotoxicity remained significantly higher for patients in the intraperitoneal arm 12 months post-treatment. Future studies to lessen the added burden associated with intraperitoneal therapy are going [42]. Recently, Vergote et al. [44] reported the results of a Gynaecologic Cancer Intergroup Collaboration Trial which compared upfront debulking followed by chemotherapy to neoadjuvant chemotherapy. This was the first randomized Phase III Trial of neoadjuvant chemotherapy in ovarian cancer using QOL as an endpoint. The two groups reported similar survival outcomes. QOL scores did not differ among the two groups [44].

The majority of ovarian cancer patients will eventually relapse. In fact, it is not uncommon for ovarian cancer patients to undergo numerous chemotherapeutics treatments. In this context, the evaluation of QOL is of utmost importance. In the management of recurrent ovarian cancer, tumour control without compromising QOL should be the goal of the therapy [50]. However, there are deficits in the measurement of general QOL data in the recurrent setting, in terms of QOL disruptions and number of studies including QOL measurements [26]. A recent trial published data pertaining the impact of early versus delayed treatment of recurrent ovarian cancer based on Ca125 measurements exceeding twice the upper limit of normal. Results showed that women did not live longer if chemotherapy was initiated earlier based on Ca125, as opposed to delaying treatment until symptoms developed. In addition, QOL was higher in women who underwent treatment at the time of clinical recurrence [47]. Despite the limitations of this study, these findings may have potential impact on clinical practice.

4.2. QOL in ovarian cancer survivors

Despite the considerable increase in the number of QOL studies carried out in ovarian cancer patients, few studies have focused, particularly, in assessing QOL in ovarian cancer survivors. Although, ovarian cancer patients do not belong to the most prevalent survivor population due to the aggressiveness of the disease and relatively low survival rates, it is of utmost importance to understand the QOL of those women who live years after the diagnosis without symptoms of the disease [9, 51, 52]. QOL has been evaluated namely among small samples of survivors by using mostly the EORTC QOL-C30, EORTC QOL-OV28 and supplemented by several other questionnaires to assess specific dimensions of QOL.

Overall, with the exception of the study conducted by Liaavaaq et al [53], available data suggests that ovarian cancer survivors have generally good QOL; however, specific deficits are reported and these are more prevalent in ovarian cancer survivors that in women without a history of cancer [52, 54-57]. Results concerning psychological functioning are inconsistent, ranging from good emotional status to psychological distress, including PTSD and depression. Below are described with more detail findings from recent studies examining QOL in ovarian cancer survivors.

Results from the study conducted by Steward et al [54] support the view that this group of survivors experiences overall good QOL. These investigators assessed 200 ovarian cancer survivors, who were at the time of the study without active disease and not on treatment, on physical, psychological and social well-being. On average, women had been diagnosed with ovarian cancer in the previous 7 years. Results showed that the majority of the survivors (89%) regarded their health as good or excellent. Participants also reported a better mental health and equivalent energy levels comparing to the general population. However, the majority of the women suffered from pelvic pain and discomfort (54%). Study findings also demonstrated that although 57% of the survivors referred that their sexual life had been negatively affected by the cancer and its treatment, their general sense of loss regarding sexual functioning was perceived as moderate to low. Unsurprisingly, women under 55 years of age reported a greater sense of loss about sexual functioning and fertility. According to these authors, the experience of surviving ovarian cancer appeared to have enriched these women, altering their life priorities and developing on them an impressive resilience [54]. Furthermore, authors highlighted that these survivors showed in general a great pleasure in life and relationships [54]. Similar findings were obtained in the study conducted by Wenzel et al [55], who examined 49 early stage ovarian cancer survivors (> 5 years). Findings revealed that survivors enjoyed a good QOL, with physical, emotional and social well-being comparable to other survivors and same aged samples without a history of cancer. Few deficits were reported, such as problems related to abdominal and gynaecological symptoms, and neurotoxicity. In the emotional domain, scores were more variable, with only one third of the survivors experiencing an excellent emotional well-being. Fears of future diagnostic tests (30%) and recurrence (20%) were also found. Investigators emphasised the resilience and growth that survivors reported in their study as a result of their ovarian cancer experience [55]. Another attempt to understand QOL in ovarian cancer survivors was carried out by Matulonis et al [56], who evaluated 55 early stage survivors. Findings demonstrated that survivors had good physical QOL, with few long-term physical symptoms (such as abdominal complaints and neurotoxicity) and few unmet needs. However, survivors reported emotional problems, such as psychological distress (40%), anxiety about Ca125 testing (54%), fear of recurrence (56%) and 26% had scores suggestive of PTSD. Better mental health was associated with less fatigue and pain, fewer stressful life events and higher social support. The authors reported as well sexual problems, namely pain during sexual intercourse (52%). Less than 10% of participants were interested in sex or were sexually active. Additionally, it was noted that younger survivors presented greater sexual problems. Similarly, Mirabeau-Beale et al [57] who conducted the first comparison between early stage (58 women) and advanced stage (42 women) survivors on QOL (> 3 years), physical, sexual and mental function, reported that survivors experienced positive overall QOL and long-term adjustment. Investigators reported no differences between early stage and advanced stage survivors on overall QOL, unmet needs, social support, complementary therapy use, physical symptoms (neurotoxicity, fatigue and comorbidities), functioning (cognitive, sexual, physical, role, emotional and sexuality), spirituality, hopelessness and psychological state. However, advanced stage survivors experienced better social functioning. Although, the majority of survivors had a good emotional functioning, scores suggestive of PTSD were noted in 7% of early stage survivors. Diagnosable PTSD scores were not found in the advance stage survivors group. Decreased sexual interest attributed to cancer, physical comorbidities, such as degenerative joint disease, gastrointestinal distress and thyroid disease, fear of recurrence, use of complementary and alternative medicines (exercise, vitamins, prayer and massage) in order to improve their QOL were reported by survivors. The most recent account on QOL in ovarian cancer survivors was given by Greimel et al [52], who attempted to fill a gap in the literature by conducting a prospective study on QOL in long-term survivors (> 10 years). This longitudinal study examined survivors at three time points: pre-treatment (baseline), 1-year after diagnosis and 10 years post-treatment using the EORTC QOL-C30. At the baseline, 33 survivors were included; of those, 22 died within 5 years post diagnosis and 11 survived beyond 10 years. In general, results corroborated previous findings reporting that survivors experienced a good physical, psychological, social and spiritual health. Despite no differences at baseline in FIGO stage, residual tumour, performance status and treatment characteristics between short-term and long-term survivors, the latter group experienced better physical functioning, role functioning, cognitive functioning and less symptoms than short-term survivors. Higher levels of symptoms and intra operative ascites were also more prevalent in the short-term survivors group. One year after treatment, the majority of the QOL dimensions were comparable among the two groups; however, long-term survivors reported better global QOL but more insomnia. Emotional functioning and global QOL improved significantly from baseline to 1 year after diagnosis and remained relatively stable in the 10 year follow-up evaluation. Long-term survivors did not experience more sleeping problems 10 years after their diagnosis than women from a general population [52].

Contradicting the trend described above, Liaavaaq et al [53] evaluated 189 ovarian cancer survivors (> 18 months after primary treatment) and found that survivors experienced poorer QOL, had more chronic fatigue and mental morbidity, used more medication and health services when compared to age-adjusted controls from the general population.

Recent studies attempted to improve methodological deficits observed in previous research, for example, by using more standardized and validate measures to assess QOL in this cancer population. However, small sample sizes, heterogeneity of samples, timing of assessment are among the difficulties posed by current research, which make problematic to reach definite conclusions. Despite this, collectively, existing studies highlight important issues and concerns experienced by ovarian cancer survivors. Beyond the expected physical and sexual sequalaes of the illness and treatment, studies highlighted, particularly, psychological difficulties faced by survivors, which may adversely affect their psychological adjustment and well-being. Findings from survivorship research are paramount to provide critical information to guide the development and design of interventions to assist survivors at risk.

The care provided to the cancer patient does not cease when the treatment ends. Survivorship is now recognized as a phase in the cancer trajectory that requires special attention and ongoing specialized care. In 2006, the Institute of Medicine (IOM) published a report on cancer survivorship entitled: 'From cancer patient to cancer survivor: Lost in transition' [58], identifying unique concerns for cancer survivors, recommending the development of a survivorship plan to be developed at the end of treatment for all people treated for cancer of any type. Examples of requirements of the survivorship care plan as recommended by the IOM include, among others, information on possible late and long term effects of treatments and symptoms of such effects, information on the possible effects of cancer on marital/partner relationship, sexual functioning, work and parenting and the potential future need for psychosocial support, referrals to specific follow-up care providers (e.g. rehabilitation, psychology), support groups, and/or the patient's primary care provider.

5. QOL in ovarian cancer: The challenges

Definitely, one of the main challenges in QOL research is to translate and apply the findings obtained in research settings to clinical practice. In fact, in order to fully take advantage of all the benefits offered by QOL research, it is imperative that QOL research provides health care professionals with clinically relevant and interpretable information that can guide treatment decisions. However, routine use of QOL measures has been limited in clinical settings [6]. Challenges of using QOL data to inform clinical practice may include the use of somewhat arbitrary cutoff points or magnitude of change in QOL scores to determine when therapeutic change is needed [26]. To optimize treatment decisions for patients with ovarian cancer, it is paramount that health care professionals are familiar with differences between treatment regimens regarding toxicity, dosage and administration but also findings from QOL measurements [11].

From the research perspective, there is a need for standardized collection and reporting of QOL data from ovarian cancer patients, such as use of common instruments that demonstrate the most sensitivity to the study hypothesis and outcomes of interest, common data collection time points, minimum expectations for data analysis and publication reporting guidelines. These would allow comparative effectiveness research to be carried out [18]. Further larger and rigorous studies are needed to fully understand QOL issues in ovarian cancer patients. Longitudinal studies examining QOL across the different phases of ovarian cancer trajectory would give valuable insights into the QOL of these patients.

As new treatment regimens for ovarian cancer continue to be developed and investigated in the hope of improving survival of patients, it is paramount that QOL is regarded as one of the most important endpoints in clinical trials. However, this is not sufficient. It is as well important to routinely assess QOL disruptions in patients in clinical settings in order to screen and identify patients at risk. Therefore, efforts should also be targeted to the development of interventions to be used in women at need, to prevent or ameliorate the negative impact of the illness on QOL. The assessment of QOL in clinical settings also allows the identification of QOL needs throughout the cancer trajectory.

6. Conclusion

Ovarian cancer patients may experience QOL disruptions and a wide range of sequalae that do not dissipate with time and may persist for a long-term period. Measuring QOL in ovarian cancer patients during the illness trajectory is of utmost importance. This is of great value to develop and design interventions to assist ovarian cancer patients at need, and as well to assist in the therapeutic decision process.

Author details

Vânia Gonçalves

Address all correspondence to: vmo.goncalves@hotmail.com

Relationships, Development and Health Research Line, Institute of Cognitive Psychology, Vocational and Social Development, Faculty of Psychology and Educational Sciences, University of Coimbra, Coimbra, Portugal

References

[1] Arriba LN, Fader AN Frasure HE, von Gruenigen. A review of issues surrounding quality of life among women with ovarian cancer. Gynecologic Oncology 2010; 119 (2): 390-396.

[2] Bottomley A. The cancer patient and quality of life. Oncologist 2002; 7(2):120–125.

[3] Higginson I. Using quality of life measures in the clinical setting. British Medical Journal 2001; 322 (7297): 1297-300.

[4] Penson RT, Wenzel LB, Vergote I, Cella D. Quality of life considerations in gynecologic cancer. FIGO 26th Annual Report on the Results of Treatment in Gynecological Cancer. International Journal of Gynaecology and Obstetrics 2006; 95 Suppl 1:S247-57.

[5] Jacobsen PB, Davis K, Cella D. Assessing quality of life in research and clinical practice. Oncology (Williston Park) 2002; 16(9 Suppl 10):133-139.

[6] Murphy BA, Ridner S, Wells N, Dietrich M. Quality of life research in head and neck cancer: a review of the current state of the science. Critical Reviews in Oncology/Hematology 2007; 62(3):251-67.

[7] Velikova G, Stark D, Selby P. Quality of life instruments in oncology. European Journal of Cancer 1999; 35 (11):1571-80.

[8] Siegel R, Naishadham D, Jemal A. Cancer statistics, 2012. CA: A Cancer Journal for Clinicians. 2012; 62 (5).

[9] Goncalves V. Long-term quality of life in gynaecological cancer survivors. Current Opinion in Obstetrics and Gynaecology 2010;22(1):30-35.

[10] Stavraka C, Ford A, Ghaem-Maghami S, Crook T, Agarwal R, Gabra H, Blagden S.A study of symptoms described by ovarian cancer survivors. Gynecologic Oncology 2012;125(1):59-64.

[11] Grzankowski KS, Carney M. Quality of Life in Ovarian Cancer. Cancer Control 2011; 18(1): 52-58.

[12] Hamilton AB. Psychological aspects of ovarian cancer. Cancer Investigation 1999; 17(5): 335-341.

[13] Bodurka-Bevers D, Basen-Engquist K, Carmack CL, Fitzgerald MA, Wolf JK, de Moor C, Gershenson DM. Depression, anxiety, and quality of life in patients with epithelial ovarian cancer. Gynecologic Oncology 2000; 78(3 Pt 1):302-308.

[14] Hipkins J, Whitworth M, Tarrier N, Jayson G. Social support, anxiety and depression after chemotherapy for ovarian cancer: a prospective study. British Journal of Health Psychology 2004; 9 (Pt 4): 569-581.

[15] Norton TR, Manne SL, Rubin S, Carlson J, Hernandez E, Edelson MI, Rosenblum N, Warshal D, Bergman C. Prevalence and predictors of psychological distress among women with ovarian cancer. Journal of Clinical Oncology 2004; 22(5): 919-926.

[16] Goncalves V, Jayson G, Tarrier N. A longitudinal investigation of psychological morbidity in patients with ovarian cancer. British Journal of Cancer 2008; 99 (11): 1794-1801.

[17] Gonçalves V, Jayson G, Tarrier N. A longitudinal investigation of posttraumatic stress disorder in patients with ovarian cancer. Journal of Psychosomatic Research 2011; 70(5):422-431.

[18] Hess LM, Stehman FB. State of the science in ovarian cancer quality of life research: a systematic review. International Journal of Gynecological Cancer 2012; 22(7): 1273-1280

[19] Huang L, Cronin KA, Johnson KA, et al. Improved survival time: what can survival cure models tell us about population-based survival improvements in late-stage colorectal, ovarian, and testicular cancer? Cancer 2008;112:2289Y2300.

[20] Cella DF, Tulsky DS, Gray G, et al. The Functional assessment of Cancer Therapy (FACT) scale : development and validation of the general measure. Journal of Clinical Oncology 1993; 11(3): 570-579.

[21] Ferrell B, Smith SL, Cullinane CA, et al. Psychological well-being and quality of life in ovarian cancer survivors. Cancer 2003; 98(5):1061–1071.

[22] WHOQOL Group. Measuring Quality of Life: The development of the World Health Organization Quality of Life Instrument (WHOQOL). Geneva: WHO; 1993.

[23] Bowling A. Health-related quality of life: conceptual meaning, use and measurement. Buckingham: Open University Press; 2001.

[24] Morris JN, Suissa S, Sherwood S, and Greer D. Last days: a study of the quality of life of terminally ill cancer patients. Journal of Chronic Diseases, 39 (1): 47-62.

[25] Langenhoff BS, Krabbe PFM, Wobbes T, Ruers TJM. Quality of life as an outcome measure in surgical oncology. British Journal of Surgery 2001;88(5):643–652.

[26] Chase DM, Wenzel L. Health-related quality of life in ovarian cancer patients and its impact on clinical management. Expert Review of Pharmacoeconomics & Outcomes Research 2011;11(4):421-31.

[27] Ware JE Jr, Sherbourne CD. The MOS 36-item short-form health survey (SF-36). I. Conceptual framework and item selection. Medical Care 1992;30(6):473-483.

[28] Aaronson NK, Ahmedzai S, Bergman B, Bullinger M, Cull A, Duez NJ, Filiberti A, Flechtner H, Fleishman SB, de Haes JC, et al. The European Organization for Research and Treatment of Cancer QLQ-C30: a quality-of-life instrument for use in international clinical trials in oncology. Journal of the National Cancer Institute 1993;85(5):365-376.

[29] Cull A, Howat S, Greimel E, Waldenstrom AC, Arraras J, Kudelka A, Chauvenet L, Gould A; EORTC Quality of Life Group [European Organization for Research and Treatment of Cancer]; Scottish Gynaecological Cancer Trials Group. Development of a European Organization for Research and Treatment of Cancer questionnaire module to assess the quality of life of ovarian cancer patients in clinical trials: a progress report. European Journal of Cancer 2001; 37(1):47-53.

[30] Greimel E, Bottomley A, Cull A, Waldenstrom AC, Arraras J, Chauvenet L, Holzner B, Kuljanic K, Lebrec J, D'haese S; EORTC Quality of Life Group and the Quality of Life Unit. An international field study of the reliability and validity of a disease-spe-

cific questionnaire module (the QLQ-OV28) in assessing the quality of life of patients with ovarian cancer. European Journal of Cancer 2003; 39(10):1402-1408.

[31] Basen-Engquist K, Bodurka-Bevers D, Fitzgerald MA, Webster K, Cella D, Hu S, Gershenson DM: Reliability and validity of the functional assessment of cancer therapyo-varian. Journal of Clinical Oncology 2001, 19(6):1809–1817.

[32] Chi D, Hoskins J, 2000. Primary Surgical Management of Ovarian Cancer. In: Bartlett JMS (ed), Ovarian Cancer: Methods and Protocols. New Jersey: Human Press; 2000. p75-88.

[33] Kaye SB. Future directions for the management of ovarian cancer. European Journal of Cancer 2001; 37 (suppl 9): S19-S23.

[34] Sun CC, Ramirez PT, Bodurka DC. Quality of life for patients with epithelial ovarian cancer. Nature Clinical Practice Oncology 2007 ;4(1):18-29.

[35] Meraner V, Gamper EM, Grahmann A, Giesinger JM, Wiesbauer P, Sztankay M, Zeimet AG, Sperner-Unterweger B, Holzner B. Monitoring physical and psychosocial symptom trajectories in ovarian cancer patients receiving chemotherapy. BMC Cancer 2012; 28,12:77.

[36] von Gruenigen VE, Frasure HE, Jenison EL, Hopkins MP, Gil KM. Longitudinal assessment of quality of life and lifestyle in newly diagnosed ovarian cancer patients: The roles of surgery and chemotherapy. Gynecologic Oncology 2006;103 (1):120–126.

[37] Minig L, Vélez JI, Trimble EL, Biffi R, Maggioni A, Jeffery DD. Changes in short-term health-related quality of life in women undergoing gynecologic oncologic laparotomy: an associated factor analysis. Supportive Care Cancer 2012 Aug 29.

[38] Mutch DG, Orlando M, Goss T, Teneriello MG, Gordon AN, McMeekin SD, Wang Y, Scribner DR Jr, Marciniack M, Naumann RW, Secord AA. Randomized phase III trial of gemcitabine compared with pegylated liposomal doxorubicin in patients with platinum-resistant ovarian cancer. Journal of Clinical Oncology 2007;25(19): 2811-2818.

[39] Carey MS, Bacon M, Tu D, Butler L, Bezjak A, Stuart GC. The prognostic effects of performance status and quality of life scores on progression-free survival and overall survival in advanced ovarian cancer. Gynecologic Oncology 2008; 108(1):100-5.

[40] Gupta D, Grutsch JF, Lis CG. Patient satisfaction with quality of life as a prognostic indicator in ovarian cancer patients treated in an integrative treatment setting. Journal of the Society for Integrative Oncology 2008; 6(3):98-104.

[41] von Gruenigen VE, Huang HQ, Gil KM, Frasure HE, Armstrong DK, Wenzel LB. The association between quality of life domains and overall survival in ovarian cancer patients during adjuvant chemotherapy: a Gynecologic Oncology Group Study. Gynecologic Oncology 2012;124(3):379-382.

[42] Wenzel LB, Huang HQ, Armstrong DK, Walker JL, Cella D; Gynecologic Oncology Group. Health-related quality of life during and after intraperitoneal versus intrave-

nous chemotherapy for optimally debulked ovarian cancer: a Gynecologic Oncology Group Study. Journal of Clinical Oncology 2007; 25(4):437-443.

[43] Vasey PA, Jayson GC, Gordon A, Gabra H, Coleman R, Atkinson R, Parkin D, Paul J, Hay A, Kaye SB; Scottish Gynaecological Cancer Trials Group. Phase III randomized trial of docetaxel-carboplatin versus paclitaxel-carboplatin as first-line chemotherapy for ovarian carcinoma. Journal of the National Cancer Institue 2004; 96(22):1682-1691.

[44] Vergote I, Tropé CG, Amant F, Kristensen GB, Ehlen T, Johnson N, Verheijen RH, van der Burg ME, Lacave AJ, Panici PB, Kenter GG, Casado A, Mendiola C, Coens C, Verleye L, Stuart GC, Pecorelli S, Reed NS; European Organization for Research and Treatment of Cancer-Gynaecological Cancer Group; NCIC Clinical Trials Group. Neoadjuvant chemotherapy or primary surgery in stage IIIC or IV ovarian cancer. The New England Journal of Medicine 2010; 363(10):943-953.

[45] du Bois A, Lück HJ, Meier W, Adams HP, Möbus V, Costa S, Bauknecht T, Richter B, Warm M, Schröder W, Olbricht S, Nitz U, Jackisch C, Emons G, Wagner U, Kuhn W, Pfisterer J; Arbeitsgemeinschaft Gynäkologische Onkologie Ovarian Cancer Study Group. A randomized clinical trial of cisplatin/paclitaxel versus carboplatin/paclitaxel as first-line treatment of ovarian cancer. The New England Journal of Medicine 2003; 95(17):1320-1329.

[46] Ferrandina G, Ludovisi M, Lorusso D, Pignata S, Breda E, Savarese A, Del Medico P, Scaltriti L, Katsaros D, Priolo D, Scambia G. Phase III trial of gemcitabine compared with pegylated liposomal doxorubicin in progressive or recurrent ovarian cancer. Journal of Clinical Oncology 2008; 26(6):890-896.

[47] Rustin GJ, van der Burg ME, Griffin CL, Guthrie D, Lamont A, Jayson GC, Kristensen G, Mediola C, Coens C, Qian W, Parmar MK, Swart AM; MRC OV05; EORTC 55955 investigators.Early versus delayed treatment of relapsed ovarian cancer (MRC OV05/ EORTC 55955): a randomised trial. Lancet 2010; 376(9747):1155-1163.

[48] Gardner GJ, Jewell EL. Current and future directions of clinical trials for ovarian cancer. Cancer Control 2011;18(1):44-51.

[49] Guastalla JP 3rd, Diéras V.The taxanes: toxicity and quality of life considerations in advanced ovarian cancer. British Journal of Cancer 2003; 89 Suppl 3:S16-22.

[50] Greimel ER, Bjelic-Radisic V, Pfisterer J, Hilpert F, Daghofer F, du Bois A; Arbeitsgemeinschaft Gynaekologische Onkologie Ovarian Cancer Study Group. Randomized study of the Arbeitsgemeinschaft Gynaekologische Onkologie Ovarian Cancer Study Group comparing quality of life in patients with ovarian cancer treated with cisplatin/paclitaxel versus carboplatin/paclitaxel. Journal of Clinical Oncology 2006;24(4): 579-586.

[51] Bloom JR, Petersen DM, Kang SH. Multi-dimensional quality of life among long-term (5+ years) adult cancer survivors. Psychooncology 2007; 16(8):691-706.

[52] Greimel E, Daghofer F, Petru E. Prospective assessment of quality of life in long-term ovarian cancer survivors. International Journal of Cancer 2011; 128(12):3005-3011

[53] Liavaag AH, Dørum A, Fosså SD, Tropé C, Dahl AA. Controlled study of fatigue, quality of life, and somatic and mental morbidity in epithelial ovarian cancer survivors: how lucky are the lucky ones? Journal of Clinical Oncology 2007;25(15): 2049-2056.

[54] Stewart DE, Wong F, Duff S, Melancon CH, Cheung AM. "What doesn't kill you makes you stronger": an ovarian cancer survivor survey. Gynecologic Oncology 2001; 83(3):537-542.

[55] Wenzel LB, Donnelly JP, Fowler JM, Habbal R, Taylor TH, Aziz N, Cella D.Resilience, reflection, and residual stress in ovarian cancer survivorship: a gynecologic oncology group study. Psychooncology 2002; 11(2):142-153.

[56] Matulonis UA, Kornblith A, Lee H, Bryan J, Gibson C, Wells C, Lee J, Sullivan L, Penson R. Long-term adjustment of early-stage ovarian cancer survivors. International Journal of Gynecological Cancer 2008; 18(6):1183-1193.

[57] Mirabeau-Beale KL, Kornblith AB, Penson RT, Lee H, Goodman A, Campos SM, Duska L, Pereira L, Bryan J, Matulonis UA. Comparison of the quality of life of early and advanced stage ovarian cancer survivors. Gynecologic Oncology 2009;114(2): 353-359.

[58] Hewitt M, Greenfield S, Stovall E. From cancer patient to cancer survivor: lost in transition. Washington, DC: National Academic Press; 2006.

Chapter 3

Preventive Strategies for Ovarian Cancer

L. Cortesi, A. Toss and E. De Matteis

Additional information is available at the end of the chapter

http://dx.doi.org/10.5772/54686

1. Introduction

According to the American Cancer Society, in 2012 ovarian cancer is expected to account for 3% (22,280) of all new cases and 6% (15,500) of all female cancer deaths in the United States. The proportion of ovarian cancer among gynaecological cancers is increasing, also because of the decrease in cervical cancer as a result of pap smear screening programmes. On the other hand, survival from ovarian cancer is the poorest of all gynaecological cancers, with a five-year relative survival rate of 44% for all stages [1,2]. The main reasons for this poor survival are the lack of early detection strategies and an unfavourable anatomical situation. Thus, the vast majority of ovarian cancer is diagnosed at an advanced stage and therapy for this pathology is very complex [3-5]. Reduction in mortality rates could be gained both with new screening strategies and with ameliorations in surgical and medical treatments. However, neither of these approaches will affect cancer incidence, thus, it is clear that the prospects for making a major impact on the mortality from ovarian cancer lie more in the area of prevention.

The purpose of this chapter is to identify the evidence for the appropriate practical strategies to prevent ovarian cancer or the detection of cancer in the early stages in order to improve the overall survival. The search was restricted to full reports and guidelines published in English between 2000 and May 2012, in an attempt to summarize the principal findings regarding primary and secondary ovarian cancer prevention.

2. Primary prevention for ovarian cancer in general population

Primary prevention aims to prevent the disease before its biological onset, thus it is based on avoiding risk factors and increasing protective factors.

A summary of the most significant risk and protective factors, with relative hazard ratio, for epithelial ovarian cancer is summarized in Tables 1a and1b,

AUTHORS	RISK FACTORS	RR (95% CI)
Schorge JO et al. [6]	White race	1.35 (1.08-1.50)
Schouten LJ et al. [7]	Height≥160 cm	1.38 (1.16-1.65)
Lahmann PH et al. [8]	BMI≥25	1.33 (1.05-1.68)
Camargo MC et al. [9]	Asbestos exposure	1.77 (1.37-2.28)
Cramer DW [10]	early age at menarche	1.74 (1.28-2.18)
Cramer DW [10]	late menopause	1.61 (1.15-2.08)
Beral V et al. [11]	HRT	1.20 (0.98-1.32)
Melin A et al. [12]	Endometriosis	1.43 (1.19-1.71)
Chen S et al. [13]	BRCA1 BRCA2	42.4 (15-119.6) 20.6 (7.75-57.2)
Watson P et al. [14]	MMR	19 (5.0-30.0)
	(a)	

AUTHORS	PROTECTIVE FACTORS	HR (95% CI)
Trudel D et al. [15]	green tea components	0.66 (0.54-0.80)
Collaborative Group on Epidemiological Studies of Ovarian Cancer [16]	hormonal contraceptive use	0.73 (0.70-0.76)
Ness RB et al. [17]	Multiparity(≥ 4 pregnancies)	0.40 (0.30-0.50)
Danforth KN et al. [18]	breastfeeding	0.98 per month (0.97-1.00)
Hankinson SE et al. [19]	bilateral tube ligation	0.33 (0.16-0.64)
Hankinson SE et al. [19]	hysterectomy	0.67 (0.45-1.00)
	(b)	

Table 1. (a) Main significant risk factors for ovarian cancer. (b) Main significant protective factors for ovarian cancer.

The average age at diagnosis is approximately 60 years, but the overall incidence of ovarian cancer rises with increasing age up to 75-84 years, due to the accumulation of random genetic alterations, before declining slightly among women beyond 84 years [20]. Women residing in North America, Northern Europe or in any industrialized Western country have a higher risk of developing ovarian cancer. Conversely, women residing in developing countries have shown the lowest rate [6]. The exact reasons for this distribution are unknown but discrepancies in parity, rates of gynaecologic surgery and dietary habits may account for some differences [21]. In particular, regarding dietary habits, a comprehensive meta-analysis of the observational studies published up to September 2011 provided no evidence of a material association between alcohol drinking and epithelial ovarian cancer risk [22]. Finally, a recent study provided some suggestion that soy and phytoestrogen consumption may decrease ovarian cancer risk, although the results did not reach statistical significance [23].

Exposure to radiation may increase the risk of ovarian cancer and the risk increases with increasing dose. The Life Span Study incidence data for ovarian cancer demonstrated a borderline significant association [24], and mortality data showed a significant positive association between exposure to radiation and ovarian cancer [25].

With regards to reproductive factors, early age at menarche and late menopause have been consistently associated with an increased risk of ovarian cancer, likely due to an increase in ovulation and in oestrogen exposure [26]. The effect of combined hormonal contraceptive use on the risk of ovarian cancer has been long discussed. In 2007, the IARC review concluded that women who had at least for a period used combined hormonal contraceptives orally had an overall reduced risk for ovarian cancer, which persists for at least 20 years after cessation of use, and an inverse relationship was observed with duration of use [27]. These results have been confirmed by the Collaborative Group on Epidemiological Studies of Ovarian Cancer [16] that reported an overall reduction in ovarian cancer risk in users versus non-users of 27%, which was not confined to any particular type of oral formulation nor to any histological type of ovarian cancer, although it was less consistent for mucinous than for other types of ovarian cancer. On this basis, the "incessant menstruation" hypothesis was postulated, which concludes that the use of oral contraceptives (OC) should be favoured for prolonged periods of time, especially in women with endometriosis, a population at doubled risk of ovarian cancer [28]. On the other hand, in the Million Women Study HRT after menopause was shown to increase the risk of ovarian cancer [11].

Women who have never had children are at increased risk of developing ovarian cancer [29]. Regarding fertility drug use, previous studies have provided conflicting results. Recent data demonstrated that fertility drug use does not significantly contribute to ovarian cancer risk among the majority of women. However, women who despite their use remain nulliparous may have an increased risk [30]. The role of breastfeeding as a protective factor against ovarian cancer has been long discussed. Finally, the risk of ovarian cancer decreases in women who underwent bilateral tube ligation or hysterectomy, probably because these surgical interventions do not allow the carcinogenic agents to enter the body from the vagina and reach the ovaries [19, 31]. For instance, a number of observational studies (largely case-control) conducted over the last two decades suggested an association between use of talc powders on the female perineum and increased risk of ovarian cancer, although the weak statistical associations observed in a number of epidemiological studies do not support a causal association between cosmetic talc use and ovarian cancer [32,33].

Endometriosis represents another considerable risk factor for epithelial ovarian cancer. In particular, self-reported endometriosis was associated with a significantly increased risk of clear-cell, low-grade serous and endometrioid invasive ovarian cancers. No association was noted between endometriosis and risk of mucinous or high-grade serous invasive ovarian cancers or borderline tumours of either subtype [34]. Also, pelvic inflammatory disease has been suggested to double the risk of epithelial ovarian cancer [35], but few studies have been done and the conclusions are inconsistent.

The most important risk factor still remains a family history of breast or ovarian cancer. Up to 10% of ovarian cancer patients may have inherited a germline mutation that places them at increased risk of the disease. Mutations in the breast and ovarian cancer-susceptibility genes *BRCA1* and *BRCA2* confer an increased lifetime risk of ovarian cancer. *BRCA1* and *BRCA2* are tumour suppressor genes involved in many cellular functions to prevent carcinogenesis [Fig.1].

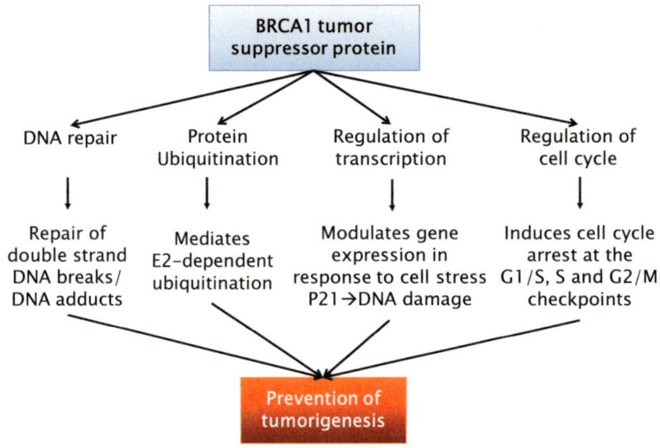

Figure 1. BrCa1 protein functions.

The mechanism to repair the double-strand DNA breaks is shown in Fig.2.

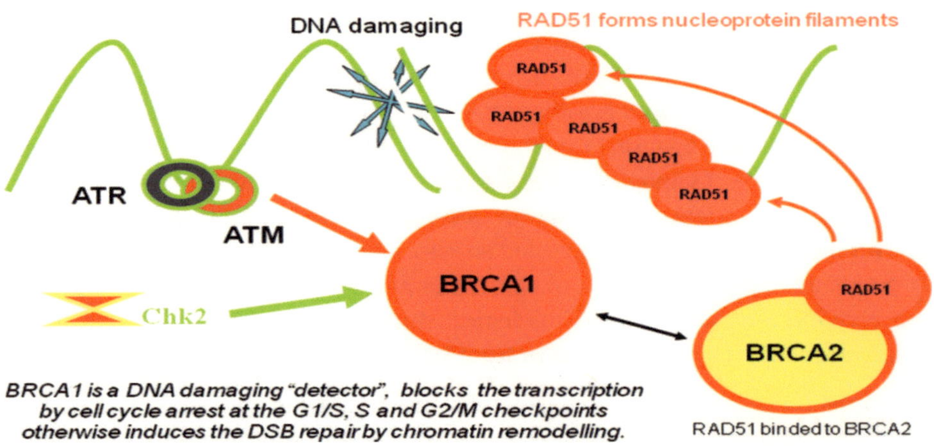

Figure 2. Repair of double-strand DNA breaks by BRCA1 and BRCA2 genes.

Heterozygous germline mutation leads to genetic instability as shown in the Fig.3, modified by Brodie *et al.* [36]

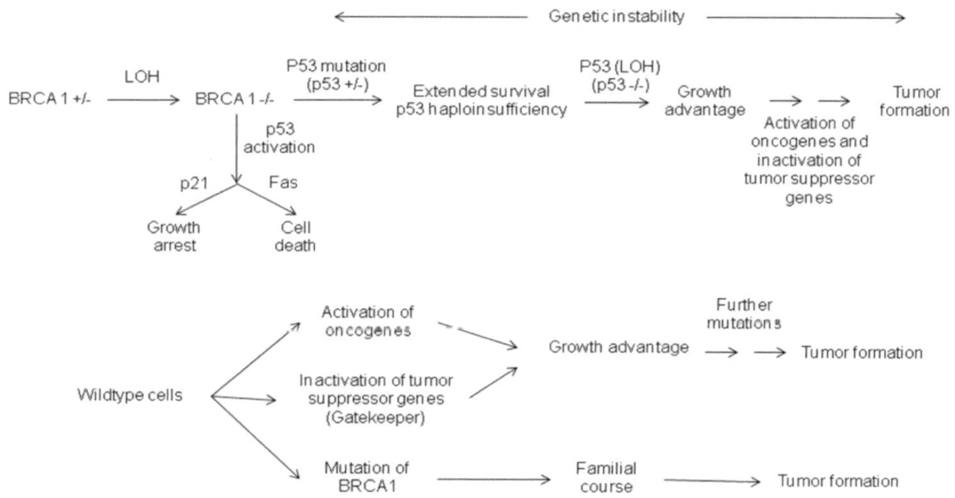

Figure 3. Genetic instability in the germline and somatic BrCa1 mutations [36].

However, *BRCA* mutations do not account for the entire range of hereditary ovarian cancer syndromes. Other hereditary epithelial ovarian cancers are attributed to Lynch syndrome. Lynch syndrome is an autosomal dominant disorder, which predisposes to colorectal cancer, endometrial cancer, ovarian, gastric, small bowel, biliary/pancreatic, urothelial, skin, and central nervous system cancers. The cumulative risk of ovarian cancer is estimated to be 8–10%, with an average age at onset of 42 years [14]. Moreover, other genes often associated with rare cancer syndromes such as *TP53* and *PTEN*, or *CHEK2* and *PALB2* confer a low to moderate risk of breast and ovarian cancer [37-39]. Recent technological advances have aided in the recognition of additional tumour suppressor genes potentially associated with hereditary breast cancer, such as *RAD51* and *BARD1* [40]. To date, at least 16 genes have been associated with hereditary ovarian cancer, mostly involved in the *FA-BRCA* pathway and the mismatch repair system. However, many families with suspicious pedigrees do not have a specific mutation identified through clinical testing, due to a currently undetectable *BRCA1/2* mutation or a mutation in another susceptibility gene. Although their cancer risks are not as well defined, these families should be considered as part of the hereditary breast and/or ovarian cancer spectrum [13].

However, most of the common risk and protective factors only slightly influence the risk of developing ovarian cancer, thus, to date; the knowledge of these factors has still not been translated into practical strategies to prevent ovarian cancer.

3. Primary prevention for ovarian cancer in high risk women

Some women have a high risk of developing ovarian cancer due to hereditary conditions associated to BRCA syndrome and Lynch syndrome. Thus, when one of these forms of hereditary or familial breast and/or ovarian cancer is suspected in clinical practice, the general practitioner should refer the patient to a cancer centre specialising in cancer-specific genetic counselling for the identification, definition and management of risk. Genetic counselling, defined by the American Society of Human Genetics as 'a communication process which deals with the human problems associated with the occurrence or risk of occurrence of a genetic disorder in a family', involves one or more professional figures to help the affected individuals or families [41-44]. Genetic counselling in the oncological setting (cancer-specific genetic counselling) should also provide sufficient information to enable the user to make a fully informed choice as to course of action, particularly with regards to prevention, in the case of the identification of a mutation or of a familial cancer risk [45, 46].

A recent review investigated the impact of cancer genetic risk assessment on outcomes, including perceived risk of inherited cancer and psychological distress. The review found favourable outcomes for patients after risk assessment for familial breast cancer, suggesting that cancer-specific genetic risk assessment services help to reduce distress, improve the accuracy of the perception of risk of ovarian cancer, and increase the knowledge of ovarian cancer and genetics. However, there were too few papers to make any significant conclusions on how best to deliver cancer genetic risk assessment services. Further research is needed, assessing the best means of delivering cancer risk evaluation, by different health professionals, in different ways and in alternative locations [47].

Women at increased risk of breast and ovarian cancer are advised to consider risk-reducing strategies; however, such methods vary in their effectiveness. These strategies include chemoprevention and prophylactic surgery (risk-reducing salpingo-oophorectomy, RRSO). Risk-reducing strategies have been shown to have associations with a lengthening of life expectancy in *BRCA1/2* carriers.

3.1. Risk-reducing salpingo-oophorectomy (RRSO)

Women who have inherited mutations in the *BRCA1* or *BRCA2* genes have substantially elevated risks of breast and ovarian cancer, with a lifetime risk of breast cancer of 56%–84% [48-51]. Breast cancer in *BRCA1/2* mutation carriers also occurs at an earlier age, particularly among the *BRCA1* mutation carriers, than in non-carriers. The risk for ovarian cancer depends on whether the mutation has occurred in *BRCA1* or *BRCA2*, with estimated risks ranging from 34% to 44% for *BRCA1* mutation carriers and from 12% to 25% for *BRCA2* mutation carriers [48, 49, 52-54]. Carriers of *BRCA1/2* mutations are counselled to help them interpret the implications of these elevated risks, choose strategies to reduce these risks, and maximize early detection of cancers. The risk of breast cancer can be reduced either with RRSO and/or mastectomy or non-surgically (i.e. with chemoprevention). However, due to the lack of effective screening for ovarian cancer, RRSO is usually strongly recommended to *BRCA1/2* mutation carriers once childbearing is complete.

RRSO has also been demonstrated to decrease the risk of both breast and ovarian cancer in *BRCA1/2* mutation carriers [55-60]. However, the studies examining the extent of risk reduction have used different designs; some are retrospective case–control studies, while others used a prospective cohort design. In a large, retrospective analysis of 551 *BRCA* carriers, RRSO was found to reduce the risk of ovarian cancer by 96% and breast cancer by 53% at a mean follow-up of 9 years [55]. A multicentre prospective study, Kauff *et al.* [56] found that, during a 3-year follow-up, RRSO was associated with an 85% reduction in BRCA1-associated gynaecologic cancer risk and a 72% reduction in BRCA2-associated breast cancer risk. Although protection against BRCA1-associated breast cancer and BRCA2-associated gynaecologic cancer was suggested, neither effect reached statistical significance. The authors postulate that the protection conferred by RRSO against breast and gynaecologic cancers may differ between the carriers of *BRCA1* and *BRCA2* mutations.

Similar findings were observed in a prospective study of 170 *BRCA* carriers. During a mean follow-up of 2 years, the incidence of ovarian or peritoneal cancer and breast cancer was significantly greater amongst those women who selected surveillance than amongst those who chose to undergo RRSO [59.] Even among prospective studies, the inclusion criteria and the definitions of follow-up time differ. In some studies, only unaffected mutation-positive women are included and followed up. In others, particularly when examining ovarian cancer risk, women with breast cancer are included. Such differences in study design can introduce biases (such as the survival bias) and can have an impact on risk reduction estimates. For example, the reported efficacy of RRSO in reducing the risk of ovarian/fallopian tube cancers varies from 71% to 96% [55-61]. Although these estimates imply a substantial reduction in risk, this variability may affect the decisions of premenopausal women who are making a decision about whether to undergo a treatment that will cause abrupt and premature menopause. Patients and their physicians need as much information as possible regarding the efficacy of RRSO in reducing cancer risk to balance this benefit with the health risks caused by premature entry into menopause.

A summary of published studies on RRSO is presented in Table 2.

Reference	Study design	With/Without RRSO	MYFU	OC Risk Reduction (%)	BC Risk Reduction (%)
Rebbeck et al., 2002 [55]	RC	261/292	8.5	96	53
Kauff et al., 2008 [56]	PC	509/283	3.2	85	72
Finch et al., 2006 [57]	RC	1041/779	3.5	80	NA
Chang-Claude et al., 2007 [58]	RC	55/1601	65,675 PY	NA	44
Rutter et al., 2003 [60]	RC	5/223	NA	67	NA
Kauff et al., 2002 [61]	PC	98/72	2.0	85	68

PC = prospective cohort; RC = retrospective cohort; MYFU = mean years of follow-up; PY = person-years; NR = not reported; and NA = not applicable; RRSO = risk-reducing salpingo-oophorectomy.

Table 2. Published studies on risk-reducing salpingo-oophorectomy in BrCa1and/ or BrCa2 mutation carriers.

A synopsis of different management strategies available for *BRCA1* and *BRCA2* mutation carriers is shown in Table 3.

Management options Gynecologic cancer	Strategy	Advantage	Limitation
Chemoprevention	OC	Likely 30-60% reduction in ovarian cancer risk	Potential increase in risk of breast cancer
Screening	TVUS, CA 125	Avoids RRSO	Unproven efficacy
Risk-reducing surgery	Bilateral salpingo-oophorectomy	Substantial decrease in risk of ovarian and fallopian tube cancers	Premature menopause and iatrogenic infertility

TVUS= Transvaginal Ultrasound; RRSO = risk-reducing salpingo-oophorectomy

Table 3. Synopsis of different prevention strategies for BRCA1 and BRCA2 mutation carriers.

The National Comprehensive Cancer Network (NCCN) guidelines and other institutions concerning this method, recommend RRSO "for women with a known BRCA1/2 mutation, ideally between 35 and 40 years or upon completion of child bearing" or at an adjusted age based on earliest age of ovarian cancer diagnosis in the family" [62].

Also ACOG, the Committee on Genetics and the Society of Gyneacologic Oncologists, recommends RRSO for women with *BRCA1/2* mutations, by the age of 40 years or when childbearing is complete [63].

The National Cancer Institute (NCI) [64] on the clinical management of *BRCA* mutation carriers considers, besides salpingo-oophorectomy, bilateral salpingectomy as an interim procedure to reduce risk in *BRCA* mutation carriers. There are no data available on the efficacy of salpingectomy as a risk-reducing procedure. The procedure preserves ovarian function and spares the premenopausal patient the adverse effects of a premature menopause. It can be performed using a minimally invasive approach, and a subsequent bilateral oophorectomy could be deferred until the patient approaches menopause. While the data make the compelling argument that some pelvic serous cancers in *BRCA* mutation carriers originate in the fallopian tube, clearly, some cancers arise in the ovary. Furthermore, bilateral salpingectomy could give patients a false sense of security that they have eliminated their cancer risk as completely as if they had undergone a bilateral salpingo-oophorectomy. A small study of 14 young *BRCA* mutation carriers documented the procedure as feasible [65]. However, efficacy and impact on ovarian function was not assessed in this study. Future prospective trials are needed to establish the validity of the procedure as a risk-reducing intervention.

For the European Society of Medical Oncology ESMO [66], RRSO is associated with a reduction in risk of breast cancer in premenopausal *BRCA* mutation carriers, a reduction in risk of ovarian cancer, and there is evidence of a reduction in overall mortality [67]. RRSO is recommended after the age of 35 and when childbearing decisions are complete.

The significantly reduced risk of breast cancer by RRSO seems to be higher in *BRCA2* mutation carriers than in *BRCA1* carriers. Several reports have addressed this question although additional research is required [56]. Short-term HRT after RRSO seems not to decrease the overall benefit of this strategy for breast cancer risk reduction [68].

However, it should be noted that the NCCN and other institutions couch these recommendations within a multidisciplinary consultative process in which reproductive desires, assessment of cancer risk, and the pros and cons of surgery along with the potential sequelae of surgery are fully discussed.

The recommendations of different organizations regarding surgical primary prevention for *BRCA1/2* mutation carriers are shown in Table 4.

Management options	NCCN [62]	ACOG Committee on Genetics and the Society of Gynecologic Oncologists [63]	National Cancer Institute (NCI) [64]	ESMO [65]
RRSO	Between 35 and 40 years or upon completion of child bearing	By the age of 40 years or when childbearing is complete	Considered but age is not indicated	After age 35 and when childbearing decisions are complete
Bilateral salpingectomy	-	-	Considered but age is not indicated	-

Table 4. Recommendations of several organizations regarding primary prevention for BRCA mutation carriers.

3.2. Chemoprevention

Women at increased risk, based on their personal or family history of breast and/or ovarian cancer including *BRCA1/2* mutation carriers, may join a cancer prevention clinical trial or a chemoprevention trial. OC have been the most widely studied chemopreventive agents in ovarian cancer. Recently, Iodice *et al.* conducted a meta-analysis updated to March 2010 on the association between OC use and breast or ovarian cancer in *BRCA1/2* mutation carriers [69]. Based on 18 studies a total of 2855 breast cancer cases and 1503 ovarian cancer cases carrying an ascertained *BRCA1/2* mutation were included. As previously noted, use of OC at any point during one's life was associated with a 50% reduction in relative risk of developing ovarian cancer for *BRCA1/2* mutation carriers. Looking specifically at duration of use, each 10-year period of OC use resulted in a 36% relative risk reduction in the development of ovarian cancer. However, the meta-analysis showed no evidence of a significant association between OC use and breast cancer risk. Notably, formulations used before 1975 correlated with an increased risk of breast cancer, but there was no correlation with the use of more recent formulations. A summary of the association between OC use and ovarian cancer risk in mutation carriers is shown in Table 5.

EXPOSURE	GENES WITH MUTATION	CATEGORIES OF EXPOSURE	No. of STUDIES	No. of CASES	HR (95% CI)
OC USERS	BRCA 1/2	Users	5	1503	0.50 (0.33-0.75)
	BRCA 1		5	1251	0.51 (0.40-0.65)
	BRCA 2		4	286	0.52 (0.31-0.87)
DURATION OF USE	BRCA 1/2	1 year	4	1336	0.96 (0.94-0.97)
		5 years			0.80 (0.73-0.88)
		10 years			0.64 (0.53-0.78)

Table 5. Summary of the association between OC use and ovarian cancer risk in mutation carriers

Another meta-analysis of cohort, case-control and case-case studies published in English up to December 2009 confirmed a significantly decreased ovarian cancer risk in *BRCA1/2* mutation carriers associated with the use of OC, while a significantly increased risk in breast cancer was only shown in a subset of cohort studies on *BRCA1* mutation carriers. To conclude, OC use can be considered as an alternative strategy in the chemoprevention of ovarian cancer in *BRCA1* mutation carriers who do not accept RRSO above the age of 30 years [70].

Other chemopreventative agents such as retinoids, vitamin D, cyclo-oxygenase inhibitors and peroxisome proliferator activated receptor-gamma ligands have shown promise in early investigations of disease prevention [71].

Retinoids, a class of compounds comprising vitamin A, its natural derivatives, and synthetic analogs, have been extensively studied in both the prevention and treatment of gynaecologic malignancies [72]. One of the most promising retinoids to be used in chemoprevention trials is the synthetic amide of retinoic acid fenretinide, *N*-4-hydroxyphenyl retinamide (4-HPR). 4-HPR has been found to have significant chemopreventive action in a large variety of in vitro and in vivo systems. Since both fenretinide and its major metabolite, 4-metoxyphenyl retinamide (MPR), selectively accumulate in the human breast, evaluation of 4-HPR as a chemopreventive agent in breast cancer has been particularly attractive [73]. The most important clinical trials with 4-HPR are mentioned in Table 6.

The most important study where 4-HPR was administrated was a multicentric phase III randomized trial, coordinated by the Istituto Nazionale dei Tumori in Milan, which started in 1987. Most notably, the younger the women were, the greater the benefit of 4-HPR. Such a benefit was associated with a remarkable 50% risk reduction in women aged 40 years or younger, whereas it disappeared after 55 years of age. Interestingly, the incidence of ovarian cancer during the 5-year intervention period was significantly lower in the treatment arm [74].

The role of analgesic drug use in the development of ovarian cancer is still widely discussed.

STUDY	DESIGN	TREATMENT	END POINTS	OUTCOMES
Costa et al., 1989 [75]	Phase I, Randomized, Placebo controlled (60)	Orally: 100, 200 and 300mg x 6 months subsequently at 200mg for another 6 months.	Tolerability	Recommended dose for chemoprevention trials of HPR is 200mg/die.
Formelli et al., 1989 [76]	Phase II, Randomized, Placebo controlled (60)	Orally: 100, 200 and 300mg x 6 months subsequently at 200mg for another 6 months.	Pharmacokinetic	HPR treatment lowers retinol and RPB plasma concentrations. Effect related to HPR levels and reversible on cessation of HPR administration.
Veronesi et al., 1999 [77]	Phase III, Randomized (2867)	Orally 200mg versus no treatment x 5 years.	Second breast cancer prevention	No statistically significant effect but a possible benefit in premenopausal women.
Veronesi et al., 2006 [78]	Phase III, Randomized, 15-year follow-up (1879)	Orally 200mg versus no treatment x 5 years: 15-years followup.	Second breast cancer prevention	4-HPR induces a significant reduction of risk of second breast cancer in premenopausal women, which is remarkable at younger ages, and persists several years after treatment cessation.

HPR: fenretinide, RBP: retinol-binding protein.

Table 6. Clinical trials with 4-HPR [74].

A recent population-based case-control study, carried out in Denmark in the period 1995-1999, analysed the association between analgesic drug use and ovarian cancer risk using multiple logistic regression models. The study showed that regular use of non-aspirin non-steroidal anti-inflammatory drugs (NA-NSAID), paracetamol or other analgesics did not decrease ovarian cancer risk. In contrast, use of any analgesics (OR = 0.72; 95% CI 0.53-0.98) or aspirin (OR = 0.60; 95% CI 0.36-1.00) resulted in a statistically significant decreased risk of serous ovarian cancer but not mucinous or other ovarian tumours [79]. On the other hand, recent data reported by the Multiethnic Cohort Study did not find compelling evidence to support an association between use of NSAID and risk of ovarian and endometrial cancers in a multiethnic population. The RR (95% CI) for ovarian cancer associated with aspirin, non-aspirin NSAID, and acetaminophen were 0.87 (0.68, 1.14), 0.97 (0.74, 1.26), and 0.86 (0.67, 1.12), respectively. No heterogeneity across ethnic groups (P's ≥0.29) or dose-response relation with increased duration of use (P's for trend ≥0.16) was observed [80]. Finally, in an attempt to review and summarize the evidence provided by longitudinal studies on the association between NSAID use and ovarian cancer risk, a comprehensive literature search for articles published up to December 2011 was performed (Table 7). The meta-analysis found no evidence of an association between aspirin or NA-NSAID use and ovarian cancer risk, based on a random-effects model or a fixed-effects model. Furthermore, the analysis did not show strong association between frequency or duration of NA-NSAID use and ovarian cancer, leading to the conclusion that there is no strong evidence of an association between aspirin/NA-NSAID use and ovarian cancer [81].

	No. Of studies	Fixed-effects model		Random-effects model		P-value
		RR	(95% CI)	RR	(95% CI)	
			ASPIRIN USE			
All studies	17	0,94	(0,87-1,01)	0,91	(0,82-1,01)	0,046
C-C studies	14	0,94	(0,87-1,02)	0,90	(0,79-1,03)	0,015
Cohort studies	3	0,92	(0,77-1,09)	0,92	(0,77-1,10)	0,456
Regular Use	7	0,86	(0,73-1,03)	0,83	(0,65-1,05)	0,119
Irregular Use	7	1,07	(0,96-1,20)	1,07	(0,96-1,21)	0,421
Duration > 5 yrs	5	0,91	(0,67-1,24)	0,89	(0,63-1,25)	0,332
			NA-NSAID use			
All studies	7	0,86	(0,76-0,98)	0,89	(0,74-1,08)	0,089
C-C studies	4	0,88	(0,75-1,03)	0,97	(0,73-1,28)	0,042
Cohort studies	3	0,82	(0,64-1,04)	0,89	(0,74-1,08)	0,283
Regular Use	3	1,45	(1,07-1,98)	1,47	(0,95-2,27)	0,153
Irregular Use	3	0,96	(0,69-1,33)	0,93	(0,49-1,76)	0,038
Duration > 5 yrs	3	1,65	(1,13-2,41)	1,56	(0,92-2,65)	0,21

NA-NSAID: non aspirin- non-steroidal anti-inflammatory drugs

Table 7. Metanalysis of longitudinal studies on the association between NSAID use and ovarian cancer risk

4. Secondary prevention for ovarian cancer

This is based on diagnosing and treating extant disease in the early stages before it causes significant morbidity. CA125 (or MUC16) glycoprotein is the most studied tumour marker, alone and/or in combination with other biomarkers, for ovarian cancer screening. However, false positive CA125 levels can occur in women with benign conditions, including menstruation, appendicitis, benign ovarian cysts, endometriosis and pelvic inflammatory disease, as well as with other malignancies, including breast, lung, endometrial and pancreatic cancers. Thus, a large number of false-positive screening tests can occur, potentially leading to unnecessary surgeries and subsequent issues of morbidity and cost [82]. Consequently, multimodal strategies, in particular the combination of CA125 with pelvic ultrasound, have been examined, in order to improve sensitivity and positive predictive value of ovarian cancer screening.

4.1. Transvaginal ultrasound

In the general population, TVUS appears to be superior to transabdominal ultrasound in the preoperative diagnosis of adnexal masses. Both techniques have lower specificity in premenopausal women than in postmenopausal women due to the cyclic menstrual changes in premenopausal ovaries (e.g., transient corpus luteum cysts) that can cause difficulty in the interpretation. The randomized prospective Prostate, Lung, Colorectal, and Ovarian Cancer Screening Trial found no reduction in mortality with the annual use of combined TVUS and CA125 in screening asymptomatic, postmenopausal women at average risk of ovarian cancer [83].

Data are limited regarding the potential benefit of TVUS in screening women at inherited risk of ovarian cancer. A number of retrospective studies have reported experiments with ovarian cancer screening in high-risk women using TVUS with or without CA125 [84-90].

However, there is little uniformity in the definition of high-risk criteria and compliance with screening, and in whether the cancers detected were incident or prevalent. One of the largest reported studies included 888 *BRCA1/BRCA2* mutation carriers who were annually screened with TVUS and CA125. Ten women developed ovarian cancer; five of the ten developed interval cancers after normal screening results within 3 to 10 months before diagnosis. Five of the ten ovarian cancers were screen-detected incident cases, which had had normal screening results within 6 to 14 months before diagnosis. Out of these five cases, four were stage IIIB or IV [85].

A similar study reported the results of annual TVUS and CA125 combined-screening in a cohort of 312 high-risk women (152 *BRCA1/BRCA2* mutation carriers) [86]. Out of four cancers detected because of abnormal TVUS and CA125, all cases were symptomatic, and three had an advanced-stage disease. Annual screening of *BRCA1/BRCA2* mutation carriers with pelvic ultrasound, TVUS, and CA125 failed to detect early-stage ovarian cancer among 241 women in a study from the Netherlands [87]. Three cancers were detected over the course of the study, all advanced stage IIIC disease. Finally, a study of 1,100 moderate- and high-risk women who underwent annual TVUS and CA125 combined screening reported that ten out of 13 ovarian tumours were detected due to screening. Only five out of ten were stage I or II [88]. There are limited data related to the efficacy of semiannual screening with TVUS and CA125 [89].

The first prospective study of TVUS and CA125 with survival as the primary outcome was completed in 2009. Out of 3,532 high-risk women screened, 981 were *BRCA* mutation carriers, of which 49 developed ovarian cancer. The 5- and 10-year survival was 58.6% (95% CI, 50.9–66.3) and 36% (95% CI, 27–45), respectively, and there was no difference in survival between carriers and non-carriers. A major limitation of the study was the absence of a control group. Despite these limitations, this study suggests that annual surveillance by TVUS and CA125 level appears to be ineffective in detecting tumours at an early stage to substantially influence survival [90].

4.2. Serum CA125

Serum CA125 screening for ovarian cancer in high-risk women has been evaluated in combination with TVUS in a number of retrospective studies, as described in the previous section [84-90].

The National Institutes of Health (NIH) Consensus Statement on Ovarian Cancer recommended against routine screening of the general population for ovarian cancer with serum CA125. The NIH Consensus Statement did, however, recommend that women at inherited risk of ovarian cancer undergo TVUS and serum CA125 screening every 6 to 12 months, beginning at the age of 35 years [91]. The Cancer Genetics Studies Consortium task force recommends that female carriers of a deleterious *BRCA1* mutation undergo annual or semi-annual screening using TVUS and serum CA125 levels, beginning at age of 25 to 35 years [92]. Both recommendations are based solely on expert opinion and best clinical judgment.

NCCN for those patients who have not chosen RRSO, consider concurrent TVUS (preferably day 1-10 menstrual cycle women in premenopausal women) + CA125 (preferably after day 5 of menstrual cycle women in premenopausal women) every 6 months starting at the age of 30 years or 5-10 years before the earliest age of first diagnosis of ovarian cancer in the family [93].

Although there are retrospective data indicating that annual ovarian cancer screening using TVUS and measurement of serum CA125 levels is neither an effective strategy for the early detection of ovarian tumours nor a reasonable substitute for a bilateral RRSO, the effectiveness of these interventions is limited to six-monthly screening. Investigational imaging and screening studies may be considered for this population.

4.3. Proton Magnetic Resonance Spectroscopy (MRS)

MRS has proved to be a reliable technique for probing metabolic patterns, biochemical effects of tumour microenvironment, and the action of therapy in cancer cells, both in vivo and in vitro [94]. In particular, an increase in the total choline-containing compounds (tCho) content allows to distinguish malignant from benign lesions in the breast [95].

Moreover, some studies have also shown alterations of the phospholipid metabolism in vitro using epithelial ovarian carcinoma cell lines [96,97], and demonstrated the feasibility of 3D CSI MRS to detect a choline peak in ovarian lesions in vivo at 1.5 T.

Then, the metabolic meaning of a high concentration of choline in ovarian tumours merits some consideration. This topic has been extensively reviewed by Podo *et al.* in 2007 [98]. The high choline concentration of ovarian tumours can be considered as the result of an inappropriate storage attributable to metabolic deregulation associated with clinical indicators of increased malignancy. The possibility of using a spatially resolved approach for MRS of ovarian masses opens an intriguing prospect for the diagnosis of early-stage tumours, with potential impact on the overall survival. This is especially true for carriers of a *BRCA* mutation, with a lifetime risk of 39% to 46% among women with the *BRCA1* mutation and a risk of 12% to 20% among those with the *BRCA2* mutation [99].

Based on peer-reviewed published data, several institutions established the Guidelines to facilitate clinical management of patients with a suggestive personal or family history of breast and/or ovarian cancer, in particular individuals from a family with a known deleterious BRCA1/2 mutation. Screening options include transvaginal ultrasonography (TVUS), and serum CA125, while prevention options include medical therapy with drugs and surgery such as RRSO. The guidelines, summarized in Table 8, include age ranges for which these options should be begun and how often screening should take place. [53].

Management options	NCCN [62]	ACOG Committee on Genetics and the Society of Gynecologic Oncologists [63]	National Cancer Institute (NCI) [64]	ESMO [65]
		Surveillance		
TVU+CA125	Every 6 months starting at age 30 years	Periodic screening beginning between the ages 30 years and 35years	Every 6 to 12 months, beginning at age 35 years	Not considered
		Surgery		
RRSO	Between 35 and 40 years or upon completion of child bearing	By age 40 years or when childbearing is complete	Considered but age is not indicated	After age 35 and when childbearing decisions are complete
Bilateral salpingectomy	-	-	Considered but age is not indicated	-
Chemoprevention	Considered	Considered	Considered	Not considered
Investigational imaging and screening studies	Considered	Considered	Considered	Not considered

Table 8. Published Guidelines/Consensus Statements for the management of BRCA mutation carriers.

4.4. Human Epididymis Protein 4 (HE4)

Additional potential serum biomarkers have been studied for the detection of ovarian cancer. For instance, human epididymis protein 4 (HE4) is a secreted glycoprotein over-expressed by serous and endometrioid ovarian cancers and expressed by 32% of ovarian cancers lacking CA125 expression.

To define the clinical utility of HE4, a comprehensive assessment of HE4 protein expression in benign and malignant ovarian and non-ovarian tissues by immunohistochemistry was performed and published in 2005. In comparison with normal surface epithelium, which does not express the protein, HE4 was widely found in cortical inclusion cysts lined by metaplastic Mullerian epithelium. These findings suggested that the formation of Mullerian epithelium is a prerequisite step in the development of some types of epithelial ovarian cancer. Moreover, the expression was restricted to certain histologic subtypes: 93% of serous and 100% of endometrioid epithelial ovarian cancers expressed HE4, while only 50% and 0% of clear cell carcinomas and mucinous tumours, respectively, were positive. HE4 protein expression is restricted in normal tissue to the reproductive tracts and respiratory epithelium. In fact, tissue microarrays revealed that the majority of non-ovarian carcinomas do not express HE4 [100].

In 2008 the Food and Drug Administration (FDA) approved HE4 to monitor disease recurrence and this marker was recently incorporated into the clinical evaluation of ovarian cancer patients. Recently, Moore *et al.* published a series of papers that used a combination of CA125, HE4 and menopausal status to predict the presence of a malignant ovarian tumour and developed the Risk of Ovarian Malignancy Algorithm (ROMA), a simple biomarker based algorithm, which requires US [101, 102].

In the last few years, several multi-modal screenings of women at high risk, combining different approaches, were carried out to improve ovarian cancer diagnostic test performance [103,104]. In 2010, a prospective case-control study was designed to evaluate the independent contributions of HE4, CA125 and the Symptom Index (SI) to predict ovarian cancer status in a multivariate model [105]. The SI is a screening tool that evaluates specific symptoms in conjunction with their frequency and duration to identify women who are at risk of ovarian cancer [106]. The SI, HE4 and CA125 all made significant independent contributions to ovarian cancer prediction. A rule for the positive cut-off based on anyone of the three tests being positive had a sensitivity of 95% with specificity of 80%. A rule based on any two of the three tests being positive had a sensitivity of 84% with a specificity of 98.5%. The SI alone had sensitivity of 64% with specificity of 88%. If the SI index is used to select women for CA125 and HE4 testing, specificity is 98.5% and sensitivity is 58% using the 2-of-3-positive positive cut-off rule. A comparison between different markers in ovarian cancer early diagnosis is presented in Table 9.

SCREENING TESTS	DESCRIPTION
Single Markers	
CA125	CA125 was dichotomized at 95th percentile in the control group. Subjects with a marker value above that threshold were considered to be positive for CA125.
HE4	HE4 was dichotomized at 95th percentile in the control group. Subjects with a marker value above that threshold were considered to be positive for HE4.
Symptom Index (SI)	The SI was considered to be positive if the patient had at least one of the following symptoms for less than one year but more than 12 times per month: bloating or increased abdominal size, abdominal or pelvic pain, difficulty eating or feeling full quickly.
Marker Combinations	
CA125 or HE4	Screen considered positive if CA125, HE4 or both were positive.
SI or CA125	Screen considered positive if either the SI or CA125 was positive, or if both were positive.
SI or HE4	Screen considered positive if either the SI or HE4 was positive, or if both were positive.
Any 1 of 3 tests positive	Screen considered positive if any one of the SI or CA125 or HE4 was positive, or if two or more tests were positive.
Any 2 of 3 tests positive	Screen considered positive if both the SI and CA125 were positive, or if both the SI and HE4 were positive, or if both CA125 and HE4 were positive, or if all three tests were positive.
SI and at least 1 additional test positive	Classified as positive if SI was positive in addition to either a positive CA125 or a positive HE4, or if all three tests were positive.

Table 9. Description of screening tests and biomarker combinations.

4.5. Proteomic profiling of ovarian cancer for biomarker discovery

Unfortunately, current diagnostic tools have had very limited success in early detection. The search for an ovarian cancer screening method with improved specificity and sensitivity has led to the examination of serum biomarker patterns using new 'omic' technologies [107-110]. In recent years, the advancing techniques for proteomics have accelerated the research for ovarian cancer biomarkers. Numerous proteomics-based molecular biomarkers/panels have been identified and hold great potential for diagnostic applications, but they need further development and validation.

Several studies have analysed the proteomic profiles of ovarian tumour tissue, cell lines, urine, ascites fluid and blood samples from ovarian cancer patients (Table 10) [111- 114].

AUTHORS	IDENTIFIED BIOMARKER	REGULATION IN CANCER
An et al.,(2006)[111]	NM23-H1	↑
	Annexin-1	↑
	Protein phosphatase-1	↑
	Ferritin light chain	↑
	Proteasome alpha-6	↑
	NAGK (N-acetyl glucosamine kinase)	↑
Petri et al., (2009) [112]	fibrinogen alpha fragment	↑
	collagen alpha 1 (III) fragment	↑
	fibrinogen beta NT fragment	↑
Li et al., (2009) [113]	prx-II	↓
	prx-III	↑
	hsp27	↑
	hsp60	↑
	mitochondrial short-chain enoyl-CoA hydratase	↑
	Prohibitin	↑
Cortesi et al.,(2011) [114]	Annexin-5 (ANXA5)	↓
	Phosphatidylethanolamine-biding protein 1 (PEBP)	↓
	glutathione S-transferase A2 (GSTA2)	↓
	galectin-3 (LEG3)	↓
	protein S100-A8-calgranulin A (S100A8)	↑
	retinol binding protein (RET1)	↓

Table 10. Promising biomarkers discovered by proteomic technology for ovarian cancer diagnosis.

An *et al.* [111] identified that different histologic subtypes of ovarian malignant epithelial tumours showed distinctly different protein expression profiles. The potential candidate biomarkers screened in ovarian tumours and found to be significantly up-regulated in comparison to normal tissues were: NM23, annexin-1, protein phosphatase-1, ferritin light chain, proteasome R-6, and NAGK (N-acetylglucosamine kinase). More recently, Petri *et al.* [112] examined whether urine could be used to measure specific ovarian cancer proteomic profiles and whether one peak alone or in combination with CA125 or other peaks had the sensitivity and specificity to discriminate between ovarian cancer pelvic mass and benign pelvic mass. Twenty-one significantly different peaks ($p<0.001$) were examined and the three most significant peaks were identified as fibrinogen alpha fragment, collagen alpha 1 (III) fragment and fibrinogen beta NT fragment. These results supported the feasibility of using urine as a diagnostic tool and suggested the enhanced prediction performance of combined marker analysis. Li *et al.* [113] performed a comparative proteomic study of normal ovarian epithelial and ovarian epithelial serous cystadenocarcinoma tissue and identified six proteins significantly differentially expressed. In particular, Prx-II expression was found to be linearly decreased from normal ovarian tissue, to benign ovarian lesions, and ovarian malignancies. No statistical difference between carcinoma groups in different clinical stages, differentiation status, and histological type was seen, suggesting that the decreased level of Prx-II is a common marker for ovarian malignancies. This was the first report on the altered expression of Prx-II in ovarian cancer.

A recent comparative proteomic study investigated and defined protein expression patterns associated with advanced stage ovarian cancer, to define a panel of diagnostic and/or prognostic markers. The study also investigated proteins secreted by the cancer cell into the interstitial fluid, as cancer growth and progression also depends on stromal factors present in the tumour microenvironment. Moreover, many biomarkers present in biopsied cancer tissues can also be found in blood serum, representing potential biomarkers of the disease. Proteomic profiling of differentially expressed proteins in cancer ovarian tissue, tumoral interstitial fluid (TIF) and ascitic fluid, compared with healthy tissue samples and normal interstitial fluid (NIF), allowed the identification of protein spots consistently differentially expressed between normal and cancer samples. Protein expression/identification was evaluated by 2-DE (two-dimensional gel electrophoresis) and MS (mass spectrometry) analysis and was confirmed by immunohistochemistry. Six proteins showed differential expression in tumoral interstitial fluid and tumour tissue compared to normal interstitial fluid and healthy tissue. Differential protein expression between tumoral and normal ovarian tissue is presented in Table 11.

PROTEIN NAME	FOLD CHANGE TUMORAL VERSUS NORMAL TISSUE	P-value	FOLD CHANGE TIF VERSUS NIF	P-value
ANXA5	-1,88 ± -0,48	<0,0001	-5,605 ± -3,29	<0,01
PEBP	-4,21 ± -2,90	<0,01	-2,82 ± -0,69	<0,0001
GSTA2	-4,67 ± -1,88	<0,0001	-27,39 ± -21,24	<0,01
LEG3	-2,19 ± -0,69	<0,0001	-5,10 ± -4,42	<0,05
S100A8	3,67 ± 1,50	<0,001	3,58 ± 1,11	<0,0001
RET1	-6,33 ± -3,30	<0,001	-5,01 ± -4,28	<0,05

The fold change indicates the direction and the magnitude of the change in expression level. Data are expressed as mean ± standard deviation.

Table 11. Modification in protein expression in tumoral tissue and interstitial fluid

Five were found to be down-regulated and identified as galectin 3, glutathione S-transferase A-2, retinol binding protein 1, phosphatidylethanolamine-binding protein and annexin 5, while the calgranulin, was significantly up-regulated in all pathological samples, including the ascitic fluid. This is the first study to report an over-expression of calgranulin by 2-DE analysis combined with MS/MS on surgical biopsy. As previously reported, the reduced expression of galectin 3 and retinol binding protein 1 in cystic fluid and serum of patients with early stage disease is confirmed in this study. The results highlight alterations in proteins that control cell-cycle progression and apoptosis, as well as factors that modulate the activity of signal transduction pathways. Moreover, this study suggests that calgranulin expression may be used as a diagnostic and/or prognostic biomarker [114].

However, critical assessment of the results has shown significant shortcomings and uncertainties with regard to the reproducibility of the findings and identity of the proteins behind the peak patterns, thus, the validation of the newly discovered biomarkers still remains the most challenging aspect of clinical proteomics. The advancing techniques for proteomics have shown promise in a variety of studies and have provided new insights into ovarian cancer diagnosis, but few have turned out to be useful in the clinic. At present, the development of an effective strategy for early detection of ovarian cancer is still a work in progress [110].

5. Discussion

Primary and secondary prevention of ovarian cancer play a crucial role in the attempt to improve the overall survival from the disease. In particular, primary prevention is based on avoiding risk factors and increasing protective factors. Despite the identification of several risk and protective factors among the general population, most of the common factors described to date only slightly influence the risk of developing ovarian cancer, thus, the knowledge of these factors has still not been translated into practical strategies to prevent ovarian cancer.

On the other hand, primary prevention could represent a good opportunity for high-risk women. Women who inherit a mutation in either the *BRCA1* or *BRCA2* gene have greatly elevated lifetime risks of ovarian cancer, fallopian tube cancer and breast cancer. Surveillance for ovarian and fallopian tube cancer has not been proven to be effective. For this reason, preventive surgical removal of the ovaries and fallopian tubes (salpingo-oophorectomy) is actively recommended to these women by the age of 35 or 40 years, often prior to natural menopause, to prevent cancer. Moreover, women at increased risk may join a cancer prevention clinical trial or a chemoprevention trial. In particular, oral contraceptive use can be considered as an alternative strategy in the chemoprevention of ovarian cancer in *BRCA1* mutation carriers who do not accept RRSO above the age of 30 years. Other chemopreventive agents such as retinoids, analgesic drugs, vitamin D, cyclo-oxygenase inhibitors and peroxisome proliferator activated receptor-gamma ligands have shown promise in early investigations of disease prevention.

Regarding radiological methods to investigate ovaries and their adnexes, new techniques besides TVUS need to be explored. Pelvic Magnetic Radiological Imaging could be of interest even if it is difficult to imagine such an expensive technique being employed in the screening of high-risk women. For high-risk women, recommended cancer screening strategies, which need to be adjusted depending on the earliest age of onset in a family, have not been assessed by randomized trials or case-control studies. Ovarian cancer screening relies on a combination of annual or semi-annual pelvic examination, annual or semi-annual transvaginal ultrasound examination with colour Doppler, and annual measurement of serum CA125 concentrations.

Current approaches are a futile attempt to detect ovarian cancer in the early stages, but future research should be directed to better characterizing critical pathways in ovarian carcinogenesis and to identifying appropriate surveillance programs based on biomarker tests and/or radiological investigations, in order to improve overall survival, which dramatically decreases in the first 5 years. Due to the fact that an analysis of potentially thousands of proteins which could be simultaneously altered is necessary, comparative proteomics is a promising mode of potential biomarker discovery for cancer detection and monitoring. A better estimation of the biological importance of certain proteins with regard to the progression from pre-neoplastic tissue alterations to malignant tumours, as well as the prediction of the metastasis-forming potential by biomarkers, will be a necessary prerequisite to provide a more detailed insight and understanding of tumour progression.

Acknowledgements

The authors thank the "Angela Serra" Association for Cancer Research (Modena, Italy) and the "Fondazione Cassa di Risparmio "of Modena, Italy for financial support. A special thanks to Dr Adriano Benedetti and Dr Daniela Manzini (C.I.G.S., University of Modena and Reggio Emilia) for skilled assistance in protein analysis by ESI-Q-TOF MS. This work was supported by grants from the Italian Minister of University and Research, PRIN 2008 (20088RFCMH).

Author details

L. Cortesi, A. Toss and E. De Matteis

Department of Oncology and Haematology, University of Modena and Reggio Emilia, Modena, Italy

References

[1] Siegel R, Naishadham D, Jemal A. Cancer statistics, 2012. CA Cancer J Clin 2012; 62(1): 10-29.

[2] Anttila A, Ronco G, Clifford G, Bray F, Hakama M, Arbyn M, Weiderpass E. Cervical cancer screening programmes and policies in 18 European countries. Br J Cancer 2004;91(5):935-41.

[3] Marth C, Hiebl S, Oberaigner W, Winter R, Leodolter S, Sevelda P. Influence of department volume on survival for ovarian cancer: results from a prospective quality assurance program of the Austrian Association for Gynecologic Oncology. Int J Gynecol Cancer 2009;19(1):94-102.

[4] Chan JK, Urban R, Cheung MK, Osann K, Shin JY, Husain A, Teng NN, Kapp DS, Berek JS, Leiserowitz GS. Ovarian cancer in younger vs older women: a population-based analysis. Br J Cancer 2006;95(10):1314-20.

[5] Nagle CM, Bain CJ, Green AC, Webb PM. The influence of reproductive and hormonal factors on ovarian cancer survival Int J Gynecol Cancer 2008;18(3):407-13.

[6] Schorge JO, Modesitt SC, Coleman RL, Cohn DE, Kauff ND, Duska LR, Herzog TJ. SGO White Paper on ovarian cancer: etiology, screening and surveillance. Gynecol Oncol. 2010;119(1):7-17.

[7] Schouten LJ, Rivera C, Hunter DJ, Spiegelman D, Adami HO, Arslan A, Beeson WL, van den Brandt PA, Buring JE, Folsom AR, Fraser GE, Freudenheim JL, Goldbohm RA, Hankinson SE, Lacey JV Jr, Leitzmann M, Lukanova A, Marshall JR, Miller AB, Patel AV, Rodriguez C, Rohan TE, Ross JA, Wolk A, Zhang SM, Smith-Warner SA. Height, body mass index, and ovarian cancer: a pooled analysis of 12 cohort studies. Cancer Epidemiol Biomarkers Prev. 2008;17(4):902-12.

[8] Lahmann PH, Cust AE, Friedenreich CM, Schulz M, Lukanova A, Kaaks R, Lundin E, Tjønneland A, Halkjaer J, Severinsen MT, Overvad K, Fournier A, Chabbert-Buffet N, Clavel-Chapelon F, Dossus L, Pischon T, Boeing H, Trichopoulou A, Lagiou P, Naska A, Palli D, Grioni S, Mattiello A, Tumino R, Sacerdote C, Redondo ML, Jakszyn P, Sánchez MJ, Tormo MJ, Ardanaz E, Arriola L, Manjer J, Jirström K, Bueno-de-Mesquita HB, May AM, Peeters PH, Onland-Moret NC, Bingham S, Khaw KT, Allen NE, Spencer E, Rinaldi S, Slimani N, Chajes V, Michaud D, Norat T, Riboli E. Anthropometric measures and epithelial ovarian cancer risk in the European Prospective Investigation into Cancer and Nutrition. Int J Cancer. 2010;126(10):2404-15.

[9] Camargo MC, Stayner LT, Straif K, Reina M, Al-Alem U, Demers PA, Landrigan PJ. Occupational exposure to asbestos and ovarian cancer: a meta-analysis. Environ Health Perspect. 2011;119(9):1211-7.

[10] Cramer DW. The epidemiology of endometrial and ovarian cancer. Hematol Oncol Clin North Am. 2012;26(1):1-12.

[11] Beral V; Million Women Study Collaborators, Bull D, Green J, Reeves G. Ovarian cancer and hormone replacement therapy in the Million Women Study. Lancet. 2007;369(9574):1703-10.

[12] Melin A, Sparén P, Persson I, Bergqvist A. Endometriosis and the risk of cancer with special emphasis on ovarian cancer. Hum Reprod. 2006;21(5):1237-42.

[13] Chen S, Parmigiani G. Meta-analysis of BRCA1 and BRCA2 penetrance. J Clin Oncol. 2007;25(11):1329-33.

[14] Watson P, Bützow R, Lynch HT, Mecklin JP, Järvinen HJ, Vasen HF, Madlensky L, Fidalgo P, Bernstein I; International Collaborative Group on HNPCC. The clinical features of ovarian cancer in hereditary nonpolyposis colorectal cancer. Gynecol Oncol. 2001;82(2):223-8.

[15] Trudel D, Labbé DP, Bairati I, Fradet V, Bazinet L, Têtu B. Green tea for ovarian cancer prevention and treatment: A systematic review of the in vitro, in vivo and epidemiological studies. Gynecol Oncol. 2012;126(3):491-8.

[16] Collaborative Group on Epidemiological Studies of Ovarian Cancer, Beral V, Doll R, Hermon C, Peto R, Reeves G. Ovarian cancer and oral contraceptives: collaborative reanalysis of data from 45 epidemiological studies including 23,257 women with ovarian cancer and 87,303 controls. Lancet 2008;371(9609):303-14.

[17] Ness RB, Cramer DW, Goodman MT, Kjaer SK, Mallin K, Mosgaard BJ, Purdie DM, Risch HA, Vergona R, Wu AH. Infertility, fertility drugs, and ovarian cancer: a pooled analysis of case-control studies. Am J Epidemiol. 2002;155(3):217-24.

[18] Danforth KN, Tworoger SS, Hecht JL, Rosner BA, Colditz GA, Hankinson SE. Breastfeeding and risk of ovarian cancer in two prospective cohorts. Cancer Causes Control. 2007;18(5):517-23.

[19] Hankinson SE, Hunter DJ, Colditz GA, Willett WC, Stampfer MJ, Rosner B, Hennekens CH, Speizer FE. Tubal ligation, hysterectomy, and risk of ovarian cancer. A prospective study. JAMA 1993;270(23):2813-8.

[20] Goodman MT, Howe HL, Tung KH, Hotes J, Miller BA, Coughlin SS, Chen VW. Incidence of ovarian cancer by race and ethnicity in the United States, 1992-1997. Cancer 2003;97(10 Suppl):2676-85.

[21] Kiani F, Knutsen S, Singh P, Ursin G, Fraser G. Dietary risk factors for ovarian cancer: the Adventist Health Study (United States). Cancer Causes Control. 2006;17(2):137-46.

[22] Rota M, Pasquali E, Scotti L, Pelucchi C, Tramacere I, Islami F, Negri E, Boffetta P, Bellocco R, Corrao G, La Vecchia C, Bagnardi V. Alcohol drinking and epithelial ovarian cancer risk. a systematic review and meta-analysis. Gynecol Oncol. 2012;125(3):758-63.

[23] Bandera EV, King M, Chandran U, Paddock LE, Rodriguez-Rodriguez L, Olson SH. Phytoestrogen consumption from foods and supplements and epithelial ovarian cancer risk: a population-based case control study. BMC Womens Health. 2011;11:40.

[24] Preston DL, Ron E, Tokuoka S, Funamoto S, Nishi N, Soda M, Mabuchi K, Kodama K. Solid cancer incidence in atomic bomb survivors: 1958-1998. Radiat Res. 2007;168(1):1-64.

[25] Preston DL, Shimizu Y, Pierce DA, Suyama A, Mabuchi K. Studies of mortality of atomic bomb survivors. Report 13: Solid cancer and noncancer disease mortality: 1950-1997. Radiat Res. 2003;160(4):381-407.

[26] Parkin DM. 10. Cancers attributable to exposure to hormones in the UK in 2010. Br J Cancer. 2011;105 Suppl 2:S42-8.

[27] International Agency for research on cancer (iarc) 2007. IARC monographs on the evaluation of carcinogenic risks to humans vol 91. Combined estrogen-progestogen contraceptives and combined estrogen-progestogen menopausal therapy.

[28] Vercellini P, Crosignani P, Somigliana E, Viganò P, Buggio L, Bolis G, Fedele L. The incessant menstruation' hypothesis: a mechanistic ovarian cancer model with implications for prevention. Hum Reprod. 2011;26(9):2262-73.

[29] Titus-Ernstoff L, Perez K, Cramer DW, Harlow BL, Baron JA, Greenberg ER. Menstrual and reproductive factors in relation to ovarian cancer risk. Br J Cancer 2001;84(5):714-21.

[30] Kurta ML, Moysich KB, Weissfeld JL, Youk AO, Bunker CH, Edwards RP, Modugno F, Ness RB, Diergaarde B. Use of fertility drugs and risk of ovarian cancer: results from a u.s.-Based case-control study. Cancer Epidemiol Biomarkers Prev. 2012;21(8):1282-92.

[31] Miracle-McMahill HL, Calle EE, Kosinski AS, Rodriguez C, Wingo PA, Thun MJ, Heath CW Jr. Tubal ligation and fatal ovarian cancer in a large prospective cohort study. Am J Epidemiol. 1997;145(4):349-57.

[32] Huncharek M, Muscat J. Perineal talc use and ovarian cancer risk: a case study of scientific standards in environmental epidemiology. Eur J Cancer Prev. 2011;20(6): 501-7.

[33] Muscat JE, Huncharek MS. Perineal talc use and ovarian cancer: a critical review. Eur J Cancer Prev. 2008;17(2):139-46.

[34] Pearce CL, Templeman C, Rossing MA, Lee A, Near AM, Webb PM, Nagle CM, Doherty JA, Cushing-Haugen KL, Wicklund KG, Chang-Claude J, Hein R, Lurie G, Wilkens LR, Carney ME, Goodman MT, Moysich K, Kjaer SK, Hogdall E, Jensen A, Goode EL, Fridley BL, Larson MC, Schildkraut JM, Palmieri RT, Cramer DW, Terry KL, Vitonis AF, Titus LJ, Ziogas A, Brewster W, Anton-Culver H, Gentry-Maharaj A, Ramus SJ, Anderson AR, Brueggmann D, Fasching PA, Gayther SA, Huntsman DG, Menon U, Ness RB, Pike MC, Risch H, Wu AH, Berchuck A; Ovarian Cancer Association Consortium. Association between endometriosis and risk of histological subtypes of ovarian cancer: a pooled analysis of case-control studies. Lancet Oncol. 2012;13(4): 385-94.

[35] Lin HW, Tu YY, Lin SY, Su WJ, Lin WL, Lin WZ, Wu SC, Lai YL. Risk of ovarian cancer in women with pelvic inflammatory disease: a population-based study. Lancet Oncol. 2011;12(9):900-4.

[36] Brodie SG, Deng CX. BRCA1-associated tumorigenesis: what have we learned from knockout mice? Trends Genet. 2001;17(10):S18-22.

[37] Walsh T, Casadei S, Coats KH, Swisher E, Stray SM, Higgins J, Roach KC, Mandell J, Lee MK, Ciernikova S, Foretova L, Soucek P, King MC. Spectrum of mutations in BRCA1, BRCA2, CHEK2, and TP53 in families at high risk of breast cancer. JAMA 2006;295(12):1379-88.

[38] Rahman N, Seal S, Thompson D, Kelly P, Renwick A, Elliott A, Reid S, Spanova K, Barfoot R, Chagtai T, Jayatilake H, McGuffog L, Hanks S, Evans DG, Eccles D; Breast Cancer Susceptibility Collaboration (UK), Easton DF, Stratton MR. PALB2, which encodes a BRCA2-interacting protein, is a breast cancer susceptibility gene. Nat Genet. 2007;39(2):165-7.

[39] Casadei S, Norquist BM, Walsh T, Stray S, Mandell JB, Lee MK, Stamatoyannopoulos JA, King MC. Contribution of inherited mutations in the BRCA2-interacting protein PALB2 to familial breast cancer. Cancer Res. 2011;71(6):2222-9.

[40] Engel NJ, Gordon P, Thull DL, Dudley B, Herstine J, Jankowitz RC, Zorn KK. A multidisciplinary clinic for individualizing management of patients at increased risk for breast and gynecologic cancer. Fam Cancer. 2012 May 27. [Epub ahead of print]

[41] Peters JA, Stopfer JE. Role of the genetic counselor in familial cancer. Oncology (Williston Park). 1996;10(2):159-66, 175; discussion 176-6, 178.

[42] American College of Medical Genetics. Genetic Susceptibility to Breast and Ovarian Cancer: Assessment, Counseling and Testing Guidelines. New York State Department of Health 1999; http://www.health.state.ny.us (accessed 19 September 2012)

[43] American Society of Clinical Oncology. American Society of Clinical Oncology Policy Statement Update: Genetic Testing for Cancer Susceptibility. J Clin Oncol 2003;21:2397-2406.

[44] Hopwood P. Genetic risk counseling for breast cancer families. Eur J Cancer 1998;34:1477-1479.

[45] Hoskins KF, Stopfer JE, Calzone KA, Merajver SD, Rebbeck TR, Garber JE, Weber BL. Assessment and counseling for women with a family history of breast cancer. A guide for clinicians. JAMA 1995;273(7):577-85.

[46] Contegiacomo A, Pensabene M, Capuano I, Tauchmanova L, Federico M, Turchetti D, Cortesi L, Marchetti P, Ricevuto E, Cianci G, Venuta S, Barbieri V, Silingardi V; Italian Network on Hereditary Breast Cancer. An oncologist-based model of cancer genetic counselling for hereditary breast and ovarian cancer. Ann Oncol. 2004;15(5):726-32.

[47] Hilgart JS, Coles B, Iredale R. Cancer genetic risk assessment for individuals at risk of familial breast cancer. Cochrane Database Syst Rev. 2012 Feb 15;2:CD003721.

[48] Ford D, Easton DF, Stratton M, Narod S, Goldgar D, Devilee P, Bishop DT, Weber B, Lenoir G, Chang-Claude J, Sobol H, Teare MD, Struewing J, Arason A, Scherneck S, Peto J, Rebbeck TR, Tonin P, Neuhausen S, Barkardottir R, Eyfjord J, Lynch H, Ponder BA, Gayther SA, Zelada-Hedman M, et al. Genetic heterogeneity and penetrance

analysis of the BRCA1 and BRCA2 genes in breast cancer families. The Breast Cancer Linkage Consortium. Am J Hum Genet. 1998;62(3):676-89.

[49] Pennington KP, Swisher EM. Hereditary ovarian cancer: beyond the usual suspects. Gynecol Oncol. 2012;124(2):347-53.

[50] Antoniou AC, Pharoah PD, Easton DF, Evans DG. BRCA1 and BRCA2 cancer risks. J Clin Oncol. 2006;24(20):3312-3.

[51] Struewing JP, Hartge P, Wacholder S, Baker SM, Berlin M, McAdams M, Timmerman MM, Brody LC, Tucker MA. The risk of cancer associated with specific mutations of BRCA1 and BRCA2 among Ashkenazi Jews. N Engl J Med 1997;336(20):1401-1408.

[52] Finch A, Evans G, Narod SA. BRCA carriers, prophylactic salpingo-oophorectomy and menopause: clinical management considerations and recommendations. Womens Health (Lond Engl) 2012;8(5):543-55.

[53] Prevalence and penetrance of BRCA1 and BRCA2 mutations in a population-based series of breast cancer cases. Anglian Breast Cancer Study Group. Br J Cancer 2000;83(10):1301-1308.

[54] Satagopan JM, Boyd J, Kauff ND, Robson M, Scheuer L, Narod S, Offit K. Ovarian cancer risk in Ashkenazi Jewish carriers of BRCA1 and BRCA2 mutations. Clin Cancer Res. 2002;8(12):3776-3781.

[55] Rebbeck TR, Lynch HT, Neuhausen SL, Narod SA, Van't Veer L, Garber JE, Evans G, Isaacs C, Daly MB, Matloff E, Olopade OI, Weber BL; Prevention and Observation of Surgical End Points Study Group. Prophylactic oophorectomy in carriers of BRCA1 or BRCA2 mutations. N Engl J Med 2002; 346(21):1616-1622.

[56] Kauff ND, Domchek SM, Friebel TM, Robson ME, Lee J, Garber JE, Isaacs C, Evans DG, Lynch H, Eeles RA, Neuhausen SL, Daly MB, Matloff E, Blum JL, Sabbatini P, Barakat RR, Hudis C, Norton L, Offit K, Rebbeck TR. Risk-reducing salpingo-oophorectomy for the prevention of BRCA1 and BRCA2 associated breast and gynecologic cancer: a multi-center, prospective study. J Clin Oncol 2008;26(8):1331-1337.

[57] Finch A, Beiner M, Lubinski J, Lynch HT, Moller P, Rosen B, Murphy J, Ghadirian P, Friedman E, Foulkes WD, Kim-Sing C, Wagner T, Tung N, Couch F, Stoppa-Lyonnet D, Ainsworth P, Daly M, Pasini B, Gershoni-Baruch R, Eng C, Olopade OI, McLennan J, Karlan B, Weitzel J, Sun P, Narod SA; Hereditary Ovarian Cancer Clinical Study Group. Salpingo-oophorectomy and the risk of ovarian, fallopian tube, and peritoneal cancers in women with a BRCA1 or BRCA2 mutation. JAMA 2006;296(2):185-192.

[58] Chang-Claude J, Andrieu N, Rookus M, Brohet R, Antoniou AC, Peock S, Davidson R, Izatt L, Cole T, Noguès C, Luporsi E, Huiart L, Hoogerbrugge N, Van Leeuwen FE, Osorio A, Eyfjord J, Radice P, Goldgar DE, Easton DF; Epidemiological Study of Familial Breast Cancer (EMBRACE); Gene Etude Prospective Sein Ovaire (GENEPSO); Genen Omgeving studie van de werkgroep Hereditiair Borstkanker Onderzoek Nederland (GEO-HEBON); International BRCA1/2 Carrier Cohort Study (IBCCS)

collaborators group. Age at menarche and menopause and breast cancer risk in the International BRCA1/2 Carrier Cohort Study. Cancer Epidemiol Biomarkers Prev 2007;16(4):740-746.

[59] Rebbeck TR, Levin AM, Eisen A, Snyder C, Watson P, Cannon-Albright L, Isaacs C, Olopade O, Garber JE, Godwin AK, Daly MB, Narod SA, Neuhausen SL, Lynch HT, Weber BL. Risk-reducing salpingo-oophorectomy in women with a BRCA1 or BRCA2 mutation. N Engl J Med 2002;346(21):1609-1615.

[60] Rutter JL, Wacholder S, Chetrit A, Lubin F, Menczer J, Ebbers S, Tucker MA, Struewing JP, Hartge P. Gynecologic surgeries and risk of ovarian cancer in women with BRCA1 and BRCA2 Ashkenazi founder mutations: an Israeli population-based case-control study. J Natl Cancer Inst 2003;95(14):1072-1078.

[61] Kauff ND, Satagopan JM, Robson ME, Scheuer L, Hensley M, Hudis CA, Ellis NA, Boyd J, Borgen PI, Barakat RR, Norton L, Castiel M, Nafa K, Offit K. Risk-reducing salpingo-oophorectomy in women with a BRCA1 or BRCA2 mutation. N Engl J Med 2002;346(21):1609-15.

[62] National Comprehensive Cancer Network. NCCN Clinical Practice Guidelines in Oncology. Genetic/Familial High-Risk Assessment: Breast and Ovarian pdf 2012.

[63] American College of Obstetricians and Gynecologists ACOG. Practice Bulletin No. 103: Hereditary breast and ovarian cancer syndrome. Obstet Gynecol 2009;13(4):957-66.

[64] http://www.cancer.gov/cancertopics/pdq/genetics/breast-and-ovarian/ (accessed 19 September 2012)

[65] Leblanc E, Narducci F, Farre I, Peyrat JP, Taieb S, Adenis C, Vennin P. Radical fimbriectomy: a reasonable temporary risk-reducing surgery for selected women with a germ line mutation of BRCA 1 or 2 genes? Rationale and preliminary development. Gynecol Oncol 2011;121(3):472-6.

[66] Balmaña J, Díez O, Rubio IT, Cardoso F; ESMO Guidelines Working Group. BRCA in breast cancer: ESMO Clinical Practice Guidelines. Ann Oncol. 2011;22 Suppl 6:vi31-4.

[67] Domchek SM, Friebel TM, Neuhausen SL, Wagner T, Evans G, Isaacs C, Garber JE, Daly MB, Eeles R, Matloff E, Tomlinson GE, Van't Veer L, Lynch HT, Olopade OI, Weber BL, Rebbeck TR. Mortality after bilateral salpingo-oophorectomy in BRCA1 and BRCA2 mutation carriers: a prospective cohort study. Lancet Oncol. 2006;7(3):223-9.

[68] Domchek SM, Weber BL. Clinical management of BRCA1 and BRCA2 mutation carriers. Oncogene 2006;25:5825-5831.

[69] Iodice S, Barile M, Rotmensz N, Feroce I, Bonanni B, Radice P, Bernard L, Maisonneuve P, Gandini S. Oral contraceptive use and breast or ovarian cancer risk in BRCA1/2 carriers: a meta-analysis. Eur J Cancer 2010;46(12):2275-84.

[70] Cibula D, Zikan M, Dusek L, Majek O. Oral contraceptives and risk of ovarian and breast cancers in BRCA mutation carriers: a meta-analysis. Expert Rev Anticancer Ther. 2011;11(8):1197-207.

[71] Zorn KK et al. Epithelial ovarian cancer. In: Kelloff GJ, Hawk ET, Sigman CC, editors. Cancer chemoprevention: strategies for cancer chemoprevention, vol. 2. Totowa (NJ): Humana; 2005.

[72] Whitworth JM, Straughn JM Jr, Atigadda VR, Muccio DD, Buchsbaum DJ. The use of retinoids in ovarian cancer: a review of the literature. Int J Gynecol Cancer 2012;22(2): 191-8.

[73] Mehta RG, Moon RC, Hawthorne M, Formelli F, Costa A. Distribution of fenretinide in the mammary gland of breast cancer patients. Eur J Cancer 1991;27(2):138-41.

[74] Cazzaniga M, Varricchio C, Montefrancesco C, Feroce I, Guerrieri-Gonzaga A. Fenretinide (4-HPR): a preventive chance for women at genetic and familial risk? J Biomed Biotechnol. 2012;2012:172897.

[75] Costa A, Malone W, Perloff M, Buranelli F, Campa T, Dossena G, Magni A, Pizzichetta M, Andreoli C, Del Vecchio M, et al. Tolerability of the synthetic retinoid Fenretinide (HPR). Eur J Cancer Clin Oncol. 1989;25(5):805-8.

[76] Formelli F, Carsana R, Costa A, Buranelli F, Campa T, Dossena G, Magni A, Pizzichetta M. Plasma retinol level reduction by the synthetic retinoid fenretinide: a one year follow-up study of breast cancer patients. Cancer Res. 1989;49(21):6149-52.

[77] Veronesi U, De Palo G, Marubini E, Costa A, Formelli F, Mariani L, Decensi A, Camerini T, Del Turco MR, Di Mauro MG, Muraca MG, Del Vecchio M, Pinto C, D'Aiuto G, Boni C, Campa T, Magni A, Miceli R, Perloff M, Malone WF, Sporn MB. Randomized trial of fenretinide to prevent second breast malignancy in women with early breast cancer. J Natl Cancer Inst. 1999; 91(21):1847-56.

[78] Veronesi U, Mariani L, Decensi A, Formelli F, Camerini T, Miceli R, Di Mauro MG, Costa A, Marubini E, Sporn MB, De Palo G. Fifteen-year results of a randomized phase III trial of fenretinide to prevent second breast cancer. Ann Oncol. 2006;17(7):1065-71.

[79] Ammundsen HB, Faber MT, Jensen A, Høgdall E, Blaakaer J, Høgdall C, Kjaer SK. Use of analgesic drugs and risk of ovarian cancer: results from a Danish case-control study. Acta Obstet Gynecol Scand. 2012;91(9):1094-102.

[80] Setiawan VW, Matsuno RK, Lurie G, Wilkens LR, Carney ME, Henderson BE, Kolonel LN, Goodman MT. Use of Nonsteroidal Anti-inflammatory Drugs and Risk of Ovarian and Endometrial Cancer: The Multiethnic Cohort. Cancer Epidemiol Biomarkers Prev. 2012;21(9):1441-9.

[81] Ni X, Ma J, Zhao Y, Wang Y, Wang S. Meta-analysis on the association between non-steroidal anti-inflammatory drug use and ovarian cancer. Br J Clin Pharmacol. 2012 Apr 3. doi: 10.1111/j.1365-2125.2012.04290.x. [Epub ahead of print]

[82] Dann RB, Kelley JL, Zorn KK. Strategies for ovarian cancer prevention. Obstet Gynecol Clin North Am. 2007;34(4):667-86.

[83] Buys SS, Partridge E, Black A, Johnson CC, Lamerato L, Isaacs C, Reding DJ, Greenlee RT, Yokochi LA, Kessel B, Crawford ED, Church TR, Andriole GL, Weissfeld JL, Fouad MN, Chia D, O'Brien B, Ragard LR, Clapp JD, Rathmell JM, Riley TL, Hartge P, Pinsky PF, Zhu CS, Izmirlian G, Kramer BS, Miller AB, Xu JL, Prorok PC, Gohagan JK, Berg CD; PLCO Project Team. Effect of screening on ovarian cancer mortality: the Prostate, Lung, Colorectal and Ovarian (PLCO) Cancer Screening Randomized Controlled Trial. JAMA 2011;305(22):2295-303.

[84] Scheuer L, Kauff N, Robson M, Kelly B, Barakat R, Satagopan J, Ellis N, Hensley M, Boyd J, Borgen P, Norton L, Offit K. Outcome of preventive surgery and screening for breast and ovarian cancer in BRCA mutation carriers. J Clin Oncol 2002;20(5):1260-8.

[85] Hermsen BB, Olivier RI, Verheijen RH, van Beurden M, de Hullu JA, Massuger LF, Burger CW, Brekelmans CT, Mourits MJ, de Bock GH, Gaarenstroom KN, van Boven HH, Mooij TM, Rookus MA. No efficacy of annual gynaecological screening in BRCA1/2 mutation carriers; an observational follow-up study. Br J Cancer 2007;96(9): 1335-42.

[86] Olivier RI, Lubsen-Brandsma MA, Verhoef S, van Beurden M. CA125 and transvaginal ultrasound monitoring in high-risk women cannot prevent the diagnosis of advanced ovarian cancer. Gynecol Oncol. 2006;100(1):20-6.

[87] Van Der Velde NM, Mourits MJ, Arts HJ, De Vries J, Leegte BK, Dijkhuis G, Oosterwijk JC, De Bock GH. Time to stop ovarian cancer screening in BRCA1/2 mutation carriers? Int J Cancer. 2009;124(4):919-23.

[88] Stirling D, Evans DG, Pichert G, Shenton A, Kirk EN, Rimmer S, Steel CM, Lawson S, Busby-Earle RM, Walker J, Lalloo FI, Eccles DM, Lucassen AM, Porteous ME. Screening for familial ovarian cancer: failure of current protocols to detect ovarian cancer at an early stage according to the international Federation of gynecology and obstetrics system. J Clin Oncol. 2005;23(24):5588-96.

[89] Laframboise S, Nedelcu R, Murphy J, Cole DE, Rosen B. Use of CA-125 and ultrasound in high-risk women. Int J Gynecol Cancer. 2002;12(1):86-91.

[90] Evans DG, Gaarenstroom KN, Stirling D, Shenton A, Maehle L, Dørum A, Steel M, Lalloo F, Apold J, Porteous ME, Vasen HF, van Asperen CJ, Moller P. Screening for familial ovarian cancer: poor survival of BRCA1/2 related cancers. J Med Genet. 2009;46(9):593-7.

[91] NCCN Clinical Practice Guidelines in Oncology. Genetic/Familial High-Risk Assessment: Breast and Ovarian. http://nccn.org (accessed 19 September 2012)

[92] Burke W, Daly M, Garber J, Botkin J, Kahn MJ, Lynch P, McTiernan A, Offit K, Perlman J, Petersen G, Thomson E, Varricchio C. Recommendations for follow-up care of

individuals with an inherited predisposition to cancer. II. BRCA1 and BRCA2. Cancer Genetics Studies Consortium. JAMA 1997;277(12):997-1003.

[93] NIH consensus conference. Ovarian cancer. Screening, treatment, and follow-up. NIH Consensus Development Panel on Ovarian Cancer. JAMA 1995;273(6):491-7.

[94] Glunde K, Artemov D, Penet MF, Jacobs MA, Bhujwalla ZM. Magnetic resonance spectroscopy in metabolic and molecular imaging and diagnosis of cancer. Chem Rev. 2010;110(5):3043-59.

[95] Sardanelli F, Fausto A, Di Leo G, de Nijs R, Vorbuchner M, Podo F. In vivo proton MR spectroscopy of the breast using the total choline peak integral as a marker of malignancy. AJR Am J Roentgenol. 2009;192(6):1608-17.

[96] Iorio E, Mezzanzanica D, Alberti P, Spadaro F, Ramoni C, D'Ascenzo S, Millimaggi D, Pavan A, Dolo V, Canevari S, Podo F. Alterations of choline metabolism in ovarian tumor progression. Cancer Res. 2005;65(20):9369-76.

[97] Spadaro F, Ramoni C, Mezzanzanica D, Miotti S, Alberti P, Cecchetti S, Iorio E, Dolo V, Canevari S, Podo F. Phosphatidylcholine-specific phospholipase C activation in epithelial ovarian cancer cells. Cancer Res. 2008;68(16):6541-9.

[98] Podo F, Sardanelli F, Iorio E, Canese R, Carpinelli G, Fausto A, Canevari S. Abnormal choline phospholipid metabolism in breast and ovary cancer: molecular bases for noninvasive imaging approaches. Curr Med Imaging Rev. 2007;3:123–137.

[99] Clarke-Pearson DL. Clinical practice. Screening for ovarian cancer. N Engl J Med. 2009;361(2):170-7.

[100] Drapkin R, von Horsten HH, Lin Y, Mok SC, Crum CP, Welch WR, Hecht JL. Human epididymis protein 4 (HE4) is a secreted glycoprotein that is overexpressed by serous and endometrioid ovarian carcinomas. Cancer Res. 2005;65(6):2162-9.

[101] Moore RG, McMeekin DS, Brown AK, DiSilvestro P, Miller MC, Allard WJ, Gajewski W, Kurman R, Bast RC Jr, Skates SJ. A novel multiple marker bioassay utilizing HE4 and CA125 for the prediction of ovarian cancer in patients with a pelvic mass. Gynecol Oncol. 2009;112(1):40-6.

[102] Van Gorp T, Cadron I, Despierre E, Daemen A, Leunen K, Amant F, Timmerman D, De Moor B, Vergote I. HE4 and CA125 as a diagnostic test in ovarian cancer: prospective validation of the Risk of Ovarian Malignancy Algorithm. Br J Cancer. 2011;104(5): 863-70.

[103] Karlsen MA, Sandhu N, Høgdall C, Christensen IJ, Nedergaard L, Lundvall L, Engelholm SA, Pedersen AT, Hartwell D, Lydolph M, Laursen IA, Høgdall EV. Evaluation of HE4, CA125, risk of ovarian malignancy algorithm (ROMA) and risk of malignancy index (RMI) as diagnostic tools of epithelial ovarian cancer in patients with a pelvic mass. Gynecol Oncol. 2012 Jul 24. [Epub ahead of print]

[104] Macuks R, Baidekalna I, Donina S. An ovarian cancer malignancy risk index composed of HE4, CA125, ultrasonographic score, and menopausal status: use in differentiation of ovarian cancers and benign lesions. Tumour Biol. 2012 Jun 14. [Epub ahead of print]

[105] Andersen MR, Goff BA, Lowe KA, Scholler N, Bergan L, Drescher CW, Paley P, Urban N. Use of a Symptom Index, CA125, and HE4 to predict ovarian cancer. Gynecol Oncol. 2010;116(3):378-83.

[106] Goff BA, Mandel LS, Drescher CW, Urban N, Gough S, Schurman KM, Patras J, Mahony BS, Andersen MR. Development of an ovarian cancer symptom index: possibilities for earlier detection. Cancer 2007;109(2):221-7.

[107] Dann RB, Kelley JL, Zorn KK. Strategies for ovarian cancer prevention. Obstet Gynecol Clin North Am. 2007;34(4):667-86.

[108] Petricoin EF, Ardekani AM, Hitt BA, Levine PJ, Fusaro VA, Steinberg SM, Mills GB, Simone C, Fishman DA, Kohn EC, Liotta LA. Use of proteomic patterns in serum to identify ovarian cancer. Lancet 2002;359(9306):572-7.

[109] Nossov V, Amneus M, Su F, Lang J, Janco JM, Reddy ST, Farias-Eisner R. The early detection of ovarian cancer: from traditional methods to proteomics. Can we really do better than serum CA-125? Am J Obstet Gynecol. 2008;199(3):215-23.

[110] Zhang B, Barekati Z, Kohler C, Radpour R, Asadollahi R, Holzgreve W, Zhong XY. Proteomics and biomarkers for ovarian cancer diagnosis. Ann Clin Lab Sci. 2010;40(3): 218-25.

[111] An HJ, Kim DS, Park YK, Kim SK, Choi YP, Kang S, Ding B, Cho NH. Comparative proteomics of ovarian epithelial tumors. J Proteome Res. 2006;5(5):1082-90.

[112] Petri AL, Simonsen AH, Yip TT, Hogdall E, Fung ET, Lundvall L, Hogdall C. Three new potential ovarian cancer biomarkers detected in human urine with equalizer bead technology. Acta Obstet Gynecol Scand. 2009;88(1):18-26.

[113] Li XQ, Zhang SL, Cai Z, Zhou Y, Ye TM, Chiu JF. Proteomic identification of tumor-associated protein in ovarian serous cystadenocarinoma. Cancer Lett. 2009; 275(1): 109-16.

[114] Cortesi L, Rossi E, Della Casa L, Barchetti A, Nicoli A, Piana S, Abrate M, La Sala GB, Federico M, Iannone A. Protein expression patterns associated with advanced stage ovarian cancer. Electrophoresis 2011;32(15):1992-2003.

Section 2

Pathology

Chapter 4

Borderline Epithelial Tumors of the Ovary

Gennaro Cormio, Vera Loizzi, Maddalena Falagario, Doriana Scardigno, Donatella Latorre and Luigi E. Selvaggi

Additional information is available at the end of the chapter

http://dx.doi.org/10.5772/54828

1. Introduction

Borderline ovarian tumors (BOT) were first described in 1929 by Taylor, which, due to the characteristics of the tumor, called it "semi malignant" or "borderline" [1]; subsequently, this group of tumors of the ovary were classified in 1973 by the World Health Organization as "low malignant potential ovarian tumor" [2] and, finally, in 2003 WHO separates them from carcinomas and call them borderline tumors. [3]

Another term accepted to designate these independent ovarian neoplasms is "atypical proliferating (or atypical proliferative) tumor". [4]

Borderline ovarian tumors represent 10-20% of epithelial ovarian neoplasm's [5] with an incidence of 1.8-4.8 out of 100.000 women per year [6] and typically have an excellent prognosis.

Unlike the invasive carcinomas, borderline ovarian tumors are characterized by cytoplasmic and nuclear atypia, (element of differential diagnosis with benign tumors), absence of stromal invasion, (element of differential diagnosis with malignant tumors), unusual degree of proliferation of the epithelial cells with cellular stratification including remarkable architectural atypia and the formation of papillary protuberances. The absence of obvious stromal invasion is a principal diagnostic criterion for BOTs. Histologically, most of them are serous or mucinous, but endometrioid, clear cell, Brenner (transitional cell) or mixed histotypes can be also seen. [7]

To date, there are still no prospective randomized trials to clinical management, although they have an excellent prognosis, with a 5-year overall survival rate of almost 100% in early-stage disease (stage I-II) and between 86% and 92% in more advanced disease (stage III-IV). [8]

2. Classification, pathology and clinical behavior

Although they might occur in every age, most of the cases are diagnosed in pre-menopausal women between 34 and 40 years [9], while malignant ovarian cancer usually is diagnosed in patients between 50 and 70 years.

Risk factors for the development of BOTs are absolutely similar to those known for ovarian cancer, menarche, age at first pregnancy, age at first delivery, menstrual history, smoking history and family history of ovarian cancer, except that BOTs seem to have a lower frequency of BRCA mutations.

Borderline ovarian tumors are staged according to the FIGO classification of ovarian cancer. In 80% of cases patients with BOTs are in FIGO stage I at the time of diagnosis, about 30% of patients are in stage II-III in the same percentages each, while stage IV BOTs are very rare. [10]

2.1. Serous borderline tumors

They represent the 70% of BOTs, and 9-15% of all serous neoplasms [11,12] the mean age at presentation is 38 years old (range 17-77). [13] According to the FIGO staging system, [14] 68% are Stage I, 11% Stage II, 21% Stage III and less than 1% Stage IV. [15]

These neoplasms can be divided in two subtypes:

- APTSs, Atypical proliferative serous tumors, behave in a benign way and show a papillary architecture with a hierarchical pattern
- Non-invasive MPSCs, micopapillary serous borderline tumors, with a non hierarchical pattern, characterized by the presence of micropapilla, they are more associated with invasive implants and a worse prognosis than APTSs.

APTSs in 25-30% of cases they are bilateral, macroscopically they appear as cysts with serous contents with friable and exuberant papillary projections. (Figure 1) These papillae are mostly observed on the inner surface of the cyst, but in 70% of cases also in the external one. Rarely these serous BOTs show solid components.

Histologically APTSs show the presence of papillae with extensive epithelial stratification and budding, the epithelial cells have low or moderate atypias, in the fluid a detachment of single cells can be seen, there must not be any sign of invasion (Figure 2), but microinvasion (not more than 10 mm^2) can be present in up to 15% of cases. F [13, 16, 17] Some patients with stage I microinvasive tumors have developed progressive disease and microinvasion for some authors can be considered as risk factor for patients with high-stage disease. [18]

The cells in APTS can show an epithelial and occasionally a mesothelial differentiation. The nuclei of these cells present more atypia than those seen in benign cystoadenomas, the nuclei are usually basally located and ovoid or rounded, the nucleoli are only occasionally prominent and the mitosis are not so common (usually less than four per ten high-power fields, HPF). [4]

APTSs are occasionally also associated to the presence of endosalpingiosis or non invasive peritoneal implants, referred as the phenomenon of autoimplantation can be observed as the presence of foci resembling non invasive desmoplastic peritoneal implants with a well-delineated border on the ovarian surface, this phenomenon does not have any clear known pathogenesis nor clinical significance. [13, 19, 20, 16, 17] Signs of necrosis are very rare. [4]

APTSs are usually positive for CK7, OC-125 and cytokeratin and express estrogen and progesterone receptors. [4]

Non-invasive MPSCs, are serous borderline tumors characterized by the presence of micro-papillae arising from central papilla, when this specific pattern constitutes either a 5 mm or grater area or 10% or greater proportion.

In invasive MPSCs (synonymous of low-grade serous carcinoma) the stromal invasion must exceed 5 mm.

Non-invasive MPSCs represent 14% of all BOTs. The mean age at diagnosis is about 42 years, in 70% of cases they are bilateral and 50% of patients are in stage I at the time of diagnosis, while the other 50% are in stage II or III.

On gross appearance, non-invasive MPSC s look like cysts with papillae without or with little necrosis just like APSTs but in contrast to them they present mostly with peritoneal implant and bilaterality; the mean size is about 8 cm.

Histologically they are neoplasm with high degree of epithelial proliferation in a non hierarchical branching architecture, with micropapillary and cribriform patterns. [4]

The differential diagnosis should be done with serous cystadenomas, serous mucinous or endometrioid borderline tumors and with malignant neoplasm.

Survival in serous BOTs differs significatively from serous invasive ovarian cancer and is characterized by an excellent prognosis.

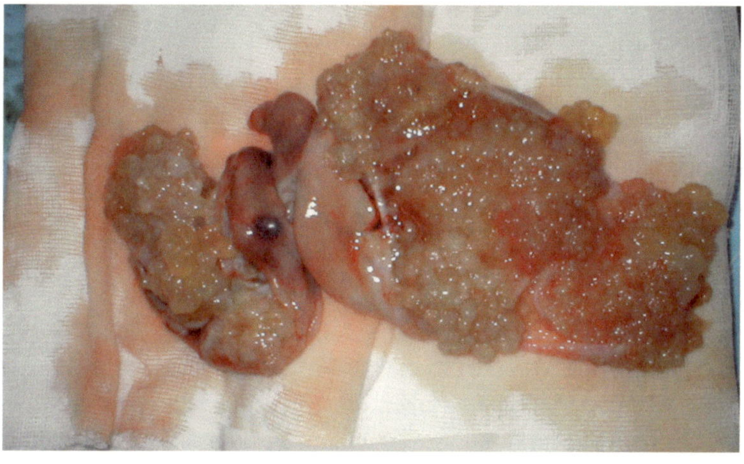

Figure 1. Serous borderline ovarian tumor

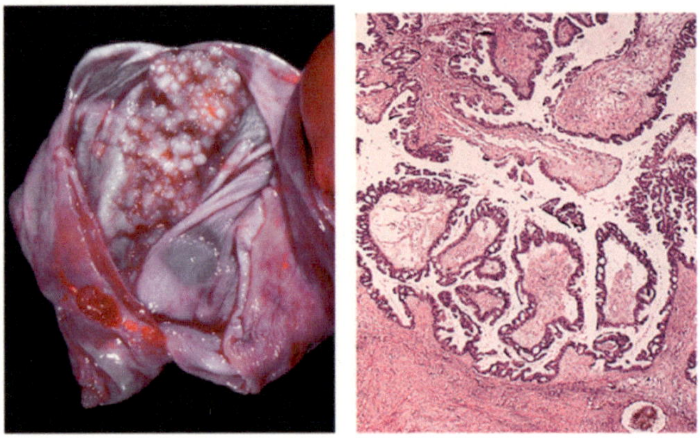

Figure 2. Serous borderline ovarian tumors

2.2. Mucinous borderline tumors

Mucinous BOTs are less common than their serous counterparts. They are also called "atypical proliferative mucinous tumor" (APMT) or "mucinous tumor of low malignant potential". They are often associated to pseudomyxoma peritonei (PMP) a condition characterized by the presence of mucinous ascites and mucoid peritoneal implant

They can be divided into two subtypes:

- Gastrointestinal type
- Endocervical-like type (müllerian or seromucinous)

The first type in 95% of cases is unilateral and appears macroscopically as a multicystic large neoplasm (mean size of about 20 cm) with a smooth capsule.

The cysts contain inside a mucinous material and their surfaces very rarely show the presence of papillary projections.

Histologically, the stromal invasion is absent, the epithelium is stratified, mucinous gastrointestinal-type, with villoglandular of papillary intraglandular growth; the cells show moderate atypia in their nuclei. [4]

Their biological behaviour is very benign with a survival rate of nearly in early stages 100%. The tumors in advanced stage have a mortality of 50%, but mostly are associated with pseudomyxoma peritonei and probably all these case can be considered of primary gastrointestinal and not ovarian origin (usually appendix but also pancreas and biliary tract). For this reason is generally accepted that the true primary APMT in advanced stage do not really exist and that those cases with mucin or benign mucinous epithelium implant on the peritoneum can be explained by the rupture of the cyst and should not be classified as PMP or as APMT with peritoneal implants. [4]

http://dx.doi.org/10.5772/54828

Atypical proliferative mucinous tumors of endocervical-like type are more frequently bilateral, smaller and are often associated with endometriosis. Macroscopically and microscopically they resemble APTS with a combination of endocervical mucinous and serous epithelium. These neoplasms very rarely present with peritoneal implants or signs of microinvasion (defined as the presence of single or small cluster of cells within the stroma) and have a benign behaviour.

In same cases these tumors can show a severe atypia and epithelial overgrowth still without any sign of stromal invasion, these cases are referred to "non invasive or intraepithelial carcinoma" and have still an excellent prognosis in stage I. [4]

The immunohistochemistry pattern of mucinous BOTs is characterized by the expression of cytokeratin (CK) 7 and 20, but no positivity for estrogen and progesterone receptors and Ca125; in the differential diagnosis with intestinal tract tumors this can be very helpful (the neoplasms of intestinal tract origin express CK20 but not CK 7). [4]

The differential diagnosis should be done with metastatic mucinous carcinomas to the ovary and benign or invasive mucinous neoplasms of ovarian origin.

2.3. Endometrioid borderline tumors

Endometrioid tumors of the ovary are usually carcinomas, while borderline forms are very rare; they can arise from endometriosis and can also be associated to endometrial hyperplasia.

Endometrioid BOTs, also called Atypical Proliferative Endometrioid Tumors (APET), account for the 0,2% of ovarian epithelial neoplasms. [4]

Macroscopically they appear as cyst sometimes with solid compounds with hemorrhagic brown fluid inside, in about 60% of cases endometriotic foci are also associated. [4]

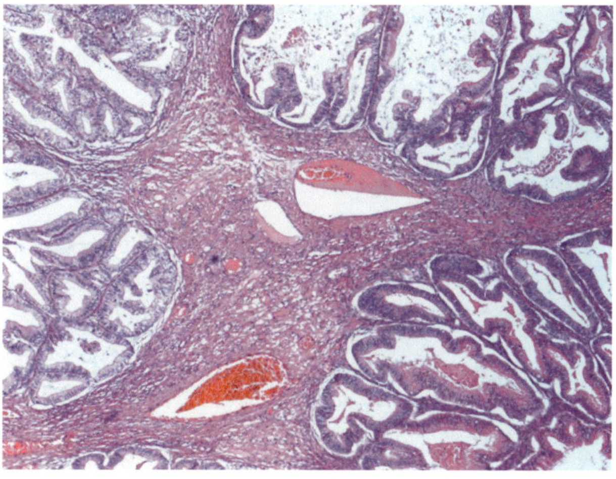

Figure 3. Endometrioid borderline ovarian tumor

Histologically they have glandular and papillary proliferation with different grade of complexity, with moderate or mild atypia in their cells, sometimes they show also squamous metaplasia and necrosis (Figure 3). A microinvasive APET can also be described if the glandular proliferation becomes confluent and the confluent area is less than 5 mm (otherwise it becomes a carcinoma) and this does not seem to be a negative prognostic factors.

Also in case of APET with intraepithelial carcinoma (referred to the presence of severely atypical cells, but without any sign of invasion) the prognosis remains benign.

The immunohistochemistry pattern of endometrioid BOTs is characterized by the expression of CK7, CK20 and p16 only focally. [4, 21]

2.4. Clear cell borderline tumors

Clear cell tumors of the ovary are usually carcinomas, while borderline forms are very rare; they are usually associated to endometriosis and sometimes to endometrial disorders.

Clear cell BOTs, also called Atypical Proliferative Clear Cell Tumors (APCCT), represent the 0,2% of ovarian epithelial neoplasm, their incidence is higher in elder people than other BOTs (mean age 60-70 years).

Macroscopically, they usually appear as cyst with a smooth lobulated surface, clear fluid inside and the cut surface has minute cyst in a rubbery stroma (honeycomb appearance). Microscopically, they are characterized by the presence of tubular glands lined by more layers of hobnail cells, with a more crowded architecture, more epithelial proliferation and more atypia in their cells, when compared to their benign counterparts (clear cell adenofibromas). [4]

As for other BOTs microinvasive APCCT or APCCT with intraepithelial carcinoma can be described, but they are actually very rare, while peritoneal implants have not been described.

The prognosis of these forms of BOTs in early stage is also very benign. [4, 22]

2.5. Borderline brenner (transitional cell) tumors

Transitional cell tumors of the ovary account for 10% of all the epithelial ovarian neoplasm, they are usually benign while malignant and borderline forms have been described but are very uncommon.

Borderline Brenner (Transitional cell) tumors are also called Atypical Proliferative Brenner (Transitional cell) tumors, the mean age at presentation is about 69 years; they are usually unilateral and in stage I at the moment of diagnosis.

Macroscopically, they are cystic, quite large (mean diameter of about 20 cm) with papillary projections in the inner surface.

Histologically, they are characterized by a transitional urothelial like epithelium, with benign areas and parts with proliferation and atypia. No cases of intraepithelial carcinoma or microinvasion have been described in literature.

In immunohistochemistry these neoplasms are usually positive for CEA, EGFR, Ras and negative for p16, p53 and cyclin d.

The prognosis is very good, with only one lethal case of recurrence occurred 50 months after the primary surgery reported in literature. [4, 23]

3. Diagnosis

The only certain diagnosis of BOT can be done by pathologists on the histological examinations, despite this, better understanding before surgery if an adnexal mass is benign, borderline or malignant is very important to decide if surgery is required and the surgical approach. The diagnosis of BOT can be suggested by the presence of certain symptoms, serum markers and image techniques patterns.

3.1. Symptoms

The range and type of symptoms claimed by BOT patients are similar to invasive cancer patients,

Most commonly [80%) patients with Borderline tumors of the ovary complain of abdominal symptoms like abdominal pain or increased abdominal size, discomfort, tense abdomen; 10-35% of these patients complain of gastrointestinal symptomatology like changes in bowel habits, nausea or constipation; 15% complain of gynaecological symptoms like abnormal vaginal bleeding and dyspareunia (more patients when compared with invasive cancer); 5-26% complain of urinary symptoms especially urinary frequency or urgency; 5-7% present with weight loss and malaise and increased urinary urgency or frequency, very few patients (around3%) complain chest pain or breathing problems. Some studies demonstrated that patients with borderline ovarian tumour are more likely to have no symptoms than patient with invasive cancer. [24, 25, 26, 27, 28, 29, 30, 31]

Olsen et al compared symptoms of women with benign, borderline and invasive ovarian tumors, and demonstrated that patients with invasive cancer reported a greater number of symptoms (3.1 and 3.6 for Stages I-II and III-IV, respectively) than women with borderline or benign tumors. (2.8 and 2.2 respectively; $p < 0.0001$). [31]

3.2. Serum markers

Many studies tried to identify a serum marker that could distinguish BOT from invasive and benign ovarian tumors.

Ca-125 increases in BOT patients, less than in women with invasive cancer; anyway this marker is not so useful in the diagnosis especially because it can overlap between patients with stage I ovarian carcinoma or benign adnexal masses like endometriomas, abscesses or myomas and BOT patients. [27, 32, 33]

Ca-125 can instead, be used in the follow up and to primarily assess the severity of the disease because several studies demonstrated that it increases more in advanced stage BOT than early ones. [34, 35, 36, 37, 38]

Ca-19.9 increases in 18,8 – 48,8% of patients, probably more in serous hystotype, [35, 39], while Carcinoembryonic antigen (CEA) levels increases in 17% of patients and more in mucinous tumor. [35, 39, 40]

Ca 72-4 increases in BOT with no differences within the hystotypes, anyway the levels of this serum marker are similar in patients with ovarian cancer. [35, 41]

3.3. Ultrasound

Transvaginal ultrasound is well known to be an effective primary screening imaging technique in patients with adnexal masses to distinguish benign from malignant conditions.

Up to 63% of patients with BOT present on the ultrasound a cyst with papillae inside, but without solid patterns, septa or any other sign of complexity. [42, 43]

BOTs appears on ultrasound images usually as:

- unilocular cyst with solid papillary projections (defined as any projections with a height greater than or equal to 3 mm) arising from the inner wall and with a positive ovarian crescent sign (Figure 4, 5)
- cyst with a "honeycomb nodule", defined as a multilocular nodule mostly with a solid pattern with cystic areas arising from the inner cyst wall. (Figure 6) [42, 43, 44, 45]

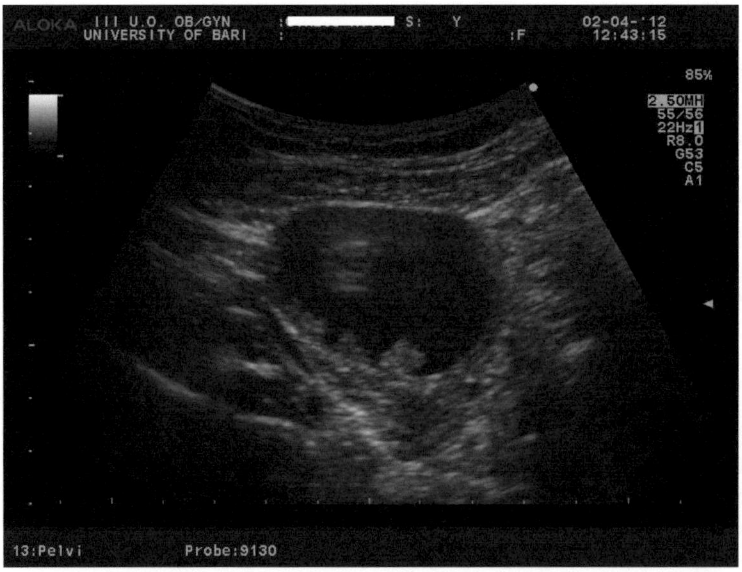

Figure 4. Unilocular cyst with solid papillary projections in BOTs

http://dx.doi.org/10.5772/54828

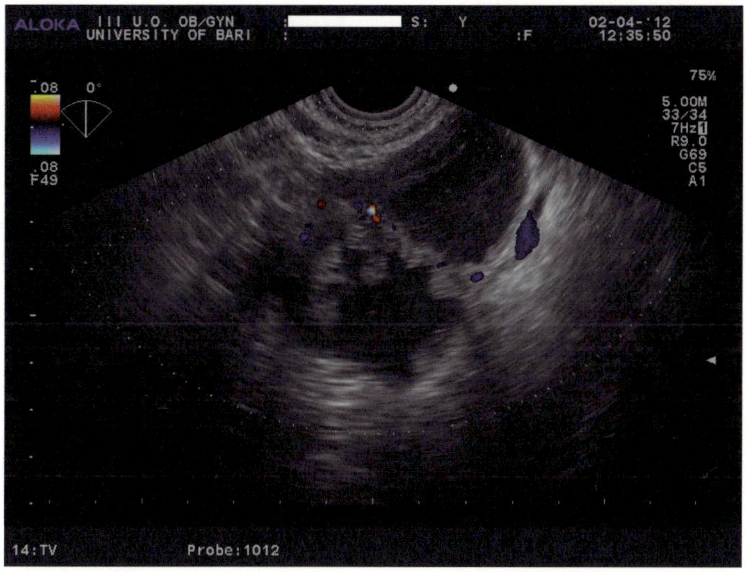

Figure 5. Papillary projections in BOTs

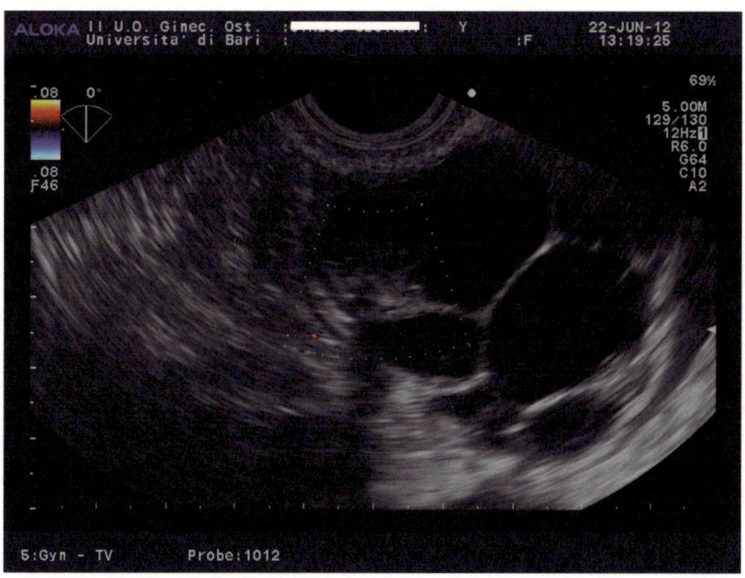

Figure 6. Honeycomb nodule in BOTs

11% of these tumors can appear as simple anechoic cysts without any papillae, and up to 30% as cysts with septa. (Figure 7) [42, 43, 45]. For these reasons, neither the presence of papillae nor septa can be considered as sensitive sonographic markers of borderline tumors, in fact it has been shown that also benign tumors can contain papillae or septa. [42, 46]

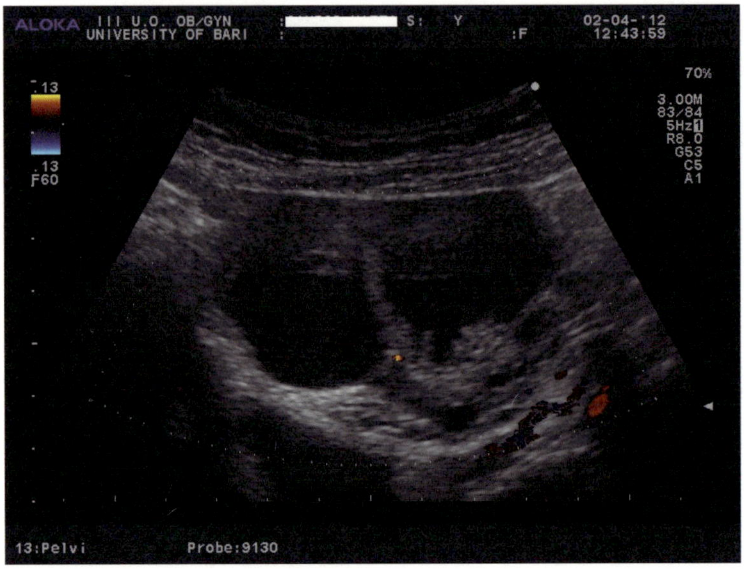

Figure 7. Cyst with septa in BOTs

The ovarian crescent sign is defined as the presence of healthy ovarian tissue adjacent to the cyst wall seen on the ultrasound images as an hypoechogenic area with or without ovarian follicles that cannot be separated from the mass when applying pressure with the transvaginal probe; it has been shown that the presence of this sign can be used to exclude the diagnosis of invasive ovarian cancer. [47]

Yazbek et al demonstrated that the presence of papillae and crescent signs are suggestive of a serous or endocervical hystotype while the presence of thick echogenic fluid and honeycomb nodules are suggestive of gastrointestinal hystotype, moreover Exacoustos et al found that the serous types seem to be smaller than mucinous. [43, 45]

Yazbek et al conclude that the diagnosis of BOT with ultrasound can be achieved in 68.6%, more in serous or endocervical (75%) than in gastrointestinal hystotype (60%). [45]

The role of Doppler ultrasound is still not clear in the diagnosis of BOTs, some authors found a difference in the resistance index and pulsatility index between BOT, benign tumors and invasive cancers, these indexes seem to gradually decrease with the grade of malignancy of the condition. [48, 49, 50]

Otherwise, Tekay et al found no statistically significative differences in the resistance and pulsatility indexes values between invasive, borderline and benign ovarian tumors. [51]

The vessel distribution within the tumor tissue has also been studied deeply but there are not still any clear conclusions, some authors demonstrated that BOT show similar vascular patterns to benign or malignant conditions. [42, 43, 49, 52]

Exacoustos et al found that the flow was present respectively in benign, borderline and malignant tumors in 80, 97 and 100% of cases and that usually a peripheral vascularization is present mostly in benign masses, while intramural or intrapapillae flow is present mostly in borderline or malignant conditions. (Figure 8, 9) [43]

The study of the distribution of the flow or the resistance and pulsatility indexes cannot be considered effective neither in the differential diagnosis between the different histotypes. [53]

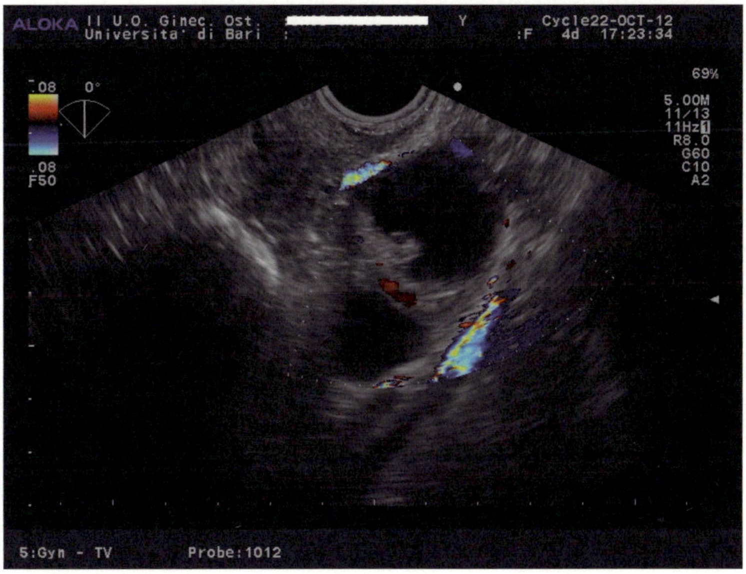

Figure 8. Flow distribution in BOTs

The use of contrast medium injected intravenously has been also suggested as a technique able to discriminate benign from borderline and malignant condition, a multicentre study including 10 cases of BOT and totally 89 patients with ovarian masses concluded that the use of second generation contrast agent like Sono Vue, Bracco, Netherland can be useful in the differential diagnosis between benign and malignant condition but not between borderline and benign ovarian masses. [54]

3.4. Computerized tomography, magnetic resonance and positron emission tomography

Computerized tomography seems not to discriminate BOT from malignant ovarian tumors, it can recognize the complex architecture of BOT, but the tissue contrast is limited so that it is not so clear the contrast between the solid and cystic components of these tumors; the role of CT scan is then mostly limited to detect the presence of metastases and to estimate the FIGO stage. [55, 56]

Magnetic Resonance is the best image technique to characterize borderline ovarian tumors. Bent et al described the appearance of BOT on MR images, and identified four morphological categories: unilocular cysts (19%), minimally septate cysts with papillae (19%), markedly septate lesions with plaque-like excrescences (45%) and predominantly solid with exophytic papillary projections (16%); they also concluded that MRI can be helpful in the differential diagnosis of BOT and in surgical planning. [57]

In T1- and T2-weighted images BOTs solid tissues are usually intermediate in signal intensity and they demonstrate also enhancement after the administration of gadolinium-based contrast media. [57, 58, 59, 60] The enhancement pattern seems to be useful in the differential diagnosis between benign, borderline and invasive ovarian tumors. [61]

In a series of 168 ovarian masses (23 BOT) Bazot et al estimated that the sensitivity and specificity of MRI for the diagnosis of BOT are 45.5% and 96.1%, respectively. [62]

Positron emission tomography can increase the accuracy of other imaging techniques in the diagnosis of BOT.

Malignant cells use glucose to survive, for this reason invasive cancer are characterized on PET images by a higher uptake of 18F-fluorodeoxyglucose than both BOT and benign tumors that do not have a high glycolitic rate. [64, 65, 66, 67]

Nam et al investigated the role of combined 18F-fluorodeoxyglucose positron emission tomography/computerized tomography (FDG-PET/CT) and found that it can be more accurate than ultrasound, CT and MRI in the differential diagnosis between BOT, benign and malignant ovarian cancer. [68]

4. Treatment and follow up

Surgery represents the gold standard treatment and a complete surgical staging is mandatory and very important. Lin et al found out that only in 12% of cases the primary surgical stadiation is actually right. Moreover, BOTs are also difficult to diagnosed in frozen section, many apparent BOTs on frozen section are found to be frankly malignant in permanent sections (the correct diagnosis is achieved in 58-86%) of patients and it depends especially on the experience of the pathologists.

The surgical approach in the management of BOT is similar to the one used in the malignant forms and includes: total abdominal hysterectomy, bilateral salpinogo-oophorectomy, omentectomy, peritoneal washings, and multiple biopsies, including pelvic and pariaortic lymph nodes sampling for the stadiation.

In mucinous BOTs is strongly recommended to perform appendectomy and to carefully analyze the entire intestinal tract to exclude a gastrointestinal tumor.

Because of the excellent prognosis and the young age of these women the treatment is becoming always more conservative and fertility sparing surgery can be considered [69, 70], it consists in ovariectomy or simple cystectomy.

Because 15% of patients who undergone unilateral salpingo oophorectomy develop a primary tumor in the preserved ovary [13, 71] the conservative approach should be considered carefully. In all cases a carefully inspection of the capsule to find any sign of rupture should be performed in case of fertility sparing surgery. Several reports suggest that the overall disease-specific survival rates between the radical e the fertility sparing surgical approaches are not different. [70, 72] Thus, it appears that young women who desire future fertility can be safety treated with fertility-sparing surgery without compromising their overall survival.

Barnhill DA et al suggested that a simple cystectomy should be performed only in selected cases if the tumor is in stage I, can be removed completely and is loosely attached. [73]

The contralateral ovary must be carefully macroscopically inspected, but performing a biopsy is not recommended in order to avoid the occurrence of adhesions that can affect the future fertility capacity of the patient. Some surgeon suggest to women with BOTs who had undergone fertility sparing surgery to complete the radical surgery after the completion of childbearing.

BOTs in advanced stage should be treated with debulking surgery.

The role of adjuvant therapy is still not clear. At this time, there is no proven benefit from adjuvant therapy, even in advanced-stage disease and with the presence of invasive implants. [74]

Generally, in absence of invasive implants, watchful expectancy should be considered, while adjuvant chemotherapy (usually platin based chemotherapy) should be offered to patients with invasive implants, with the persistence of residual tumor after surgery and in clinically progressive disease.

The follow up of these patients must be performed for more than 10 years after the primary treatment since long term recurrence (even after 20 years) have been observed especially in women who underwent a conservative surgical approach. The follow up should include pelvic and gynecological examinations, ultrasound and measurement of serum markers.

5. Our experience: 55 cases

Fifty-five women with borderline ovarian tumors were identified a tour institution from 1991 to 2011, median age at diagnosis was 40 years (range 13-79). The most common symptoms complained by patients at the moment of diagnosis were abdominal-or pelvic pain and discomfort. The tumor diameter ranged between 0.5 and 10 cm and 5.4% of patients presented ascites at the time of diagnosis.

Only in the 47% patients, [26] tumor markers were evaluated before primary surgery, specifically CA125 was higher in 13 (23.6%), CA19.9 in 2 (3.6%) and 4 patients (7.3%) presented with both of these markers increased.

Our expert pathologist in Gynecological oncology pathology found 33 serous, 18 mucinous, 1 endometrioid and 3 mixed borderline ovarian tumors.

All women underwent surgery as primary treatment, 72,8% with laparotomic approach, whereas 13 women (23.6%) underwent a laparoscopic one; in particular 20 patients (36.4%) had a total abdominal hysterectomy with bilateral salpingo-oophorectomy, 2 patients (3.6%)

had a bilateral salpingo-oophorectomy with uterus sparing and the remaining 33 women [60%) performed a procedure strictly interested the ovary. Omentectomy was performed in 32 patients [58%) whereas para aortic lymph node dissection in only 1 patient and appendectomy in 17 patients (31%). Peritoneal biopsies were performed in 27 women (49%), peritoneal cytology in 29 cases (53%) and positive in only 2 (7%).

Forty-seven patients were in FIGO stage I (85.4%), most of these in IA stage (41 patients, 74.5%), 4 patients were in stage II (7.3%) and the last 4 patients in stage III (7.3%).

Fifty-four patients (98.2%) had no residual tumor after surgical procedure, while 1 patient (1.8%) had macroscopic residual tumor ≤2 cm in the ovary and peritoneal carcinomatosis.

After surgery only 2 patients (3.7%) were treated with adjuvant platinum-based combination chemotherapy for their stage IIC and IIIC; both patients achieved a complete response after treatment.

The other patients did not received any other treatment.

The median disease free survival and the 5-year survival rate of our patient population were 42 months (range 16-84) and 97%, respectively.

The statistical analysis performed with Kaplan Meier method and log rank test showed that the survival in patients who underwent fertility-sparing surgery did not differ from those who had a complete surgical staging (p=0.08). No significative differences were observed when comparing the different stages (Stage I-II vs Stage III; p=0.7), histological type (serous versus mucinous, endometrioid and mixed tumor; p=0.15), tumor size (> 10 cm vs < 10 cm; p=0.39), surgical approach (laparotomy vs laparoscopy; p=0.56), elevation of CA125 at diagnosis (positive vs negative marker; p=0.55).

Six patients developed a recurrence of the disease. All of them underwent a secondary laparotomy, four with a conservative approach and two with a complete surgical staging because of the presence of invasive implants. These two patients received then also chemotherapy. All the six women were alive with no evidence of disease with a median survival of 39 months.

We were able to obtain the fertility status of 16 patients who underwent a fertility-sparing surgery. Four of these women became pregnant and the rest of them had not a desire of childbearing at the time of their last follow up. One of these pregnancies was obtained by in vitro fertilization techniques, while the rest of them were spontaneous.

6. Conclusions

In conclusion, BOTs have an excellent prognosis of nearly 100% of survival rate.

Conservative fertility sparing surgery should be considered for women in the reproductive age group who desire preservation of fertility.

In any case, a long-term follow-up is highly recommended for these tumors because recurrences can occur several years after primary treatment.

Author details

Gennaro Cormio, Vera Loizzi, Maddalena Falagario*, Doriana Scardigno, Donatella Latorre and Luigi E. Selvaggi

*Address all correspondence to: mad.falagario@gmail.com

Department of Gynaecology, Obstetric and Neonatology, University of Bari, Italy

References

[1] Taylor, H. Malignant and semi-malignant tumors of the ovary. Surg Gynecol Obstet, (1929). , 48, 204-230.

[2] FIGOInternational Federation of Gynecology and Obstetrics. Classification and staging of malignant tumours in the female pelvis. Acta Obstet Gynecol Scand (1971). , 50, 1-7.

[3] Tavassoli, F. A. Devilee P (eds). World Health Organization Classification of Tumours. Pathology and Genetics. Tumours of the Breast and Female Genital Organs. IARC Press: Lyon, (2003).

[4] Russell, P. Surface epithelial-stromal tumors of the ovary. In: Kurman RJ (ed). Blaustein's Pathology of the Female Genital Tract, 4th edn. Springer-Verlag: New York, (1994). , 705-782.

[5] Crispens, M. A. Borderline ovarian tumours: a review of the recent literature. Curr Opin Obstet Gynecol, (2003). , 15, 39-43.

[6] Skirnisdottir, I, Garmo, H, Wilander, E, & Holmberg, L. Borderline ovarian tumors in Sweden 1960-2005: trends in incidence and age at diagnosis compared to ovarian cancer. Int J Cancer, (2008). , 123, 1897-1901.

[7] Bostwick, D. G, Tazelaar, H. D, Ballon, S. C, Hendrickson, M. R, & Kempson, R. L. Ovarian epithelial tumors of borderline malignancy. A clinical and pathologic study of 109 cases. Cancer, (1986). , 58, 2052-2065.

[8] Benedet, J. L, Bender, H, & Jones, H. rd, Ngan, H. Y., and Pecorelli, S. FIGO staging classifications and clinical practice guidelines in the management of gynecologic cancers. FIGO Committee on Gynecologic Oncology. Int J Gynaecol Obstet, (2000). , 70, 209-262.

[9] Sherman, M. E, Mink, P. J, Curtis, R, Cote, T. R, Brooks, S, Hartge, P, & Devesa, S. Survival among women with borderline ovarian tumors and ovarian carcinoma: a population-based analysis. Cancer, (2004). , 100, 1045-1052.

[10] DiSaia PJCreasman WT. The adnexal mass and early ovarian cancer. Clinical Gynecologic Oncology. Mosby Inc. 6th edn. Mosby Inc. USA, (2002). , 259-288.

[11] Katzenstein, A. A, Mazur, M. T, Morgan, T. E, et al. Proliferative serous tumors of the ovary: histologic features and prognosis. Am J Surg Pathol (1978). , 2, 339-355.

[12] Russell, P. The pathological assessment of ovarian neoplasms. I. Introduction to the common'epithelial' tumours and analysis of benign'epithelial' tumours. Pathol (1979). , 11, 5-26.

[13] Kennedy, A. W, & Hart, W. R. Ovarian papillary serous tumors of low malignant potential (serous borderline tumors): a long term follow-up study, including patients with microinvasion, lymph node metastasis, and transformation to invasive serous carcinoma. Cancer (1996). , 78, 278-286.

[14] Scully, R. E, Young, R. H, & Clement, P. B. Tumors of the ovary, maldeveloped gonads, fallopian tube, and broad ligament. In: Rosai J (ed). Atlas of Tumor Pathology, Third Series, Fascicle 23. Armed Forces Institute of Pathology: Washington, DC, (1998).

[15] Hart, W. A. Borderline epithelial tumors of the ovary Modern Pathology ((2005). SS50. doi:10.1038/modpathol.3800307, 33.

[16] Bell, D. A, & Scully, R. E. Ovarian serous borderline tumors with stromal microinvasion: a report of 21 cases. Hum Pathol (1990). , 21, 397-403.

[17] Tavassoli, F. A. Serous tumor of low malignant potential with early stromal invasion (serous LMP with microinvasion). Mod Pathol (1988). , 1, 407-414.

[18] Mckenney, J. K, Balzer, B. L, & Longacre, T. A. Ovarian serous tumors of low malignant potential with stromal microinvasion: a clinicopathologic study of 36 cases. Mod Pathol (2004). A-206A.

[19] Prat, J, & De Nictolis, M. Serous borderline tumors of the ovary: a long-term follow-up study of 137 cases, including 18 with a micropapillary pattern and 20 with microinvasion. Am J Surg Pathol (2002). , 26, 1111-1128.

[20] Eichhorn, J. H, Bell, D. A, Young, R. H, et al. Ovarian serous borderline tumors with micropapillary and cribriform patterns: a study of 40 cases and comparison with 44 cases without these patterns. Am J Surg Pathol (1999). , 23, 397-409.

[21] Uzan, C, Berretta, R, Rolla, M, Gouy, S, Fauvet, R, Darai, E, & Duvillard, P. Morice P Management and prognosis of endometrioid borderline tumors of the ovary. Surg Oncol. (2012). Sep;, 21(3), 178-84.

[22] Uzan, C, Dufeu-lefebvre, M, Fauvet, R, Gouy, S, Duvillard, P, Darai, E, & Morice, P. Management and prognosis of clear cell borderline ovarian tumor. Int J Gynecol Cancer. (2012). Jul;, 22(6), 993-9.

[23] Uzan, C, Dufeu-lefebvre, M, Fauvet, R, Gouy, S, Duvillard, P, Darai, E, & Morice, P. Management and prognosis of borderline ovarian brenner tumors. Int J Gynecol Cancer. (2012). Oct;, 22(8), 1332-6.

[24] Goff, B. A, Mandel, L. S, Melancon, C. H, et al. (2004). Frequency of symptoms of ovarian cancer in women presenting to primary care clinics. JAMA , 291, 2705-2712.

[25] Hamilton, W, Peters, T. J, Bankhead, C, et al. (2009). Risk of ovarian ancer in women with symptoms in primary care: population based case-control study. BMJ 339:b2998

[26] Ranney, B, & Ahmad, M. I. (1979). Early identification, differentiation and treatment of ovarian neoplasia. Int J Gynaecol Obstet , 17, 209-218.

[27] Eltabbakh, G. H, Yadav, P. R, & Morgan, A. (1999). Clinical picture of women with early stage ovarian cancer. Gynecol Oncol , 75, 476-479.

[28] Vine, M. F, Ness, R. B, Calingaert, B, et al. (2001). Types and duration of symptoms prior to diagnosis of invasive or borderline ovariantumor. Gynecol Oncol Arch Gynecol Obstet (2012) 285:1103-1112, 83, 466-471.

[29] Webb, P. M, Purdie, D. M, Grover, S, et al. (2004). Symptoms and diagnosis of borderline, early and advanced epithelial ovarian cancer. Gynecol Oncol , 92, 232-239.

[30] Olsen, C. M, Cnossen, J, Green, A. C, et al. (2007). Comparison of symptoms and presentation of women with benign, low malignant potential and invasive ovarian tumors. Eur J Gynaecol Oncol , 28, 376-380.

[31] Lenhard, M. S, Nehring, S, Nagel, D, et al. (2009). Predictive value of CA 125 and CA 72-4 in ovarian borderline tumors. Clin Chem Lab Med , 47, 537-542.

[32] Van Calster, B, Timmerman, D, Bourne, T, et al. (2007). Discrimination between benign and malignant adnexal masses by specialist ultrasound examination versus serum CA-125. J Natl Cancer Inst , 99, 1706-1714.

[33] Rice, L. W, Lage, J. M, Berkowitz, R. S, et al. (1992). Preoperative serum CA-125 levels in borderline tumors of the ovary. Gynecol Oncol , 46, 226-229.

[34] Tamakoshi, K, Kikkawa, F, Shibata, K, et al. (1996). Clinical value of CA125, CA19-9, CEA, CA72-4, and TPA in borderline ovarian tumor. Gynecol Oncol , 62, 67-72.

[35] Gotlieb, W. H, Soriano, D, Achiron, R, et al. (2000). CA 125 measurement and ultrasonography in borderline tumors of the ovary. Am J Obstet Gynecol , 183, 541-546.

[36] Kolwijck, E, Thomas, C. M, Bulten, J, et al. (2009). Preoperative CA-125 levels in 123 patients with borderline ovarian tumors: a retrospective analysis and review of the literature. Int J Gynecol Cancer , 19, 1335-1338.

[37] Tempfer, C. B, Polterauer, S, Bentz, E. K, et al. (2007). Accuracy of intraoperative frozen section analysis in borderline tumors of the ovary: a retrospective analysis of 96 cases and review of the literature. Gynecol Oncol , 107, 248-252.

[38] Darai, E, Teboul, J, Walker, F, et al. (1996). Epithelial ovarian carcinoma of low malignant potential. Eur J Obstet Gynecol Reprod Biol , 66, 141-145.

[39] Engelen, M. J, De Bruijn, H. W, Hollema, H, et al. (2000). Serum CA125, carcinoembryonic antigen, and CA 19-9 as tumor markers in borderline ovarian tumors. Gynecol Oncol , 78, 16-2017.

[40] Gotlieb, W. H, Soriano, D, Achiron, R, et al. (2000). CA 125 measurement and ultrasonography in borderline tumors of the ovary. Am J Obstet Gynecol , 183, 541-546.

[41] Lenhard, M. S, Nehring, S, Nagel, D, et al. (2009). Predictive value of CA 125 and CA 72-4 in ovarian borderline tumors. Clin Chem Lab Med , 47, 537-542.

[42] Pascual, M. A, Tresserra, F, Grases, P. J, et al. (2002). Borderline cystic tumors of the ovary: gray-scale and color Doppler sonographic findings. J Clin Ultrasound , 30, 76-82.

[43] Exacoustos, C, Romanini, M. E, Rinaldo, D, et al. (2005). Preoperative sonographic features of borderline ovarian tumors. Ultrasound Obstet Gynecol , 25, 50-59.

[44] Fruscella, E, Testa, A. C, Ferrandina, G, et al. (2005). Ultrasound features of different histopathological subtypes of borderline ovarian tumors. Ultrasound Obstet Gynecol , 26, 644-650.

[45] Yazbek, J, Raju, K. S, Ben-nagi, J, et al. (2007). Accuracy of ultrasound subjective 'pattern recognition' for the diagnosis of borderline ovarian tumors. Ultrasound Obstet Gynecol , 29, 489-495.

[46] Alca´zar JLErrasti T, Mı´nguez JA et al ((2001). Sonographic features of ovarian cystadenofibromas: spectrum of findings. J Ultrasound Med , 20, 915-919.

[47] Yazbek, J, Aslam, N, Tailor, A, Hillaby, K, Raju, K. S, & Jurkovic, D. A comparative study of the risk of malignancy index and the ovarian crescent sign for the diagnosis of invasive ovarian cancer. Ultrasound Obstet Gynecol (2006). , 28, 320-324.

[48] Wu, C. C, Lee, C. N, Chen, T. M, et al. (1994). Incremental angiogenesis assessed by color Doppler ultrasound in the tumorigenesis of ovarian neoplasms. Cancer , 73, 1251-1256.

[49] Tepper, R, Lerner-geva, L, Altaras, M. M, et al. (1995). Transvaginal color flow imaging in the diagnosis of ovarian tumors. J Ultrasound Med , 14, 731-734.

[50] Reles, A, Wein, U, & Lichtenegger, W. (1997). Transvaginal color Doppler sonography and conventional sonography in the preoperative assessment of adnexal masses. J Clin Ultrasound , 25, 217-225.

[51] Zanetta, G, Lissoni, A, Cha, S, et al. (1995). Pre-operative morphological and colour Doppler features of borderline ovarian tumours. Br J Obstet Gynaecol , 102, 990-996.

[52] Tekay, A, & Jouppila, P. (1992). Validity of pulsatility and resistance indices in classification of adnexal tumors with transvaginal color

[53] Emoto, M, Udo, T, Obama, H, et al. (1998). The blood flow characteristics in borderline ovarian tumors based on both color Doppler ultrasound and and histopathological analyses. Gynecol Oncol , 70, 351-357.

[54] Testa, A. C, Timmerman, D, Van Belle, V, et al. (2009). Intravenous contrast ultrasound examination using contrast-tuned imaging(CnTI) and the contrast medium SonoVue for discrimination between benign and malignant adnexal masses with solid components. Ultrasound Obstet Gynecol , 34, 699-710.

[55] Lalwani, N, Shanbhogue, A. K, Vikram, R, et al. (2010). Current update on borderline ovarian neoplasms. AJR Am J Roentgenol , 194, 330-336.

[56] Buy, J. N, Ghossain, M. A, Sciot, C, et al. (1991). Epithelial tumors of the ovary: CT findings and correlation with US. Radiology , 178, 811-818.

[57] Bent, C. L, Sahdev, A, Rockall, A. G, et al. (2009). MRI appearances of borderline ovarian tumours. Clin Radiol , 64, 430-438.

[58] Desouza, N. M, Neill, O, & Mcindoe, R. GA et al ((2005). Borderline tumors of the ovary: CT and MRI features and tumor markers in differentiation from stage I disease. AJR Am J Roentgenol , 184, 999-1003.

[59] Bazot, M, Darai, E, Nassar-slaba, J, et al. (2008). Value of magnetic resonance imaging for the diagnosis of ovarian tumors: a review. J Comput Assist Tomogr , 32, 712-723.

[60] Van Vierzen, P. B, Massuger, L. F, Ruys, S. H, et al. (1998). Borderline ovarian malignancy: ultrasound and fast dynamic MR findings. Eur J Radiol , 28, 136-142.

[61] Thomassin-naggara, I, Bazot, M, Darai, E, et al. (2008). Epithelial ovarian tumors: value of dynamic contrast-enhanced MR imaging and correlation with tumor angiogenesis. Radiology , 248, 148-159.

[62] Bazot, M, Nassar-slaba, J, Thomassin-naggara, I, et al. (2006). MR imaging compared with intraoperative frozen-section examination for the diagnosis of adnexal tumors; correlation with final histology. Eur Radiol , 16, 2687-2699.

[63] Lapela, M, Leskinen-kallio, S, Varpula, M, et al. (1995). Metabolic imaging of ovarian tumors with carbon-11-methionine: a PET study. J Nucl Med , 36, 2196-2200.

[64] Grab, D, & Flock, F. Sto°hr I et al ((2000). Classification of asymptomatic adnexal masses by ultrasound, magnetic resonance imaging, and positron emission tomography. Gynecol Oncol , 77, 454-459.

[65] Rieber, A. Nu°ssle K, Sto°hr I et al ((2001). Preoperative diagnosis of ovarian tumors with MR imaging: comparison with transvaginal sonography, positron emission tomography, and histologic findings. AJR Am J Roentgenol , 177, 123-129.

[66] Ju, W, & Kim, S. C. (2007). Discrepancy between magnetic resonance and 18F-fluorodeoxyglucose positron emission tomography imaging in a case of borderline ovarian tumor. Int J Gynecol Cancer , 17, 1031-1033.

[67] Yamamoto, Y, Oguri, H, Yamada, R, et al. (2008). Preoperative evaluation of pelvic masses with combined 18F-fluorodeoxyglucose positron emission tomography and computed tomography. Int J Gynaecol Obstet , 102, 124-127.

[68] Nam, E. J, Yun, M. J, Oh, Y. T, et al. (2010). Diagnosis and staging of primary ovarian cancer: correlation between PET/CT, Doppler US, and CT or MRI. Gynecol Oncol , 116, 389-394.

[69] Morice, P, Camatte, S, El Hassan, J, Pautier, P, Duvillard, P, & Castaigne, D. Clinical outcomes and fertility after conservative treatment of ovarian borderline tumors. Fertil Steril, (2001). , 75, 92-96.

[70] Morris, R. T, Gershenson, D. M, Silva, E. G, Follen, M, Morris, M, & Wharton, J. T. Outcome and reproductive function after conservative surgery for borderline ovarian tumors. Obstet Gynecol, (2000). , 95, 541-547.

[71] Bostwick, D. G, Tazelaar, H. D, Ballon, S. C, et al. Ovarian epithelial tumors of borderline malignancy: a clinical and pathologic study of 109 cases. Cancer (1986). , 58, 2052-2065.

[72] Tazelaar, H. D, Bostwick, D. G, Ballon, S. C, Hendrickson, M. R, & Kempson, R. L. Conservative treatment of borderline ovarian tumors. Obstet Gynecol, (1985). , 66, 417-422.

[73] Barnhill, D. A, Kurman, R. J, Brady, M. F, et al. Preliminary analysis of the behavior of stage I ovarian serous tumors of low malignant potential: a Gynecologic Oncology Group study. J Clin Oncol (1995). , 13, 2752-2756.

[74] Trope, C, Kaern, J, Vergote, I. B, Kristensen, G, & Abeler, V. Are borderline tumors of the ovary overtreated both surgically and systemically? A review of four prospective randomized trials including 253 patients with borderline tumors. Gynecol Oncol, (1993). , 51, 236-243.

Chapter 5

Implication of Clear Cell and Mucinous Histology

Jun Naniwa, Hiroaki Itamochi and Junzo Kigawa

Additional information is available at the end of the chapter

http://dx.doi.org/10.5772/54931

1. Introduction

The incidence of ovarian cancer in 2008 was projected to be 225,500 new cases and 140,200 deaths worldwide, representing 3.7% of all female cancers and 4.2% of all cancer deaths in women [1]. Ovarian cancer, one of the major causes of death from cancer in women, is commonly diagnosed at an advanced stage. Cytoreductive surgery followed by chemotherapy combining platinum and taxane is currently the standard treatment for ovarian cancer [2]. Ovarian cancer is one of the most sensitive solid tumors, with objective responses ranging from 60 to 80% even in patients with advanced stage. However, most patients ultimately recur and develop resistance to platinum and taxane.

Resistance to chemotherapy presents a major obstacle in attempting to improve the prognosis of patients with ovarian cancer. Accordingly, it is important to elucidate the mechanisms of chemoresistance to manage ovarian cancer. Recently, the biological characteristics of ovarian cancer have been clarified. It has long been known that ovarian cancers of serous histology appear to be more sensitive to chemotherapy than other histological subtypes. Patients with clear cell carcinoma or mucinous adenocarcinoma of the ovary showed a significantly worse prognosis in a retrospective review of several Gynecologic Oncology Group (GOG) trials [3]. Therefore, it is important to determine optimal regimens based on histological subtype. In this chapter, clear cell carcinoma and mucinous adenocarcinoma of the ovary are discussed.

2. Clear cell carcinoma

Clear cell carcinoma (CCC) has unique clinical and biological features [4]. In North America and Europe, CCC is the third most common histological subtype of epithelial ovarian cancer (EOC), with an estimated prevalence of 1-12% [5, 6]. For unknown reason, CCC comprises more than

20% of such cancers in Japan [7-9]. Interestingly, among Asian women living in the United States, CCC was diagnosed twice as frequently (11.1%) compared to Caucasians (4.8%) [10].

Several studies have analyzed the risk factors for ovarian cancer by histologic subtype. CCC was associated (odds ratio: 2.2-2.3) with an increased body mass index (BMI 30) [11, 12]. However, in the NIH-AARP Diet and Health Study BMI was correlated only with endometrioid histology [13].

It has long been recognized that CCC often is associated with endometriosis (22-70%), whereas hobnail cells bear a very strong morphological resemblance to endometrial Aria-Stella cells [14, 15]. Several studies have reported that endometriosis frequently shows a sequential change to EOC, including CCC. Therefore, atypical endometriosis is considered to be a precancerous change. Ovarian cancers associated with endometriosis tend to occur in younger women, and present 5-6 years earlier, on average, than high-grade serous carcinoma (HGSC) [16]. In National Cancer Institute Surveillance, Epidemiology and End Results (SEER) data, women with CCC were younger than patients with serous adenocarcinoma (SAC) (55 vs. 64 years; median age) [10].

An increased incidence of vascular thromboembolic complications is seen in patients with CCC [17, 18]. Up to 40% of patients with CCC may develop thromboembolic disease and this rate is double that in matched non-CCC controls with ovarian cancers [19].

3. Clinicopathological features

Ovarian CCC usually presents as a large pelvic mass [20, 21]. The size of masses range from 3 to 20 cm, with most tumors detected preoperatively either by clinical examination or imaging. Recent reports involving large institutional cohorts compared early-stage (I/II) to advanced-stage ovarian cancers (III/IV) and showed that 57-81% of CCC were diagnosed at an early stage [9, 22]. In SEER data, 56% of CCC were stage I, compared to 19% for SAC [10]. Combining the low overall incidence of CCC and their early stage propensity, CCC may make up only 1-5% of advanced stage patients in chemotherapy trials, largely due to their overall low incidence and tendency for early stage distribution at the time for initial diagnosis [6].

Sugiyama, et al. [9] retrospectively reviewed 101 patients with CCC in Japan who underwent complete surgical staging to determine clinicopathological features of CCC. Histologic evaluation was performed under central pathological review. Tumors were diagnosed as CCC if the following appeared in 90% or more of all specimens: a small to large sheet of polyhedral clear cells with delicate fibrovascular septa, tubules and papillae, clear or hobnail, or eosinophilic cells of organoid appearance, or clear cells with coalescent vacuoles containing "targetoid" eosinophilic PAS-positive globules. Of the 662 patients with EOC, 101 (15.3%) had CCC and 235 (35.5%) SAC. All patients underwent complete surgical staging, including intraperitoneal cytology, bilateral salpingo-oophorectomy, hysterectomy, omentectomy, pelvic-/paraaortic lymphadenectomy, and aggressive cytoreductive surgery for advanced cases. Ninety-seven (96%) of 101 patients with CCC and 229 (97%) of 235 with SAC underwent platinum-based chemotherapy after initial surgery.

The median age did not differ between patients with CCC and those with SAC. The percentage of patients at stage I was significantly higher in CCC than SAC (16.6%), while significantly fewer patients were at stage III had CCC than SAC (61.7%). By contrast, the incidence of stage III was significantly lower in CCC than in SAC. Recurrence in patients with CCC occurred in 29% of stage I patients, 30% of stage II, 62% of stage III, and 73% at stage IV. Although none of the patients with stage Ia CCC relapsed, 14 of 38 patients (37%) with stage Ic did relapse.

In stage III disease the median survival time was significantly shorter for patients with CCC than those with SAC. The survival rate for patients at stage III was significantly lower in the CCC group than in the SAC group. Although estimated survival rates at 3 and 5 years in patients with no gross tumor did not differ significantly between CCC and SAC, survival rates in both patients with <2 cm and >2 cm residual disease were significantly lower in CCC than in SAC. Jenison, et al. [23] showed that the survival rates for CCC were consistently lower in each of the FIGO stages compared with SAC, although there was no statistical significance. In their study, median survival time for stage I patients with CCC was significantly shorter than that for those with SAC. Similarly, the survival rate for patients with stage Ic CCC was lower compared with patients with stage Ic SAC. Additionally, the median survival time for stage I patients with CCC was worse than those with SAC (31.8 months vs 42.3 months) and the time to recurrence in patients with stage I/II CCC was definitely shorter (12.2 months) [9]. Twenty-seven patients with stage III/IV CCC had measurable disease after initial surgery. The overall clinical response rate for SAC was 72.5%. In contrast, only three (11.1%) of 27 patients responded to platinum-based chemotherapy in CCC. Patients with CCC showed a very low rate of response and a high incidence of progressive disease. Another authors demonstrated that platinum-based chemotherapy did not appear to improve the survival of patients with CCC, compared with survival after non-platinum-based chemotherapy [24]. Additionally, CCC patients with residual tumor showed a high recurrence rate (Fig 1). CCC has a more aggressive course and a more malignant behavior than SAC. Therefore, new treatment strategies for CCC, including alternative regimens of chemotherapy, should be established.

4. Mechanisms of platinum resistance in CCC of the ovary

There is general acceptance of CCC that is insensitive to conventional platinum-based chemotherapy lead to a poor prognosis. Resistance to cisplatin (CDDP) is an important factor in the poor prognosis of patients with CCC. Several mechanisms involved in drug resistance have been proposed as explanations, including decreased drug accumulation, increased drug detoxification, increased DNA repair activity, and activation of receptor tyrosine kinases and its downstream signaling pathways [25-29].

Adenosine 5′-triphosphate (ATP)-binding cassette (ABC) transporters, such as ABCB1 (also known as P glycoprotein), ABCC1 (multidrug resistance associated protein-1) and ABCC3, are known to lower intracellular drug concentrations and are important multidrug resistance factors [30]. An immunohistochemical study of ABCB1 and ABCC1 in CCC and SAC tumors revealed that their expression of these transporters did not differ between CCC and SAC [31].

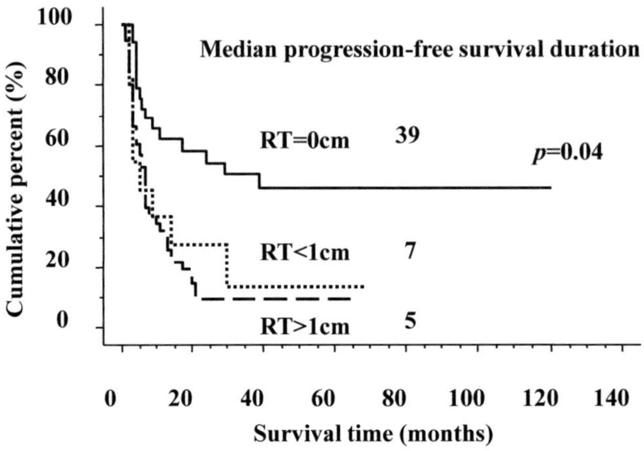

Figure 1. Progression free survival rate for stage III and IV patients, and residual tumor diameter. Progression free survival rates for the patients without residual disease were significantly greater, but there was no significant difference between those with <1 cm residual disease and with >1 cm. RT: residual tumor diameter

In addition, no significant differences were observed in the expression of ABCB1 and ABCC1 between responders and non-responders to platinum-based chemotherapy in both tumor types. These results suggest that multidrug resistance proteins do not contribute to chemoresistance in CCC. Ohishi, et al. [32] examined the expression of mRNA by ABCC superfamily members, ABCC1, ABCC2, and ABCC3, in CCC and SAC tumors. They found that only ABCC3 genes were expressed significantly more in CCC than SAC. Therefore, they concluded that increased expression of ABCC3 may, at least in part, be associated with the chemoresistant phenotype of CCC.

Several drug detoxification systems also can diminish intracellular drug activity. Cellular detoxification via the glutathione system is known to be involved in the metabolism of various cytotoxic agents, including the platinum agents, etoposide (VP-16), and mitomycin C (MMC) [27, 28, 33, 34]. Indeed, the glutathione concentrations in CCC cell lines increased significantly after exposure to CDDP or MMC [35]. A gene expression study showed that glutathione peroxidase 3 (GPx3), glutaredoxin (GLRX), and superoxide dismutase (SOD2) were expressed highly in CCC tumors and that the elevated levels of these, and perhaps other, antioxidant proteins may render the tumors more resistant to chemotherapy [36].

Nucleotide excision repair (NER) is a multienzyme DNA repair pathway in eukaryotes that has been implicated in drug resistance in human tumor cells [37]. Reed, et al. [38] examined the mRNA expression of two key genes, excision repaircross-complementing rodent repair deficiency, complementation group 1 (ERCC1) and xeroderma pigmentosum group B (XPB), that are involved in the NER pathway of EOC tumors. Expression of ERCC1 and XPB were higher in CCC tumors than in other histological tumor types. This phenomenon may be related to de novo drug resistance against chemotherapeutic agents in CCC. DNA mismatch repair systems (MMR), which correct errors that occur during DNA replication, also play a critical role in the sensitivity of DNA damaging agents. In experimental systems, cells deficient in

MMR are highly tolerant to the methylating chemotherapeutic drugs streptozocin and temozolomide and, to a lesser extent, CDDP and doxorubicin [39]. Loss of MMR may be caused either by a germline mutation of two major MMR genes, hMLH1 or hMSH2, or by somatic MMR gene inactivation through epigenetic silencing via methylation of the hMLH1 promoter. Cai, et al. [40] reported that elevated expression of hMLH1 and hMSH2 proteins are involved in the development of a subset of CCC, and that there is a strong correlation between alterations in the expression of hMLH1 and hMSH2 and the presence of MSI in CCC tumors.

Epidermal growth-factor receptor (EGFR) and v-erb-b2 erythroblastic leukemia viral oncogene homolog 2 (ERBB2; HER2) are cell-surface-receptor tyrosine kinases and can activate both the signaling pathways of mitogen-activated protein kinase and phosphatidylinositol 3'-kinase (PI3K)-Akt [41]. Activating these pathways leads to phosphorylated Bc1-2 antagonist cell death (BAD) and B-cell leukemia/lymphoma (Bcl)-2, thereby inhibiting chemotherapy-induced apoptosis [42]. An immunohistochemical study showed found EGFR in 61% of CCC tumors [43]. Molecular analyzes of various types of ovarian tumors showed HER2 to be overexpressed in CCC relative to other major histological types of EOC [44]. In ovarian cancer, the HER2 protein is overexpressed as a consequence of HER2 gene amplification in 20 to 25% of cases and predicts a poor prognosis [45, 46].

Cell proliferation is controlled by cyclin-dependent kinases (CDK), which are regulated by cyclin binding, phosphorylation, and CDK inhibitors (e.g. p16, p21, and p27) [47]. p53, known as a tumor suppressor protein, also up-regulates expression of p21 and causes cell the cycle to arrest at G1. Changes in the p53 gene are seen in 50 to 70% of cases of advanced serous adenocarcinoma [48, 49]. In contrast, the p53 mutation is rare in CCC, and immunohistochemical staining shows that CCC tends to express little or no p53 protein [50]. Cytotoxic drugs are primarily effective against proliferating cells; therefore, quiescent cells show a degree of resistance relative to cycling cells [51]. Dimanche-Boitrel, et al. [52] reported that less intracellular drug accumulates in resting cells. Itamochi et al. examined the proliferation activity and CDDP sensitivity of 11 CCC and 5 SAC cell lines, and this found that the doubling time for CCC cells was significantly longer than for SAC (61.4 vs 29.8 h) [7]. There was a significant reverse correlation between the S-phase fraction and the response to CDDP. These findings may relate to the high incidence of stage I patients with CCC, and also suggests that the resistance of CCC to CDDP may be caused by low cell proliferation. In addition, Ki-67, a nuclear antigen expressed in all states of the cell cycle except in resting cells in G0, has a significantly lower labeling index in CCC than in SAC [31]. Furthermore, a significantly higher Ki-67 labeling index (LI) is observed in responders than in non-responders in both CCC and SAC tumors.

The 5-year survival rate for high LI patients (over 18.4%; mean value for CCC) was significantly greater than that for low LI (less than 18.4%) (46.3% vs. 9.2%, $p<0.05$) (Fig. 2). A multivariable analysis revealed that the Ki-67 labeling index and residual tumor size were independent prognostic factors. Other authors have reported that immunohistochemical staining of CCC reveals a low expression of Ki-67, p53, and cyclin A, and significantly increased expression of both p21 and cyclin E, which are other histological subtypes [53]. These results suggest that

CCC has low tumor proliferation activity and that this low proliferation activity in CCC could be associated with chemoresistance.

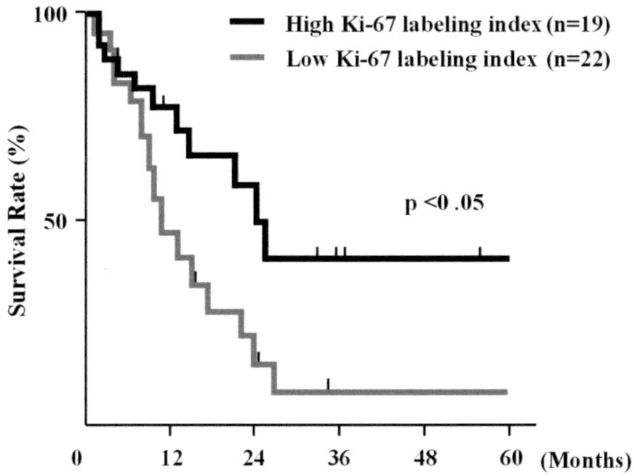

Figure 2. Estimated survival rates for patient with clear cell carcinoma. When the cut-off value of Ki-67 labeling index (LI) was set at 18.4% (the mean value of clear cell carcinoma), the estimated 5-year survival rate for elevated Ki-67 LI patients was significantly greater than that for low Ki-67 LI (46.3% vs. 9.2%).

5. Future directions

The clinicopathological features of CCC suggest that a new strategy for chemotherapy in CCC should be adopted, focusing on new agents without cross-resistance to platinum agents. Several anticancer agents with no cross-resistance to platinum analogues, such as paclitaxel (PTX), VP-16, and camptothecin (CPT-11) have been developed.

Activating the PI3K/Akt pathway and its downstream signaling mammalian target of rapamycin (mTOR) seems to indicate drug resistance and poor prognosis in many cancers. It has been reported that CCC has a high frequency of activating mutations of PIK3CA [54]. Because it is known well that activation of Akt signaling results in hypersensitivity to mTOR inhibition, CCC may be a good candidate for therapy with an mTOR inhibitor. Several clinical trials have shown potential antitumor activities for mTOR inhibitors (everolimus, deforolimus, and temsirolimus) in solid tumors. Temsirolimus (CCI779, a synthetic, ester analog of rapamycin) is indicated to treat advanced renal cell carcinoma. A phase II study is ongoing to evaluate the safety and efficacy of temsirolimus in combination with carboplatin and PTX followed by temsirolimus consolidation as first-line therapy for patients with stage III-IV CCC in the ovary (NCT01196429, ClinicalTrials.gov). We hope this combination therapy will improve the survival of patients with ovarian CCC.

http://dx.doi.org/10.5772/54931

6. Mucinous adenocarcinoma

Ovarian mucinous adenocarcinoma (MAC) is divided into intraepithelial and invasive carcinomas (Fig. 3). Intraepithelial mucinous carcinoma is characterized by marled epithelial atypia in the absence of stromal invasion. Invasive mucinous carcinoma is diagnosed once stromal invasion measuring more than 5 mm or more than 10 mm² is detected. Two types of invasive mucinous caricinoma are recognized: expansile and infiltrative. The former is characterized by conflicted glandular growth uninterrupted by normal ovarian parenchyma, while the latter demonstrates a presence of small glands, nests or individual cells infiltrating the stroma.

Mucinous tumor of borderline malignancy	Mucinous intraepithelial carcinoma	Mucinous invasive carcinoma
Complex architecture	Basically borderline tumor	Expansile type or infiltrative type
No stromal invasion	No definite stromal invasion	Obvious invasion (>5mm)
Grade 1 atypia	Grade 2-3 atypia	

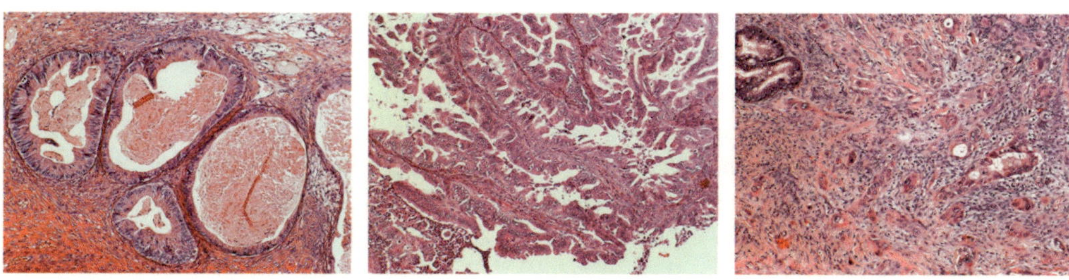

Figure 3. Criteria for central pathological review.

Intraepithelial mucinous carcinoma, FIGO stage I, has a recurrence rate of 5.8% [55]. Invasive mucinous carcinoma, FIGO stage I, has a 5-year survival rate of 91%. Patients with advanced tumors usually die of the disease [56]. Invasive mucinous carcinoma with an infiltrative pattern has a more aggressive course than mucinous carcinoma with an expansile pattern. Interestingly, invasive mucinous caricinoma of the ovary often coexistes alongside areas of mucinous borderline lesions and benign mucinous cystadenomas, suggesting that these lesions may be precursors to invasive tumors [57].

Winter, et al. [3] reviewed the data from 6 GOG phase III trials of adjuvant chemotherapy with CDDP and PTX in women with stage III EOC after primary debulking surgery, both optimal and suboptimal. Of the 1,895 patients included in these 6 studies, 74% had SAC, while only 2% had MAC. The authors found that women with mucinous tumors had a progression-free survival of 10.5 months, compared to 16.9 months for women with serous tumors. Women with MAC had a relative risk of progression of 2.18 compared their serous counterparts

($p<0.001$) [69]. The relative risk of death from MAC for compared to SAC was 4.14 ($p<0.001$). Shimada, et al. [58] compared 24 women with primary MAC to 189 women with SAC and found response rates to platinum-based regimens of 12.5 % and 37.7% respectively. Pectasides, et al. [59] compared 47 women with advanced stage primary MAC to 94 with advanced-stage SAC, all of whom had received a platinum-based regimen in 1 of 9 Hellenic Cooperative Oncology Group studies. The authors found a better response rate in women with SAC (70% for serous vs 38.5 % for mucinous), although this did not translate into survival differences between the 2 groups.

7. Clinicopathological features

Seidman, et al. [60] carefully reviewed the pathology of 220 consecutive cases of epithelial ovarian cancer. After excluding carcinosarcomas and primary peritoneal cancers, they found the incidence of primary MAC to be 3.4%. Other authors reviewed 1400 cases of EOC from 14 centers in Japan [58]. In this large group, 16% patients had an initial diagnosis of invasive primary mucinous ovarian cancer. However, after a careful pathologic review, only 4.9% had invasive primary ovarian cancer, with the remainder reclassified as either mucinous intraepithelial carcinoma, mucinous borderline tumors, or metastases from another site. Seidman and colleagues argue that these lower estimates are likely a more accurate reflection of the incidence of mucinous ovarian cancer because the following problems were likely in the literature: (1) misclassification of a gastrointestinal primary tumor as an ovarian primary tumor (80% of mucinous epithelial tumors found in the ovary are extraovarian in origin); (2) misclassification of a mucinous borderline tumor as an invasive cancer; and (3) classification of pseudomyxoma peritoneii as being of ovarian origin when it is now standard to consider all such cases as intestinal in origin.

Mutations in KRAS, BRCA, and p53 are the most frequently studied single gene alterations in ovarian cancer pathogenesis. Some investigators have gone beyond analysis of single gene mutations and have used gene expression analysis to evaluate differences between serous and mucinous ovarian carcinomas. Marchini, et al.[61] carried out genomic analyses using a microarray chip with 16,000 genes and found that serous and mucinous tumors were easily distinguished on the basis of expression profiles. Using a probe set of 59,000 genes, Heinzelmann-Schwarz, et al. [62] likewise found clear separation in expression profiles between serous and mucinous tumors of the ovary.

The role of the KRAS oncogene has been explored extensively in EOC. The RAS family of G proteins is part of the pathway that signals cell division. Mutations in the RAS genes have been found to stimulate cell growth [63]. In the literature, 50% of MAC had KRAS mutations, compared to only 5% of SAC, 10% of endometrioid ovarian caricinomas, and no CCC [64]. Interestingly, the same KRAS mutations found in invasive mucinous tumors also are found in adjacent borderline and benign mucinous lesions in the same specimens [65].

Mutations of BRCA1 and BRCA2 are thought to play a significant role in developing SAC but not MAC. BRCA1 and BRCA2 are tumor suppressor genes that help to repair damaged DNA and are commonly mutated not only in inherited SAC but also in many cases of sporadic SAC. Tonin, et al. [66] reviewed the histopathologic subtypes of ovarian carcinomas in 58 families with hereditary breast and ovarian carcinomas. In those patients with known BRCA mutations, 64% had SAC, and only 2% had MAC. In contrast, among women with ovarian cancer negative for BRCA mutation, 29% had MAC, and this proportion was significantly higher than among women with BRCA mutation. Similarly, in a review of the literature that included 636 BRCA mutation-positive women with ovarian cancer, only 2% were found to have mucinous subtypes. p53 also seems to play a prominent role in carcinogenesis of serous ovarian tumors but not mucinous ovarian tumors [70]. Mutations in p53 have been found in almost 60% of serous tumors but in only 16% of mucinous tumors.

The expression of multiple individual proteins has been examined in serous and mucinous tumor specimens using immunohistochemical stains. Compared to serous tumors, mucinous tumors are more likely to express E-cadherin (62% vs. 4%, $p<0.001$) and less likely to stain positive for N-cadherin (8% vs. 68%, $p<0.001$). The cadherin family of glycoproteins helps cells establish contact with other cells and stabilize tissue architecture. The matrix metalloproteinases, which also play a role on cell migration and adhesion, have also been found to be expressed differently between serous and mucinous tumors. Kobel, et al. evaluated 21 proteins with immunohistochemistry in 500 ovarian cancer specimens. They found different expression between serous and mucinous subtypes in 20 of the 21 biomarkers they examined, including p53, cadherin, metalloproteinase, CA125, and WT-1. Collectively, these and other molecular studies point toward a distinct pathogenesis of MAC compared to other histological subtypes of ovarian cancer.

The majority of MAC are either well or moderately differentiated and this contributes to the low risk of relapse for FIGO stage I tumors. It also is known that patients at an early stage show good outcomes. On the other hand, patients with advanced mucinous adenocarcinoma are recognized to have poorer outcomes. There was no significant difference in survival between mucinous invasive adenocarcinoma and SAC in patients with optimal surgical management [58]. In contrast, patients with suboptimal therapy showed a significantly worse prognosis than those with SAC (Fig 4).

When a mucinous tumor is grossly limited to the ovary, there is little chance of occult lymph node metastasis. Cho, et al. [71] reviewed 26 cases of MAC noted to be grossly stage I intraoperatively. All of these patients underwent lymphadenectomy as part of their staging procedures, and none were found to have lymph node disease. In contrast, 10% of patients with apparent stage I SAC of the ovary have been reported to have occult nodal metastasis at the time of diagnosis. Using the Swedish Family Canter Database of over 6,000 women with a diagnosis of ovarian cancer showed that the average overall survival was 34 months in women with serous subtypes, compared to 70 months for women with mucinous subtypes [72]. In addition, the hazard ratio for cause-specific survival from MAC compared to SAC was 0.49 (95% confidence interval, 0.41-0.57); the corresponding hazard ratio for overall survival was 0.56 (95% confidence interval, 0.48-0.64).

Patients with advanced-stage MAC had a worse prognosis than women with nonmucinous EOC [73]. The authors matched 27 patients with MAC to 54 patients with nonmucinous ovarian

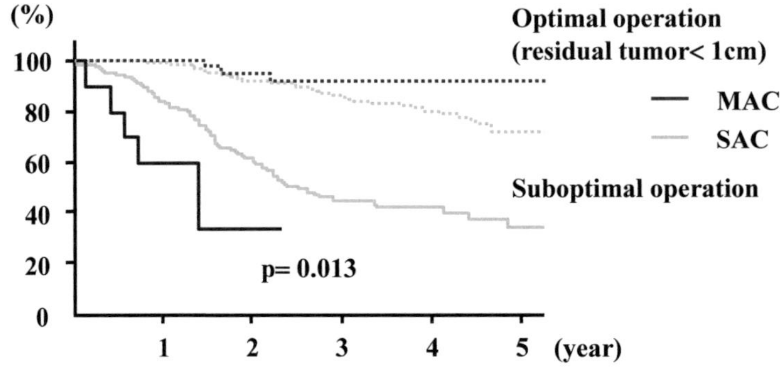

Figure 4. Overall survival and residual tumor in mucinous adenocarcinoma (MAC). There was no significant difference in survival between mucinous invasive adenocarcinoma and serous adenocarcinoma (SAC) in patients with optimal surgical management. In contrast, patients with suboptimal surgery showed a significantly worse prognosis than those with serous adenocarcinoma.

cancer (2:1), all of whom had stage III or IV disease and had undergone primary therapy. There was no difference between patients with the mucinous tumors and nonmucinous with regard to histological grade, stage, optimal or suboptimal debulking, chemotherapy regimen, or length of follow-up. Patients with advanced MAC had a progression-free survival of 5.7 months, compared to 14.1 for patients with nonmucinous ovarian cancer, and an overall survival of 12.0 compared to 36.7 months.

8. Pathological diagnosis for MAC

Most MAC involving the ovary prove to be metastases, as opposed to ovarian primary carcinomas. Therefore, surgeons and pathologists must have a high suspicion toward metastatic disease when considering the origin of MAC found in the ovary. Seidman, et al.[74] found that only 23% of invasive mucinous carcinomas of the ovary were primary ovarian cancer. Most clinicians assume that metastases to the ovary have a gastrointestinal origin. However, although gastrointestinal tract tumors are the most common source of ovarian metastases, accounting for 45% of such tumors, they also see ovarian metastases from primary tumors of the pancreas (accounting for 20% of ovarian metastases), cervix (13%), breast (8%), and uterus (5%). The remaining 10% of ovarian metastases are from unknown primary tumors [68].

At surgical exploration a working differential diagnosis can be developed on the basis of tumor size and laterality. Among unilateral tumors, more than 80% of those larger than 10 cm are ovarian primary tumors, while 88% of those smaller than 10 cm are metastases. This division has been retrospectively validated by other investigators, who showed it to be correct 84% of the time in differentiating primary from metastatic mucinous carcinomas of the ovary [74]. Other authors also have found this algorithm is useful in predicting the site of origin for ovarian carcinomas [75, 76]. In addition, primary ovarian carcinomas tend to have a smooth capsule, while ovarian metastases often involve the gross ovarian surface. However, the algorithm presented above and the status of the ovarian surface should be used clinically with caution: in one study, up to 24 % of the cases of colonic adenocarcinoma metastatic to the ovary showed unilateral ovarian involvement with tumor measurements of at least 10 cm [77]. In the same study, 46% of the cases with available information on gross intraoperative appearance had a smooth capsule.

Although gross examination of the adnexae can often predict the site of origin, both ovarian and extraovarian sources of primary disease should be explored. Intraoperatively, the surgeon should perform a careful exploration of potential gatrointestinal sources, including palpating the pancreas and running the entire small and large bowel. Postoperatively, the surgeon should consider a colonoscopy and mammogram if these screening tests have not been performed within the year prior to diagnosis.

Although the presence of certain histological features can favor a diagnosis of primary MAC over metastasis, there are cases where a definitive diagnosis cannot be provided due to the presence of discordant or overlapping features. Microscopic features that favor the diagnosis of primary ovarian MAC include a coexisting borderline and benign mucinous components, an expansile pattern of invasion, and a coexisting ovarian teratoma, Brenner tumor, or mural nodule. In contrast, the following microscopic features favor the diagnosis of metastatic adenocarcinoma to the ovary: (1) prominent desmoplastic response, (2) nodular pattern of invasion (i.e., tumor nodules among structures indigenous to the ovarian parenchyma), (3) small clusters of tumor cell within the corpora lutea or albicantia, (4) numerous pools of mucin dissecting the ovarian stroma (i.e., pseudomyxoma ovarii) in the absence of a coexistent ovarian teratoma, (5) an extensive signet ring cell pattern, (6) ovarian surface involvement, (7) vascular invasion, (8) hilar involvement, and (9) an extensive infiltrative pattern of invasion.

Immunohistochemistry may help determine the primary site of a mucinous carcinoma. Primary ovarian mucinous carcinomas tend to be positive for CK7 and CK20 with a predominance of CK7 expression, while colorectal primaries tend to express CK20 only. In addition, colorectal cancers usually express racemase and beta-catenin while primary mucinous ovarian cancers do not. In regard to other gynecological primaries metastatic to the ovary, it is worth mentioning that Human Papilloma Virus (HPV) in situ hybridization can confirm an endocervical origin because most of the endocervical adenocarcinoma are related to HPV. p16 immunostagining is useful only in well differentiated adenocarcinoma cases where a diffuse staining will be in keeping with an endocercvical origin.

Attention must be paid to the fact that high-grade ovarian mucinous or endometrioid adenocarcinomas can be positive for p16. Estrogen and progesterone receptors usually are expressed in endometrioid carcinomas, metastasizing from the endometrium or primary to the ovary. Metastatic endocervical adenocarcinomas in ovaries cannot be distinguished from a primary mucinous carcinoma of the ovary because both tumors are progesterone receptor negative and usually negative for estrogen receptors, although they can have variable expression for the latter (weak/diffuse or strong/focal staining) [78]. The presence of mesothelin, fascin, and prostate stem cell antigen (PSCA) favor a pancreatic primary, while the presence of expressed Dpc4 favors an ovarian primary for differentiating primary ovarian tumors from metastasis from the pancreas [79]. Most breast cancers are CK7-positive/CK20-negative, unlike ovarian primaries which typically express both. In addition, breast cancers almost always express estrogen receptors as well as gross cystic disease fluid protein (GCDFP)- 15 [80]. Mucinous ovarian carcinomas are unlikely to express these markers.

Carcinoembryonic antigen (CEA) is a well known serum tumor marker for gastrointestinal carcinomas. CEA has been noted to be elevated in almost one third of all ovarian carcinomas. However, CEA is much more likely to be elevated in mucinous ovarian carcinomas than in nonmucinous ovarian carcinomas (88% vs 19%) [81, 82]. Nolen, et al. [83] compared the levels of 58 serum biomarkers in serous ovarian carcinomas to mucinous, clear cell, and endoterioid ovarian carcinomas. Using immunoassays, they found significant differences between the 2 groups for 10 of the biomarkers examined. SAC had significantly higher levels of CA125, follicle-stimulating hormone, luteinizing hormone, and SMRP. Mucinous tumors had higher levels of CA72-4, matrixmetalloproteinase-9, CD40L, insulin-like growth factor-binding protein-1, myeloperoxidase, and tissue plasminogen activator-1.

9. Future directions

Realizing that MAC is a disease distinct from SAC, several collaborative groups have proposed innovative prospective chemotherapy protocols for patients with advanced or recurrent MAC. Sato, et al. [84] evaluated 6 different cytotoxic agents in 5 different primary mucinous ovarian cancer cell lines. All 5 cell lines resisted platinum agents and taxanes given as single agents. However, 2 of the 5 cell lines were sensitive to oxaliplatin, VP-16, and 5-fluorouracil (5-FU) as single agents. The investigators then treated the cell lines with oxaliplatin plus VP-16 and oxaliplatin plus 5-FU. They found that oxaliplatin with 5-FU had was significant inhibition in 4 of the 5 cell lines, whereas the combination of oxaliplatin plus VP-16 was active in only 1 of the 5 cell lines. Moreover, the combination of oxaliplatin plus 5-FU appeared to be synergistic by providing significantly more inhibition than either drug alone. The authors then applied the cell line results to a mouse model of mucinous ovarian cancer xenograft and found that mice treated with oxaliplatin plus 5-FU survived significantly longer than mice treated with either agent alone or control mice treated with placebo (Fig 5).

These basic studies led to a single-arm phase II trial of S-1 and oxaliplatin that currently is enrolling women with advanced or recurrent mucinous ovarian cancer in. S-1 is an orally active drug made by Taiho Pharmaceuticals that combines 3 separate molecules. The first is tegafur, a prodrug that is converted to fluorouracil in cells. Next is gimeracil, an inhibitor of dihydropurimidine dehydrogenase, an enzyme that degrades fluorouracil. The third component is oteracil, a molecule that inhibits the phosphorylation of fluorouracil in the gastrointestinal tract, reducing gastrointestinal toxicities. The primary endpoint of the study is response rate; secondary endpoints are toxicity, progression-free survival, and overall survival.

The GOG and the Gynecologic Cancer Intergroup (GCIG) are about to begin accrual to a 4-arm, phase III, randomized study comparing carboplatin and PTX with and without bevacizumab to oxaliplatin and capecitabine with and without bevacizumab in women with stage II-IV or recurrent, untreated, stage I, primary, mucinous ovarian or fallopian tube cancer. The

http://dx.doi.org/10.5772/54931

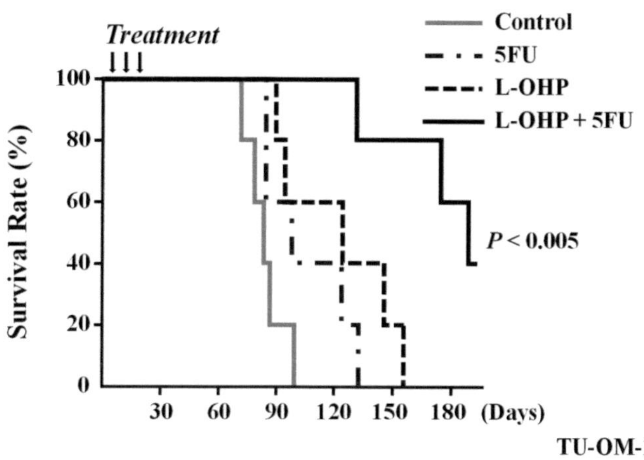

Figure 5. Survival in mice with mucinous adenocarcinoma cells (TU-OM-1 cell). Mice treated with oxaliplatin and 5-FU survived significantly longer than mice treated with either agent alone or control mice.

primary endpoint will be overall survival; secondary endpoints will be progression-free survival, response rate, toxicity, and quality of life. The study also assesses the translational endpoint, KRAS mutations and expression of vascular endothelial growth factor and epidermal growth factor. The targeted accrual for the study is 322 patients.

Based on the similarity of biological characteristics, the standard chemotherapy regimen for colorectal cancer has been given in patients with MAC. Therefore, the first phase-II chemotherapy study of oral S-1, a 5FU derivative, combined with oxaliplatin (SOX) for advanced or recurrent patients with MAC was conducted in the Japan ovarian mucinous adenocarcinoma study group.

We hope that future research in this field will enable to develop an effective strategy for conquest of chemoresistance in EOC.

	Clear cell	Serous	
No	101	235	
Median age	51 (31-72)	54 (23-82)	
FIGO stage			
Ia	49 (48.5%)	39 (16.6%)	
Ib	11 (10.9%)	15 (6.5%)	
Ic	0	2 (0.9%)	
II	38 (37.6%)	22 (9.4%)	
III	10 (9.9%)	145 (61.7%)	*P<0.0001*
IV	31 (30.7%)	38 (16.2%)	

Table 1. Patients Characteristics

Author details

Jun Naniwa, Hiroaki Itamochi and Junzo Kigawa

Tottori University Hospital Cancer Center, Japan

References

[1] http://wwwcancerorg/Research/CancerFactsFigures/GlobalCancerFactsFigures/global-facts-figures-2nd-ed

[2] Heintz AP, Odicino F, Maisonneuve P, et al. Carcinoma of the ovary. FIGO 26th Annual Report on the Results of Treatment in Gynecological Cancer. Int J Gynaecol Obstet (2006). Suppl 1) S, 161-192.

[3] Winter, W. E. rd, Maxwell GL, Tian C, et al. Prognostic factors for stage III epithelial ovarian cancer: a Gynecologic Oncology Group Study. J Clin Oncol (2007). , 25(24), 3621-3627.

[4] Kobel, M, Kalloger, S. E, Boyd, N, et al. Ovarian carcinoma subtypes are different diseases: implications for biomarker studies. PLoS Med (2008). e232.

[5] Kobel, M, Kalloger, S. E, Huntsman, D. G, et al. Differences in tumor type in low-stage versus high-stage ovarian carcinomas. Int J Gynecol Pathol (2010). , 29(3), 203-211.

[6] Mackay, H. J, Brady, M. F, Oza, A. M, et al. Prognostic relevance of uncommon ovarian histology in women with stage III/IV epithelial ovarian cancer. Int J Gynecol Cancer (2010). , 20(6), 945-952.

[7] Itamochi, H, Kigawa, J, Akeshima, R, et al. Mechanisms of cisplatin resistance in clear cell carcinoma of the ovary. Oncology (2002). , 62(4), 349-353.

[8] Rauh-hain, J. A, Winograd, D, Growdon, W. B, et al. Prognostic determinants in patients with uterine and ovarian clear carcinoma. Gynecol Oncol (2012). , 125(2), 376-380.

[9] Sugiyama, T, Kamura, T, Kigawa, J, et al. Clinical characteristics of clear cell carcinoma of the ovary: a distinct histologic type with poor prognosis and resistance to platinum-based chemotherapy. Cancer (2000). , 88(11), 2584-2589.

[10] Chan, J. K, Teoh, D, Hu, J. M, et al. Do clear cell ovarian carcinomas have poorer prognosis compared to other epithelial cell types? A study of 1411 clear cell ovarian cancers. Gynecol Oncol (2008). , 109(3), 370-376.

[11] Olsen, C. M, Nagle, C. M, Whiteman, D. C, et al. Body size and risk of epithelial ovarian and related cancers: a population-based case-control study. Int J Cancer (2008). , 123(2), 450-456.

[12] Nagle, C. M, Olsen, C. M, Webb, P. M, et al. Endometrioid and clear cell ovarian cancers: a comparative analysis of risk factors. Eur J Cancer (2008). , 44(16), 2477-2484.

[13] Yang, H. P, Trabert, B, Murphy, M. A, et al. Ovarian cancer risk factors by histologic subtypes in the NIH-AARP Diet and Health Study. Int J Cancer (2012). , 131(4), 938-948.

[14] Campbell, I. G, & Thomas, E. J. Endometriosis: candidate genes. Hum Reprod Update (2001). , 7(1), 15-20.

[15] Kennedy, A. W, Biscotti, C. V, Hart, W. R, et al. Ovarian clear cell adenocarcinoma. Gynecol Oncol (1989). , 32(3), 342-349.

[16] Aris, A. Endometriosis-associated ovarian cancer: A ten-year cohort study of women living in the Estrie Region of Quebec, Canada. J Ovarian Res (2010).

[17] Goff, B. A. Sainz de la Cuesta R, Muntz HG, et al. Clear cell carcinoma of the ovary: a distinct histologic type with poor prognosis and resistance to platinum-based chemotherapy in stage III disease. Gynecol Oncol (1996). , 60(3), 412-417.

[18] Eltabbakh, G. H, Mount, S. L, Beatty, B, et al. Clinical and molecular differences between clear cell and papillary serous ovarian carcinoma. J Surg Oncol (2006). , 93(5), 379-386.

[19] Duska, L. R, Garrett, L, Henretta, M, et al. When'never-events' occur despite adherence to clinical guidelines: the case of venous thromboembolism in clear cell cancer of the ovary compared with other epithelial histologic subtypes. Gynecol Oncol (2010). , 116(3), 374-377.

[20] Anglesio, M. S, Carey, M. S, Kobel, M, et al. Clear cell carcinoma of the ovary: a report from the first Ovarian Clear Cell Symposium, June 24th, 2010. Gynecol Oncol (2011). , 121(2), 407-415.

[21] Pectasides, D, Pectasides, E, Psyrri, A, et al. Treatment issues in clear cell carcinoma of the ovary: a different entity? Oncologist (2006). , 11(10), 1089-1094.

[22] Kobel, M, Kalloger, S. E, Santos, J. L, et al. Tumor type and substage predict survival in stage I and II ovarian carcinoma: insights and implications. Gynecol Oncol (2010). , 116(1), 50-56.

[23] Jenison, E. L, Montag, A. G, Griffiths, C. T, et al. Clear cell adenocarcinoma of the ovary: a clinical analysis and comparison with serous carcinoma. Gynecol Oncol (1989). , 32(1), 65-71.

[24] Takano, M, Kikuchi, Y, Yaegashi, N, et al. Clear cell carcinoma of the ovary: a retrospective multicentre experience of 254 patients with complete surgical staging. Br J Cancer (2006). , 94(10), 1369-1374.

[25] Andrews, P. A, & Howell, S. B. Cellular pharmacology of cisplatin: perspectives on mechanisms of acquired resistance. Cancer Cells (1990). , 2(2), 35-43.

[26] Andrews, P. A, Velury, S, Mann, S. C, et al. cis-Diamminedichloroplatinum(II) accumulation in sensitive and resistant human ovarian carcinoma cells. Cancer Res (1988). , 48(1), 68-73.

[27] Fujiwara, Y, Sugimoto, Y, Kasahara, K, et al. Determinants of drug response in a cisplatin-resistant human lung cancer cell line. Jpn J Cancer Res (1990). , 81(5), 527-535.

[28] Godwin, A. K, Meister, A, & Dwyer, O. PJ, et al. High resistance to cisplatin in human ovarian cancer cell lines is associated with marked increase of glutathione synthesis. Proc Natl Acad Sci U S A (1992). , 89(7), 3070-3074.

[29] Kasahara, K, Fujiwara, Y, Nishio, K, et al. Metallothionein content correlates with the sensitivity of human small cell lung cancer cell lines to cisplatin. Cancer Res (1991). , 51(12), 3237-3242.

[30] Borst, P, Evers, R, Kool, M, et al. A family of drug transporters: the multidrug resistance-associated proteins. J Natl Cancer Inst (2000). , 92(16), 1295-1302.

[31] Itamochi, H, Kigawa, J, Sugiyama, T, et al. Low proliferation activity may be associated with chemoresistance in clear cell carcinoma of the ovary. Obstet Gynecol (2002). , 100(2), 281-287.

[32] Ohishi, Y, Oda, Y, Uchiumi, T, et al. ATP-binding cassette superfamily transporter gene expression in human primary ovarian carcinoma. Clin Cancer Res (2002). , 8(12), 3767-3775.

[33] Kigawa, J, Minagawa, Y, Cheng, X, et al. Gamma-glutamyl cysteine synthetase upregulates glutathione and multidrug resistance-associated protein in patients with chemoresistant epithelial ovarian cancer. Clin Cancer Res (1998). , 4(7), 1737-1741.

[34] Sharma, M, He, Q. Y, & Tomasz, M. Effects of glutathione on alkylation and crosslinking of DNA by mitomycin C. Isolation of a ternary glutathione-mitomycin-DNA adduct. Chem Res Toxicol (1994). , 7(3), 401-407.

[35] Itamochi, H, Kigawa, J, Sultana, H, et al. Sensitivity to anticancer agents and resistance mechanisms in clear cell carcinoma of the ovary. Jpn J Cancer Res (2002). , 93(6), 723-728.

[36] Schwartz, D. R, Kardia, S. L, Shedden, K. A, et al. Gene expression in ovarian cancer reflects both morphology and biological behavior, distinguishing clear cell from other poor-prognosis ovarian carcinomas. Cancer Res (2002). , 62(16), 4722-4729.

[37] Xu, Z, Chen, Z. P, Malapetsa, A, et al. DNA repair protein levels vis-a-vis anticancer drug resistance in the human tumor cell lines of the National Cancer Institute drug screening program. Anticancer Drugs (2002). , 13(5), 511-519.

[38] Reed, E, Yu, J. J, Davies, A, et al. Clear cell tumors have higher mRNA levels of ERCC1 and XPB than other histological types of epithelial ovarian cancer. Clin Cancer Res (2003). , 9(14), 5299-5305.

[39] Claij, N. te Riele H. Microsatellite instability in human cancer: a prognostic marker for chemotherapy? Exp Cell Res (1999). , 246(1), 1-10.

[40] Cai, K. Q, Albarracin, C, Rosen, D, et al. Microsatellite instability and alteration of the expression of hMLH1 and hMSH2 in ovarian clear cell carcinoma. Hum Pathol (2004). , 35(5), 552-559.

[41] Agus, D. B, & Bunn, P. A. Jr., Franklin W, et al. HER-2/neu as a therapeutic target in non-small cell lung cancer, prostate cancer, and ovarian cancer. Semin Oncol (2000). Suppl 11) 53-63; discussion , 92-100.

[42] Johnstone, R. W, Ruefli, A. A, & Lowe, S. W. Apoptosis: a link between cancer genetics and chemotherapy. Cell (2002). , 108(2), 153-164.

[43] Fujimura, M, Hidaka, T, & Saito, S. Selective inhibition of the epidermal growth factor receptor by ZD1839 decreases the growth and invasion of ovarian clear cell adenocarcinoma cells. Clin Cancer Res (2002). , 8(7), 2448-2454.

[44] Rowinsky, E. K, Donehower, R. C, Jones, R. J, et al. Microtubule changes and cytotoxicity in leukemic cell lines treated with taxol. Cancer Res (1988). , 48(14), 4093-4100.

[45] Wang, Z. R, Liu, W, Smith, S. T, et al. c-myc and chromosome 8 centromere studies of ovarian cancer by interphase FISH. Exp Mol Pathol (1999). , 66(2), 140-148.

[46] Slamon, D. J, Godolphin, W, Jones, L. A, et al. Studies of the HER-2/neu proto-oncogene in human breast and ovarian cancer. Science (1989). , 244(4905), 707-712.

[47] Sherr, C. J. G. phase progression: cycling on cue. Cell (1994). , 79(4), 551-555.

[48] Marks, J. R, Davidoff, A. M, Kerns, B. J, et al. Overexpression and mutation of in epithelial ovarian cancer. Cancer Res (1991). , 53.

[49] Righetti, S. C. Della Torre G, Pilotti S, et al. A comparative study of gene mutations, protein accumulation, and response to cisplatin-based chemotherapy in advanced ovarian carcinoma. Cancer Res (1996). , 53.

[50] Ho, E. S, Lai, C. R, Hsieh, Y. T, et al. mutation is infrequent in clear cell carcinoma of the ovary. Gynecol Oncol (2001). , 53.

[51] Shah, M. A, & Schwartz, G. K. Cell cycle-mediated drug resistance: an emerging concept in cancer therapy. Clin Cancer Res (2001). , 7(8), 2168-2181.

[52] Dimanche-boitrel, M. T, Pelletier, H, Genne, P, et al. Confluence-dependent resistance in human colon cancer cells: role of reduced drug accumulation and low intrinsic chemosensitivity of resting cells. Int J Cancer (1992). , 50(5), 677-682.

[53] Shimizu, M, Nikaido, T, Toki, T, et al. Clear cell carcinoma has an expression pattern of cell cycle regulatory molecules that is unique among ovarian adenocarcinomas. Cancer (1999). , 85(3), 669-677.

[54] Kuo, K. T, Mao, T. L, Jones, S, et al. Frequent activating mutations of PIK3CA in ovarian clear cell carcinoma. Am J Pathol (2009). , 174(5), 1597-1601.

[55] Lee, K. R, & Scully, R. E. Mucinous tumors of the ovary: a clinicopathologic study of 196 borderline tumors (of intestinal type) and carcinomas, including an evaluation of 11 cases with'pseudomyxoma peritonei'. Am J Surg Pathol (2000). , 24(11), 1447-1464.

[56] Riopel, M. A, Ronnett, B. M, & Kurman, R. J. Evaluation of diagnostic criteria and behavior of ovarian intestinal-type mucinous tumors: atypical proliferative (borderline) tumors and intraepithelial, microinvasive, invasive, and metastatic carcinomas. Am J Surg Pathol (1999). , 23(6), 617-635.

[57] Rodriguez, I. M, & Prat, J. Mucinous tumors of the ovary: a clinicopathologic analysis of 75 borderline tumors (of intestinal type) and carcinomas. Am J Surg Pathol (2002). , 26(2), 139-152.

[58] Shimada, M, Kigawa, J, Ohishi, Y, et al. Clinicopathological characteristics of mucinous adenocarcinoma of the ovary. Gynecol Oncol (2009). , 113(3), 331-334.

[59] Pectasides, D, Fountzilas, G, Aravantinos, G, et al. Advanced stage mucinous epithelial ovarian cancer: the Hellenic Cooperative Oncology Group experience. Gynecol Oncol (2005). , 97(2), 436-441.

[60] Seidman, J. D, Horkayne-Szakaly I, Haiba M, et al. The histologic type and stage distribution of ovarian carcinomas of surface epithelial origin. Int J Gynecol Pathol (2004). , 23(1), 41-44.

[61] Marchini, S, Mariani, P, Chiorino, G, et al. Analysis of gene expression in early-stage ovarian cancer. Clin Cancer Res (2008). , 14(23), 7850-7860.

[62] Heinzelmann-schwarz, V. A, Gardiner-garden, M, Henshall, S. M, et al. A distinct molecular profile associated with mucinous epithelial ovarian cancer. Br J Cancer (2006). , 94(6), 904-913.

[63] Bos, J. L. ras oncogenes in human cancer: a review. Cancer Res (1989). , 49(17), 4682-4689.

[64] Gemignani, M. L, Schlaerth, A. C, Bogomolniy, F, et al. Role of KRAS and BRAF gene mutations in mucinous ovarian carcinoma. Gynecol Oncol (2003). , 90(2), 378-381.

[65] Mok, S. C, Bell, D. A, Knapp, R. C, et al. Mutation of K-ras protooncogene in human ovarian epithelial tumors of borderline malignancy. Cancer Res (1993). , 53(7), 1489-1492.

[66] Tonin, P. N, Maugard, C. M, Perret, C, et al. A review of histopathological subtypes of ovarian cancer in BRCA-related French Canadian cancer families. Fam Cancer (2007). , 6(4), 491-497.

[67] Evans, D. G, Young, K, Bulman, M, et al. Probability of BRCA1/2 mutation varies with ovarian histology: results from screening 442 ovarian cancer families. Clin Genet (2008). , 73(4), 338-345.

[68] Schuijer, M, & Berns, E. M. TP53 and ovarian cancer. Hum Mutat (2003). , 21(3), 285-291.

[69] Sarrio, D, Moreno-bueno, G, Sanchez-estevez, C, et al. Expression of cadherins and catenins correlates with distinct histologic types of ovarian carcinomas. Hum Pathol (2006). , 37(8), 1042-1049.

[70] Brun, J. L, Cortez, A, Commo, F, et al. Serous and mucinous ovarian tumors express different profiles of MMP-2,-7,-9, MT1-MMP, and TIMP-1 and-2. Int J Oncol (2008). , 33(6), 1239-1246.

[71] Cho, Y. H, Kim, D. Y, Kim, J. H, et al. Is complete surgical staging necessary in patients with stage I mucinous epithelial ovarian tumors? Gynecol Oncol (2006). , 103(3), 878-882.

[72] Ji, J, Forsti, A, Sundquist, J, et al. Survival in ovarian cancer patients by histology and family history. Acta Oncol (2008). , 47(6), 1133-1139.

[73] Hess, V, Hern, A, & Nasiri, R. N, et al. Mucinous epithelial ovarian cancer: a separate entity requiring specific treatment. J Clin Oncol (2004). , 22(6), 1040-1044.

[74] Seidman, J. D, Kurman, R. J, & Ronnett, B. M. Primary and metastatic mucinous adenocarcinomas in the ovaries: incidence in routine practice with a new approach to improve intraoperative diagnosis. Am J Surg Pathol (2003). , 27(7), 985-993.

[75] Stewart, C. J, Brennan, B. A, Hammond, I. G, et al. Accuracy of frozen section in distinguishing primary ovarian neoplasia from tumors metastatic to the ovary. Int J Gynecol Pathol (2005). , 24(4), 356-362.

[76] Yemelyanova, A. V, Vang, R, Judson, K, et al. Distinction of primary and metastatic mucinous tumors involving the ovary: analysis of size and laterality data by primary site with reevaluation of an algorithm for tumor classification. Am J Surg Pathol (2008). , 32(1), 128-138.

[77] Lewis, M. R, Deavers, M. T, Silva, E. G, et al. Ovarian involvement by metastatic colorectal adenocarcinoma: still a diagnostic challenge. Am J Surg Pathol (2006). , 30(2), 177-184.

[78] Ronnett, B. M, Yemelyanova, A. V, Vang, R, et al. Endocervical adenocarcinomas with ovarian metastases: analysis of 29 cases with emphasis on minimally invasive cervical tumors and the ability of the metastases to simulate primary ovarian neoplasms. Am J Surg Pathol (2008). , 32(12), 1835-1853.

[79] Cao, D, Ji, H, & Ronnett, B. M. Expression of mesothelin, fascin, and prostate stem cell antigen in primary ovarian mucinous tumors and their utility in differentiating primary ovarian mucinous tumors from metastatic pancreatic mucinous carcinomas in the ovary. Int J Gynecol Pathol (2005). , 24(1), 67-72.

[80] Oien, K. A. Pathologic evaluation of unknown primary cancer. Semin Oncol (2009). , 36(1), 8-37.

[81] Tholander, B, Taube, A, Lindgren, A, et al. Pretreatment serum levels of CA-125, carcinoembryonic antigen, tissue polypeptide antigen, and placental alkaline phosphatase, in patients with ovarian carcinoma, borderline tumors, or benign adnexal masses: relevance for differential diagnosis. Gynecol Oncol (1990). , 39(1), 16-25.

[82] Tuxen, M. K, Soletormos, G, & Dombernowsky, P. Tumor markers in the management of patients with ovarian cancer. Cancer Treat Rev (1995). , 21(3), 215-245.

[83] Nolen, B, Marrangoni, A, Velikokhatnaya, L, et al. A serum based analysis of ovarian epithelial tumorigenesis. Gynecol Oncol (2009). , 112(1), 47-54.

[84] Sato, S, Itamochi, H, Kigawa, J, et al. Combination chemotherapy of oxaliplatin and 5-fluorouracil may be an effective regimen for mucinous adenocarcinoma of the ovary: a potential treatment strategy. Cancer Sci (2009). , 100(3), 546-551.

Chapter 6

Demographic and Clinical Characteristics of Mucinous Epithelial Ovarian Cancer, and Survival Following a Mucinous Epithelial Ovarian Cancer Diagnosis

Sherri L. Stewart, Jennifer M. Wike,
Trevor D. Thompson, Rosemary D. Cress,
Amy R. Kahn, Cynthia D. O'Malley and
Maria J. Schymura

Additional information is available at the end of the chapter

http://dx.doi.org/10.5772/53740

1. Introduction

Ovarian cancer is the fifth leading cause of cancer death in the United States, and contributes significantly to the worldwide cancer burden [1]. The lack of gynecologic-specific symptoms and effective early detection methods for ovarian cancer leads to a preponderance of late-stage diagnoses. Ovarian cancer is a surgically-staged and treated disease, and the application of appropriate, guidelines-based treatment is currently the only option to reduce ovarian cancer mortality [2].

The National Comprehensive Cancer Network (NCCN) [3] and the National Institutes of Health (NIH) [4] publish widely used treatment guidelines for ovarian cancer cases in the United States. Both NCCN and NIH's Physician Data Query (PDQ) incorporate tumor histology into treatment guidelines. While the NCCN publishes guidelines for the three main types of ovarian cancer, epithelial, sex cord-stromal, and germ cell tumors [5]; the PDQ offers guidelines only for the most common epithelial tumors. While epithelial tumors account for about 90% of all ovarian neoplasms, they are not a homogenous group [5]. The four main epithelial subtypes (serous, mucinous, clear cell, and endometrioid) can have very different clinical and pathologic patterns.

Among epithelial ovarian cancer subtypes is mucinous epithelial ovarian cancer (mEOC), a relatively rare subtype accounting for approximately 14% of invasive ovarian cancer cases [6]. mEOC has a distinct natural history compared to other epithelial subtypes, especially the most common serous subtype. mEOCs are more often diagnosed in younger women [6] than other epithelial tumors, and epidemiologic studies have shown a lack of protective effect from parity and oral contraceptive use [7-11]. Pathologic studies have determined that mutations in the K-ras oncogene are more common in mEOC compared to other subtypes [12], while mutations in the BRCA1 tumor suppressor gene are less common [13]. Despite their distinctive nature, mEOCs are included in overall epithelial ovarian cancer treatment guidelines, as standard care for all epithelial subtypes is defined in the same manner [3,4].

Because of the differences in risk factors and presentation, a few studies have examined differences in outcomes of mEOC compared to other epithelial subtypes. Many have found lower response rates to chemotherapy and inferior outcomes compared to other subtypes [14-16]. Based on these results, it has been suggested that mEOC be treated as a different entity and not grouped along with epithelial tumors in standard treatment and also in clinical trials for epithelial ovarian cancer [17]; however, these suggestions have yet to be widely adopted or implemented. While the existing evidence seems consistent, studies producing this evidence have contained small numbers and generally represent the experience of individual institutions.

1.1. Objectives

The objective of this chapter is to fully characterize mEOC using a population-based approach. We add to the paucity of existing literature on mEOC with an analysis that utilizes ovarian cancer medical record data from two large populations in the United States, New York and Northern California. We comprehensively examine demographics, pathologic characteristics, and the outcomes of treatment for mEOC. We compare these characteristics to other epithelial subtypes in order to determine whether clinical presentation or outcomes differ among epithelial subtypes. Finally, we discuss the results of this research in the context of published studies on mEOC.

2. Study design

2.1. Setting and population

The data presented and analyzed here are from the Ovarian Cancer Treatment Patterns and Outcomes (OCTPO) study, funded by the Centers for Disease Control and Prevention (CDC), and conducted by the New York State and the California Cancer Registries [18-20]. The New York State Cancer Registry (NYSCR) conducts surveillance on all 19 million New York state residents, and the two components of the California Cancer Registry (CCR) that were funded for this study serve the contiguous geographical area of Greater San Francisco-San Jose and Sacramento regions, providing surveillance for a population of 9 million residents in California. Both the NYSCR and the CCR conduct high quality, population-based cancer surveillance, and routinely review medical records to abstract demographics, tumor characteristics and treatment data as part of state-mandated cancer surveillance. For this retrospective study, additional detailed patient, tumor, and treatment data were collected by these registries from multiple sources including hospital, outpatient facility and physician records. Vital status was determined by linkage with the National Death Index http://www.cdc.gov/nchs/ndi.htm. The study population included patients with invasive epithelial ovarian cancer diagnosed between 1998 and 2000. Only invasive cases of epithelial ovarian cancer were included; benign and low malignant potential tumors were excluded. Primary peritoneal cancers and fallopian tube cancers were also excluded. Subjects diagnosed at autopsy or by death certificate were ineligible. All cases included were histologically confirmed. Cases were followed up for six years for vital status information.

2.2. Data classification

Histology was collected according to World Health Organization International Classification of Diseases for Oncology, third edition (ICD-O-3) morphology codes [21]. All epithelial histologies collected were collapsed into categories for analysis according to Table 1.

Epithelial Ovarian Cancer (EOC) Subtype	ICD-O-3 Codes
Mucinous (mEOC)	8470, 8471, 8480, 8481
Serous	8441,8442,8460,8461,8462
Other (includes endometrioid, clear cell, Brenner, mixed, undifferentiated, and unspecified or other epithelial tumors)	8380,8940,8950,8951,8310,9000,8323,8020,8050,8052, 8070,8120,8130,8140,8260, 8330,8340,8440,8450,8490,8560,8570,8980,8981

Table 1. Histologic definitions by epithelial ovarian cancer subtype

Race and ethnicity was categorized as white non-Hispanic, black non-Hispanic, Asian non-Hispanic, and Hispanic. A total of 34 cases were excluded from the analysis on the basis of race or ethnicity data. Three of the 34 cases were classified as American Indian/Alaska Native race; these were excluded because of the inability to draw any conclusions from this race because of the very small number. The remaining 31 cases were excluded because race or ethnicity information was unspecified or missing. Stage was defined using the International Federation of Gynecology and Obstetrics (FIGO) system, with categories I, II, III IV, or unknown. Grade was collapsed into four categories defined as Grade I (well differentiated tumors), Grade II (moderately differentiated tumors), Grade III/IV (poorly differentiated and undifferentiated tumors) and unknown grade. Laterality was collapsed into unilateral (single ovary involved at diagnosis: right, left, or unspecified), or bilateral (both ovaries involved at diagnosis) categories. Comorbidity was defined using the Deyo-Charlson Comorbidity Index [22, 23], a commonly used measure of disease burden. Comorbidity information was collected via linkage with state hospital discharge data. Any comorbidity present in the 12 months prior to or 4 months following an ovarian cancer diagnosis was included. Type of treatment was defined to distinguish patients who received various combinations of surgery and chemotherapy. In descriptive analyses, chemotherapy was further categorized by receipt of specific agents. These categories consisted of surgery and platinum agent (cisplatin or carboplatin) receipt, surgery and platinum agent and paclitaxel receipt (standard treatment for EOC) [24], and surgery and any chemotherapy agent or combination of agents other than cisplatin, carboplatin, or paclitaxel.

2.3. Analyses

Statistical testing was performed using the likelihood ratio chi-square test for discrete variables. The Kruskal-Wallis test was used to test for differences among continuous variables. A generalized logits model was fit to determine the characteristics associated with epithelial subtype. Variables included in the model were age, race/ethnicity, stage, grade, and laterality. Age was transformed in all models using restricted cubic spline functions to allow for nonlinearity [25]. Due to the lack of availability of grade and stage information for some cases (31% for grade; 15% for stage), missing indicator variables were included for each variable in all models. Because of potential issues with using missing indicator variables, separate models that imputed missing data were fit (data not shown) [26,27]. These models yielded consistent results with the un-imputed models. Six-year survival curves are presented as Kaplan-Meier estimates. Statistical testing for differences in unadjusted survival rates across epithelial subtypes was performed using the log-rank test. For adjusted survival, a time-dependent Cox model was used to determine the predictors of six-year survival. Age, race/ethnicity, stage, grade, epithelial subtype, comorbidity, laterality, surgery, and chemotherapy were included as covariates in the survival model. Time-dependent covariates for surgery and chemotherapy were used to prevent an artificial inflation of the association between treatment and survival. Cases were considered as not receiving treatment until the date of the procedure; they were considered as having received treatment after the date of the procedure. Interactions between epithelial subtype and treatment were included to determine if the effects of surgery and chemotherapy varied across subtypes. The proportional hazards assumption was assessed using time-dependent covariates and the Schoenfeld residual correlation test. Laterality was found to violate the proportional hazards (PH) assumption. Stratified log[-log S(t)] plots were used to help determine time intervals within which the PH assumption held. An interaction between laterality and time was included in the final model to satisfy the PH assumption.

3. Results

3.1. Demographic and clinical characteristics of mucinous epithelial ovarian cancer

The characteristics of ovarian cancer cases in New York and Northern California are presented by epithelial subtype in Table 2. Overall, 230 (8.7%) tumors were mEOC, 1195 (45.3%) tumors were serous EOC, and 1211 (45.9%) were other EOC. mEOCs were diagnosed at younger ages (57 years) compared to other subtypes (62 years for serous, 63 years for other EOCs). Relatively higher percentages of mEOCs were found among black non-Hispanic

(8.0% vs. 5.9 and 6.7%) and Asian non-Hispanic (14.2% vs. 5.4 and 9.8%) populations compared to serous and other EOCs. Lower percentages of mEOCs (5.8%) were found among Hispanics compared to serous and mEOCs (7.5 and 7.7%). mEOCS were more likely to be diagnosed at FIGO stage I (45.2%) compared to serous (10.0%) and other mEOCs (24.9%). Higher percentages of low grade tumors and unilateral ovarian involvement at diagnosis were also present with mEOCs compared to other EOC types. A little under half of mEOC patients (46.3%) were treated with surgery only and 39.0% were treated with surgery plus a platinum agent and paclitaxel.

Characteristic	Mucinous (n=230)	Serous (n=1195)	Other Epithelial (n=1211)	**P-value**
Age at diagnosis*	57 (45, 72)	62 (52, 72)	63 (51, 75)	<0.001
Race/Ethnicity				<0.001
White Non-Hispanic	162 (72.0%)	956 (81.3%)	910 (75.8%)	
Black Non-Hispanic	18 (8.0%)	69 (5.9%)	80 (6.7%)	
Asian Non-Hispanic	32 (14.2%)	63 (5.4%)	118 (9.8%)	
Hispanic	13 (5.8%)	88 (7.5%)	93 (7.7%)	
FIGO Stage				<0.001
I	104 (45.2%)	119 (10.0%)	302 (24.9%)	
II	26 (11.3%)	66 (5.5%)	125 (10.3%)	
III	62 (27.0%)	747 (62.5%)	380 (31.4%)	
IV	19 (8.3%)	153 (12.8%)	225 (18.6%)	
Unknown	19 (8.3%)	110 (9.2%)	179 (14.8%)	
Grade				<0.001
I	73 (31.7%)	80 (6.7%)	92 (7.6%)	
II	69 (30.0%)	223 (18.7%)	193 (15.9%)	
III/IV	30 (13.0%)	730 (61.1%)	493 (40.7%)	
Unknown	58 (25.2%)	162 (13.6%)	433 (35.8%)	
Laterality				<0.001
Unilateral	167 (77.7%)	410 (36.7%)	634 (67.7%)	
Bilateral	48 (22.3%)	707 (63.3%)	302 (32.3%)	
Comorbidity				0.0257
None	161 (74.5%)	847 (77.6%)	814 (74.9%)	
1	38 (17.6%)	181 (16.6%)	170 (15.6%)	
2 or more	17 (7.9%)	63 (5.8%)	103 (9.5%)	

Characteristic	Mucinous (n=230)	Serous (n=1195)	Other Epithelial (n=1211)	**P-value**
Treatment				<0.001
Surgery only	95 (46.3%)	132 (12.2%)	196 (17.9%)	
Surgery+Platinum	7 (3.4%)	46 (4.3%)	28 (2.6%)	
Surgery+Platinum+ Paclitaxel	80 (39.0%)	826 (76.5%)	565 (51.6%)	
Surgery+other chemotherapy	2 (1.0%)	21 (1.9%)	12 (1.1%)	
Chemotherapy only	12 (5.9%)	32 (3.0%)	169 (15.4%)	
No surgery/no chemotherapy	9 (4.4%)	23 (2.1%)	124 (11.3%)	

Table 2. Demographic and clinical characteristics of invasive epithelial ovarian cancer cases by subtype, New York and Northern California. * Continuous variable presented as median (25th percentile, 75th percentile).

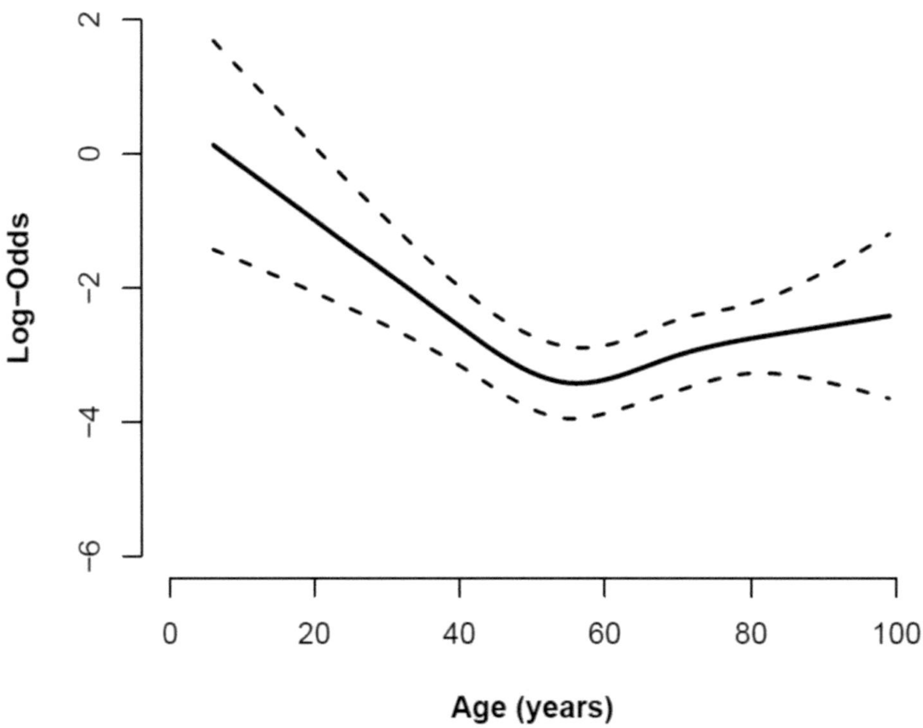

Figure 1. Adjusted relationship between age and risk of mucinous epithelial compared to serous epithelial ovarian cancer. Solid line indicates log-odds ratio, dotted lines indicated confidence intervals.

Table 3, Figure 1 and Figure 2 show the demographic and clinical characteristics significantly associated with mEOCs compared to other epithelial ovarian cancers, after adjusting for other factors. mEOCs were more often associated with Asian non-Hispanic race/ethnicity compared to serous tumors (odds ratio [OR] 1.94, 95% confidence interval [CI] 1.13-3.35). The relationship between age and epithelial subtype was nonlinear; ages 55 years and younger were more often associated with mEOC compared to both serous and other EOCs (Figures 1 and 2). Less advanced stage was associated with mEOCs compared to serous EOC (OR 0.29, 95% CI 0.18-0.47 for stage III and 0.39, 0.19-0.78 for stage IV). mEOCs were less likely to be grade III/IV compared to serous (OR 0.11, 95% CI 0.07-0.20) and other EOC (OR 0.10, 95% CI 0.06-0.16). Bilateral ovarian cancer at diagnosis was less often associated with mEOCs compared to serous EOC (OR = 0.32, 95% CI 0.22-0.49).

Characteristic	P-value	Mucinous vs. Serous Odds Ratio 95% CI	Mucinous vs. Other Epithelial Odds Ratio 95% CI
Age at diagnosis*	0.0008	Nonlinear	Nonlinear
Nonlinear	0.0002		
Race/Ethnicity	0.0723		
White non-Hispanic		1.00	1.00
Black non-Hispanic		1.36 (0.73-2.54)	1.52 (0.82-2.80)
Asian non-Hispanic		1.94 (1.13-3.35)	1.17 (0.72-1.90)
Hispanic		0.77 (0.40-1.50)	0.76 (0.40-1.44)
FIGO Stage	<.0001		
I		1.00	1.00
II		0.89 (0.50-1.60)	0.96 (0.57-1.63)
III		0.29 (0.18-0.47)	1.10 (0.70-1.72)
IV		0.39 (0.19-0.78)	0.68 (0.35-1.32)
Unknown		0.41 (0.21-0.83)	0.80 (0.41-1.57)
Grade	<.0001		
I		1.00	1.00
II		0.62 (0.38-1.00)	0.49 (0.31-0.77)
III/IV		0.11 (0.07-0.20)	0.10 (0.06-0.16)
Unknown		0.92 (0.55-1.55)	0.31 (0.19-0.49)
Laterality	<.0001		
Unilateral		1.00	1.00
Bilateral		0.32 (0.22-0.49)	0.80 (0.53-1.21)

Table 3. Adjusted odds ratios and 95% confidence intervals for demographic and clinical characteristics of invasive epithelial ovarian cases by subtype, New York and Northern California. *The relationship between age and histologic subtype is shown in Figures 1 and 2.CI=confidence interval

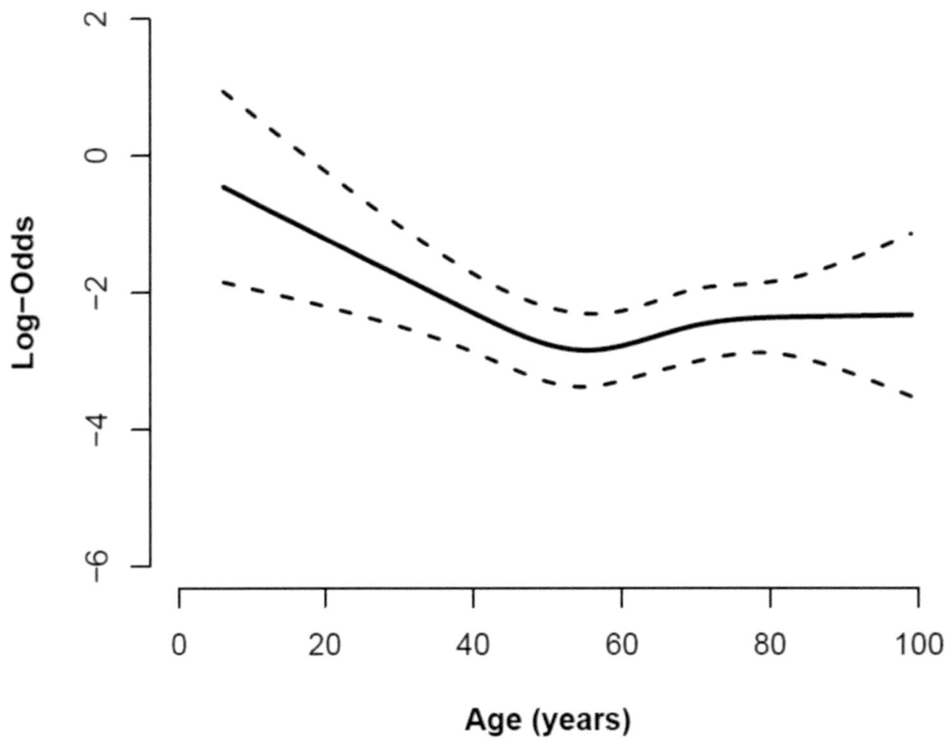

Figure 2. Adjusted relationship between age and risk of and mucinous epithelial ovarian cancer compared to other epithelial ovarian cancer. Solid line indicates log-odds ratio, dotted lines indicated confidence intervals.

3.2. Survival following a mucinous ovarian cancer diagnosis

Unadjusted Kaplan-Meier estimates showed that survival following an epithelial ovarian cancer diagnosis was initially worse for mEOC and other EOC compared to serous EOC (Figure 3). At approximately 38-40 months post-diagnosis, mEOC and other EOC tumor survival rates stabilized, whereas survival from serous EOC continually decreased. At the end of the 6 year follow-up period, survival was significantly different among the epithelial subtypes (log rank p<0.001). Unadjusted survival was 49.8% among women with mEOC, 39.0% among women with other EOC, and 30.8% among women serous EOC.

The results of the multivariable Cox model predicting 6-year survival are shown in Table 4 and Figure 4. After adjustment, black race, advanced stage, higher grade, and the presence of comorbidities were all associated with increased mortality from EOC (Table 4), as was increasing age (especially age > 60, Figure 4). By epithelial subtype, mEOC conferred a worse prognosis and was associated with increased mortality compared to both serous EOC (Hazard ratio [HR] 0.51, 95% CI 0.40-0.65), and other EOC (HR 0.56, 95% CI 0.44-0.72). Significant interactions were found between epithelial subtype and both surgery (p=0.0064) and chemotherapy (p=0.0340). In all cases, mEOC was associated with increased mortality. Significant

http://dx.doi.org/10.5772/53740

associations occurred among those who received both surgery and chemotherapy; women with serous EOC and other EOC had better survival than those with mEOC in this group (serous HR 0.45, 05% CI 0.33-0.62; other EOC HR 0.44, 95% CI 0.32-0.61). This was also the case for women who were treated with chemotherapy alone (serous EOC HR 0.16, 95% CI 0.07-0.38; other EOC HR 0.40, 95% CI 0.20-0.81). In women who received only surgery or did not receive treatment, those with serous EOC had better survival than those with mEOC (HR 0.65, 95% CI 0.42-1.00, HR 0.23, 95% CI 0.10-0.53, respectively).

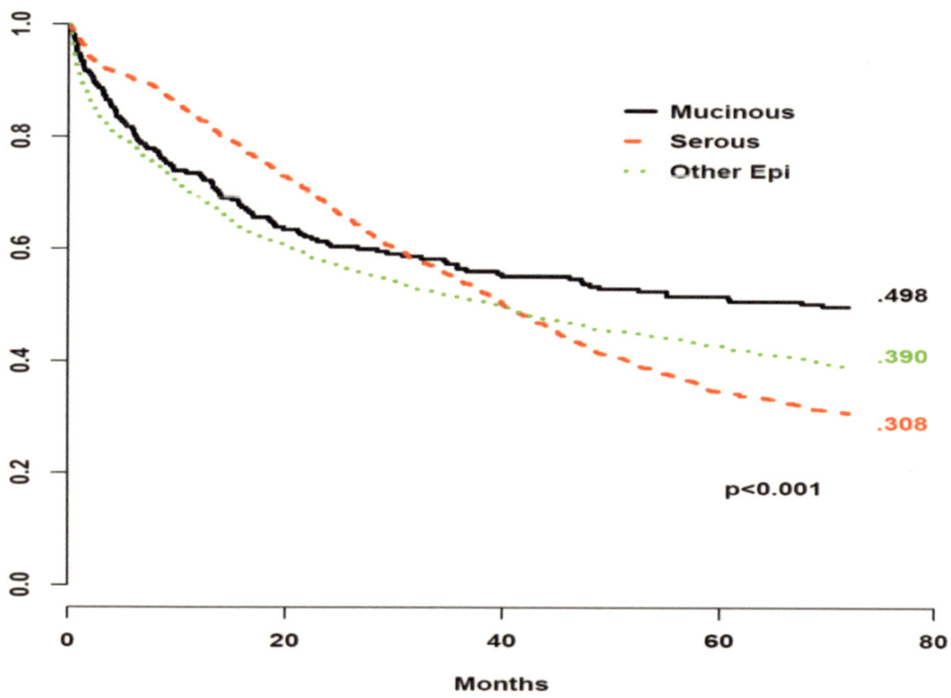

Figure 3. Six-year survival following an invasive epithelial ovarian cancer diagnosis by subtype, New York and Northern California

Characteristic	Wald χ^2	DF*	P-value	Hazard Ratio (95% CI)
Age at diagnosis*	99.68	2	<0.0001	
Nonlinear	10.75	1	0.0010	
Race/Ethnicity	26.63	3	<0.0001	
White non-Hispanic				1.00
Black non-Hispanic				1.47 (1.17-1.86)

Characteristic	**Wald χ^2**	**DF***	**P-value**	Hazard Ratio (95% CI)
Asian non-Hispanic				0.62 (0.45-0.84)
Hispanic				0.76 (0.59-0.98)
FIGO Stage	239.24	4	<0.0001	
I				1.00
II				1.40 (0.96- 2.04)
III				4.96 (3.77- 6.51)
IV				8.02 (5.93-10.84)
Unknown				5.36 (3.93- 7.31)
Grade	12.83	3	0.0050	
I				1.00
II				1.36 (1.01-1.84)
III/IV				1.50 (1.13-2.00)
Unknown				1.69 (1.25-2.29)
Laterality	38.41	2	<0.0001	
0 – 2 years				
Bilateral vs. Unilateral				1.04 (0.87-1.23)
"/>2 years – 6 years				
Bilateral vs. Unilateral				1.86 (1.53-2.27)
Comorbidity	20.04	2	<0.0001	
0				1.00
1				1.26 (1.08-1.48)
2 or more				1.59 (1.26-2.01)
Epithelial subtype**	48.68	6	<0.0001	
Mucinous				1.0
Serous				0.51 (0.40-0.65)
Other Epithelial				0.56 (0.44-0.72)
Surgery+Chemotherapy				

http://dx.doi.org/10.5772/53740

Characteristic	Wald χ^2	DF*	P-value	Hazard Ratio (95% CI)
Mucinous				1.0
Serous				0.45 (0.33-0.62)
Other Epithelial				0.44 (0.32-0.61)
Surgery/No chemotherapy				
Mucinous				1.0
Serous				0.65 (0.42-1.00)
Other Epithelial				0.83 (0.55-1.26)
Chemotherapy/No Surgery				
Mucinous				1.0
Serous				0.16 (0.07-0.38)
Other Epithelial				0.40 (0.20-0.81)
No Surgery/ No Chemotherapy				
Mucinous				1.0
Serous				0.23 (0.10-0.53)
Other Epithelial				0.75 (0.38-1.49)
Surgery (Yes vs. No)	34.93	3	<0.0001	
Mucinous				0.38 (0.20-0.75)
Serous				1.06 (0.63-1.79)
Other Epithelial				0.42 (0.31-0.58)
Chemotherapy (Yes vs. No) 11.05 3 0.0115				
Mucinous				1.25 (0.79-1.97)
Serous				0.88 (0.68-1.14)
Other Epithelial				0.67 (0.51-0.87)

Table 4. Multivariate proportional hazards results of invasive epithelial ovarian cancer cases, New York and Northern California. *The relationship between age and risk of death is shown in Figure 4. **The overall epithelial subtype comparisons are from a model excluding the subtype and treatment interactions. These are presented to show the "average" effect across treatments. All other hazard ratios in the model are calculated from the model including the interactions.

4. Discussion

This large, population-based study adds further, definitive evidence for demographic and clinical characteristics previously associated with mEOC: Asian race, early stage, low grade, and unilateral ovarian involvement at diagnosis [9,16,28]. Regardless of the large proportion of stage I diagnoses (about 45%), mEOC appears to be a particularly deadly subtype of ovarian cancer. These patterns seen in mEOC are consistent with clear cell EOC, which also tends to be diagnosed at early stages [29], and has poor overall survival compared to other EOCs [29,30]. Patterns of other epithelial subtypes vary: endometrioid EOC is often diagnosed at early stages, but generally has better overall survival compared to other EOCs [31]; serous EOC is most often diagnosed at late stages (stage III and IV), and survival from these tumors appears to be significantly associated with grade [32]. These divergent patterns suggest that EOC is an extremely heterogeneous group, and histologic subtype should be considered in addition to stage before and during treatment.

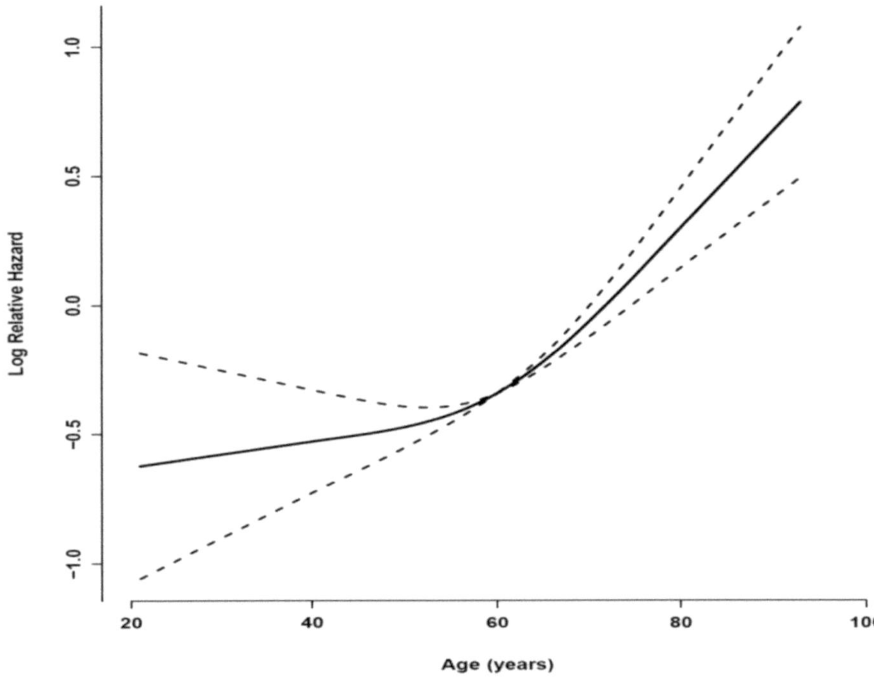

Figure 4. Adjusted relationship between age and risk of death within six years following an epithelial ovarian cancer diagnosis. Solid line indicates log-hazard ratio, dotted lines indicate 95% confidence intervals.

The poor survival from mEOC shown here is consistent with other studies [14,16,33] and may be due to a decreased response to chemotherapy. Our study results are consistent with these findings, in that chemotherapy did not appear to have a beneficial effect in women with mEOC. Evidence suggests that mEOC response rates to platinum-based chemotherapy are low overall (13-26%) [14,34]. This decreased response could be related to a lack of sensitivity of mEOCs to standard platinum-containing chemotherapy regimens [17]. It is well-established that platinum sensitivity varies by pathologic and clinical characteristics including tumor type [34,35]. Relatively recently, some groups in the United States have suggested that different treatment strategies should be considered for mEOC, and that future clinical trials should be redesigned to 1) exclude women with mEOC and other rare EOC types [36], and 2) assist with the development of novel agents more targeted to mEOC that can be used in the front-line and recurrent settings [17, 37]. Several barriers exist to such clinical trials, including decreased availability of funding [38], as well as potential lack of enrollment and participation due to the rarity and deadly nature of mEOC. Despite these limitations however, a phase III clinical trial comparing standard carboplatin and paclitaxel regimen (with and without bevacizumab) to oxalitlatin and capecitabine (with and without bevacizumab) in women with stages II-IV or recurrent untreated stage I primary mEOC was recently announced [39].

Some groups have suggested additional chemotherapeutic agents that may be more effective in the treatment of mEOC. Based on studies with mEOC cell lines, combination chemotherapy consisting of oxaliplatin and 5-fluorouracil may be beneficial for mEOCs [40]. The suggested use of fluorouracil, a chemotherapy agent used in the treatment of colon cancer [41], has gained additional support because of the similarities between mEOC and mucinous tumors of the colon [16,42]. A recent review comparing characteristics of these two tumor types concluded that there are multiple similarities with respect to mutational patterns, clinical presentation, therapy response, and outcomes [43]. The review further proposes that the search for new and more effective chemotherapeutic agents for mucinous tumors might be more successful if comparisons are made across organs [43]. However, there are clear differences in the cellular localization of mucin in these two types, and further research is needed to substantiate the usefulness of this approach.

Regardless of the availability of and evidence for alternative treatment regimens, the results presented here underscore the need for precise pathologic assessment of all EOCs with respect to site of tumor origin, histologic type and subtype, behavior and grade. The vast majority of histologic-specific analyses using medical record data (including this one) are limited by the fact that there is no central pathology review of included cases. Because of this, a few studies have retrospectively reviewed stored specimens and medical records to examine concordance of pathologic characteristics of ovarian cancer. In a population-based study using Surveillance Epidemiology and End Results (SEER) data, there was 98% concordance on site of origin, and 97% concordance on overall epithelial histologic type [44]. Concordance varied by histologic subtype; it was 100% for clear cell EOC, 87% for mEOC, 80% for serous EOC, and 73% for endometrioid EOC. For tumor behavior, there was 85% concordance for invasive ovarian tumors. In most cases (90%), tumors originally diagnosed as invasive were thought to be low malignant potential upon review. Another study examining pathology in the Gilda Radner Familial Ovarian Cancer Tumor Registry reported

95.3% concordance on primary site [45]. The agreement by histologic subtype was lower, with disagreement on 38.3% of cases. The vast majority of differences were related to differences in classification of serous EOC, either by the initial or reviewing pathologist. Concordance by grade was slightly better than that by histologic subtype, with disagreement on 31.2% of cases. The majority of differences centered on the differential assignment of grade II versus grade III. Few cases (a total of 7.6%) were upgraded or downgraded in a way that would have potential implications for treatment. While these pathologic review findings are encouraging overall and provide support for analyses of mEOC such as this one, they may not be exact enough to support the prescription of alternative treatment regimens based solely on histologic subtype.

5. Conclusions

The results presented here provide definitive evidence that mEOC is associated with different demographic and clinical characteristics than other EOC subtypes, and women diagnosed with mEOC have worse adjusted survival compared to those with other EOC subtypes. A particular strength of this study is the population-based approach, which reflects the experience of two U.S. populations of women with ovarian cancer, as opposed to that of a single institution or those participating in clinical research. This study yields several implications for future research. First and foremost, the continued characterization of the heterogeneity of ovarian cancer through basic, clinical, and population research is necessary. Second, the need for precision in pathologic assessments is paramount, and pathologists, oncologists and scientists all have a role in assisting with this through research and education. Finally, assessment of provider knowledge and awareness regarding treatment recommendations, and proposed or enacted changes to these recommendations, would be beneficial for ensuring appropriate use of evidence-based practices in the treatment of ovarian cancer.

Acknowledgments

This work was supported by cooperative agreements (U58/CCU920352 and U58/CCU220322) with the Centers of Disease Control and Prevention. The collection of cancer incidence data used in this study was supported by the California Department of Public Health as part of the statewide cancer reporting program mandated by California Health and Safety Code Section 103885; the National Cancer Institute's Surveillance, Epidemiology and End Results Program under contract N01-PC-35136 awarded to the Northern California Cancer Center and contract N01-PC-45025 awarded to the Public Health Institute; the Centers for Disease Control and Prevention's National Program of Cancer Registries, under agreement #U58/DP00080 awarded to the Public Health Institute, and agreement #U58/DP000783 awarded to the New York State Department of Health; and the New York State Department of Health as part of the statewide cancer reporting mandate specified in New York State Public Health Law Section 2401. The findings and conclusions in this report are those of the authors and do not necessarily represent the official position of the Centers for Disease Control and Prevention, the State of California Department of Public Health, and the New York State Department of Health.

Author details

Sherri L. Stewart[1], Jennifer M. Wike[2], Trevor D. Thompson[1], Rosemary D. Cress[3], Amy R. Kahn[5], Cynthia D. O'Malley[4] and Maria J. Schymura[5]

*Address all correspondence to: Sstewart2@cdc.gov

1 Division of Cancer Prevention and Control, Centers for Disease Control and Prevention, Atlanta, GA, USA

2 Centers for Disease Control and Prevention, NPCR-Contractor, Atlanta, GA, USA

3 Public Health Institute, Sacramento, CA and University of California, Davis, USA

4 Amgen, Inc, South San Francisco, CA, USA

5 New York State Registry, Albany, NY, USA

References

[1] Stewart SL (2012). Ovarian Cancer Incidence: Current and Comprehensive Statistics, Ovarian Cancer - Clinical and Therapeutic Perspectives, Samir A. Farghaly (Ed.), ISBN: 978-953-307-810-6, InTech, Available from: http://www.intechopen.com/books/ovarian-cancer-clinical-and-therapeutic-perspectives/ovarian-cancer-incidence-current-and-comprehensive-statistics-

[2] Stewart SL, Rim SH, Richards TB. Gynecologic oncologists and ovarian cancer treatment: avenues for improved survival. J Womens Health (Larchmt) 2011; 20(9): 1257-60.

[3] National Comprehensive Cancer Network Guidelines. Epithelial Ovarian Cancer (including Fallopian Tube Cancer and Primary Peritoneal Cancer). www.nccn.com/files/cancer-guidelines/ovarian/index.html (accessed Sept 5, 2012).

[4] National Cancer Institute. Ovarian Epithelial Cancer Treatment (PDQ®). http://www.cancer.gov/cancertopics/pdq/treatment/ovarianepithelial/HealthProfessional/page1 (accessed Sept 5, 2012)

[5] Scully RE. Ovarian tumors. Am. J of Pathol. 1977; 87(3): 686-720.

[6] Quirk JT, Natarajan N. Ovarian cancer incidence in the United States, 1992-1999. Gynecol Oncol. 2005;97(2):519-23.

[7] Soegaard M, Jensen A, Høgdall E, et al. Different risk factor profiles for mucinous and nonmucinous ovarian cancer: results from the Danish MALOVA study. Cancer Epidemiol Biomarkers Prev. 2007;16(6):1160-6.

[8] Kurian AW, Balise RR, McGuire V, et al. Histologic types of epithelial ovarian cancer: have they different risk factors? Gynecol Oncol. 2005; 96(2):520-30.

[9] Tung KH, Goodman MT, Wu AH, et al. Reproductive factors and epithelial ovarian cancer risk by histologic type: a multiethnic case-control study. Am J Epidemiol. 2003;158(7):629-38.

[10] Purdie DM, Webb PM, Siskind V, et al. The different etiologies of mucinous and nonmucinous epithelial ovarian cancers. Gynecol Oncol. 2003;88(1 Pt 2):S145-8.

[11] Risch HA, Marrett LD, Jain M, et al. Differences in risk factors for epithelial ovarian cancer by histologic type. Results of a case-control study. Am J Epidemiol. 1996;144(4):363-72.

[12] Gemignani ML, Schlaerth AC, Bogomolniy F, et al. Role of KRAS and BRAF gene mutations in mucinous ovarian carcinoma. Gynecol Oncol. 2003;90(2):378-81.

[13] Lakhani SR, Manek S, Penault-Llorca F, et al. Pathology of ovarian cancers in BRCA1 and BRCA2 carriers. Clin Cancer Res. 2004;10(7):2473-81.

[14] Pectasides D, Fountzilas G, Aravantinos G, et al. Advanced stage mucinous epithelial ovarian cancer: the Hellenic Cooperative Oncology Group experience. Gynecol Oncol. 2005;97(2):436-41.

[15] Pignata S, Ferrandina G, Scarfone G. Activity of chemotherapy in mucinous ovarian cancer with a recurrence free interval of more than 6 months: results from the SOCRATES retrospective study. BMC Cancer. 2008;8:252.

[16] Hess V, A'Hern R, Nasiri N, et al. Mucinous epithelial ovarian cancer: a separate entity requiring specific treatment. J Clin Oncol. 2004 15;22(6):1040-4.

[17] Gershenson DM, Birrer M. Time for action: a "sea change" in treatment strategies for rare types of epithelial ovarian cancer. Gynecol Oncol. 2007;106(1):1-3.

[18] Eheman CR, Peipins L, Wynn M, et al. Development of a public health research program for ovarian cancer. J Womens Health (Larchmt) 2006;15(4):339-45

[19] Cress RD, Bauer K, O'Malley CD, et al. Surgical staging of early stage epithelial ovarian cancer: results from the CDC-NPCR ovarian patterns of care study. Gynecol Oncol. 2011;121(1):94-9.

[20] O'Malley CD, Shema SJ, Cress RD, et al. The implications of age and comorbidity on survival following epithelial ovarian cancer: summary and results from a centers for disease control and prevention study. J Womens Health (Larchmt) 2012;21(9):887-94.

[21] Fritz A, Percy C, Jack A, et al., editors. International Classification of Diseases for Oncology, third edition. Geneva: World Health Organization 2000.

[22] Charlson ME, Pompei P, Ales KL, et al. A new method of classifying prognostic comorbidity in longitudinal studies: Development and validation. J Chronic Dis 1987;40:373–383.

[23] Deyo RA, Cherkin DC, Ciol MA. Adapting a clinical comorbidity index for use with ICD-9-CM administrative databases. J Clin Epidemiol 1992;45:613–619.

[24] Ozols, R.F. Optimum chemotherapy for ovarian cancer. Int. J. Gyn. Cancer 2000; 10(s1):33-37.

[25] Harrell, FE. Regression Modeling Strategies: With Applications to Linear Models, Logistic Regression, and Survival Analysis. New York: Springer, 2001

[26] Harrell FE et al (2008). Hmisc: Harrell Miscellaneous. R package version 3.5-2.

[27] R Development Core Team (2008). R: A language and environment for statistical computing. R Foundation for Statistical Computing, Vienna, Austria. ISBN 3-900051-07-0, URL http://www.R-project.org.

[28] Seidman JD, Horkayne-Szakaly I, Haiba M, et al. The histologic type and stage distribution of ovarian carcinomas of surface epithelial origin. Int J Gynecol Pathol. 2004;23(1):41-4.

[29] Chan JK, Teoh D, Hu JM, et al. Do clear cell ovarian carcinomas have poorer prognosis compared to other epithelial cell types? A study of 1411 clear cell ovarian cancers. Cancer 2008 15;112(10):2202-10.

[30] Pectasides D, Pectasides E, Psyrri A, et al. Treatment issues in clear cell carcinoma of the ovary: a different entity? Oncologist 2006;11(10):1089-94.

[31] Storey DJ, Rush R, Stewart M, et al. Endometrioid epithelial ovarian cancer : 20 years of prospectively collected data from a single center. Cancer 2008 15;112(10):2211-20.

[32] Diaz-Padilla I, Malpica AL, Minig L, et al. Ovarian low-grade serous carcinoma: a comprehensive update. Gynecol Oncol. 2012;126(2):279-85.

[33] Bamias A, Psaltopoulou T, Sotiropoulou M, et al. Mucinous but not clear cell histology is associated with inferior survival in patients with advanced stage ovarian carcinoma treated with platinum-paclitaxel chemotherapy. Cancer. 2010 15;116(6):1462-8.

[34] Shimada M, Kigawa J, Ohishi Y, et al. Clinicopathological characteristics of mucinous adenocarcinoma of the ovary. Gynecol Oncol. 2009;113(3):331-4.

[35] Högberg T, Glimelius B, Nygren P, et al. A systematic overview of chemotherapy effects in ovarian cancer. Acta Oncol. 2001;40(2-3):340-60.

[36] Gershenson DM. The heterogeneity of epithelial ovarian cancer: getting it right. Cancer. 2010 15;116(6):1400-2.

[37] Harrison ML, Jameson C, Gore ME. Mucinous ovarian cancer. Int J Gynecol Cancer 2008;18(2):209-14.

[38] Kramer JM, Schulman KA. Transforming the Economics of Clinical Trials. A tale of two citations. Institute of Medicine; 2012. http://www.iom.edu/~/media/Files/Perspectives-Files/2012/Discussion-Papers/HSP-Drugs-Transforming-the-Economics. (accessed Sept 5, 2012)

[39] Frumovitz M, Schmeler KM, Malpica A, et al. Unmasking the complexities of mucinous ovarian carcinoma. Gynecol Oncol. 2010;117(3):491-6.

[40] Sato S, Itamochi H, Kigawa J, et al. Combination chemotherapy of oxaliplatin and 5-fluorouracil may be an effective regimen for mucinous adenocarcinoma of the ovary: a potential treatment strategy. Cancer Sci. 2009;100(3):546-51.

[41] Andre T, de Gramont A, et al. An overview of adjuvant systemic chemotherapy for colon cancer. Clin Colorectal Cancer 2004; 4(Suppl 1):S22-8.

[42] Zaino RJ, Brady MF, Lele SM, et al. Advanced stage mucinous adenocarcinoma of the ovary is both rare and highly lethal: a Gynecologic Oncology Group study. Cancer 2011;117(3):554-62

[43] Kelemen LE, Köbel M. Mucinous carcinomas of the ovary and colorectum: different organ, same dilemma. Lancet Oncol. 2011;12(11):1071-80.

[44] Tyler CW Jr, Lee NC, Robboy SJ, et al. The diagnosis of ovarian cancer by pathologists: how often do diagnoses by contributing pathologists agree with a panel of gynecologic pathologists? Am J Obstet Gynecol. 1991;164(1 Pt 1):65-70.

[45] Piver MS, Tsukada Y, Werness BA, et al. Comparative study of ovarian cancer histopathology by registry pathologists and referral pathologists: a study by the Gilda Radner Familial Ovarian Cancer Registry. Gynecol Oncol. 2000;78(2):166-70.

Chapter 7

The Genetics of Ovarian Cancer

Constantine Gennatas

Additional information is available at the end of the chapter

http://dx.doi.org/10.5772/54541

1. Introduction

Health Care providers managing patients with Epithelial Ovarian Cancer (EOC) must be familiar not only with the diagnosis, staging, treatment and follow-up of this disease, but also with the current knowledge on carcinogenesis, genetics and prevention/early diagnosis. This knowledge is needed in order to provide the best possible care to the patients and at the same time to provide the best possible advice to their relatives.

For the general population of women, the lifetime risk of developing ovarian cancer is 1.4%, which means that a woman's average risk of developing ovarian cancer during her lifetime is about one in 70. The lifetime risk of dying from ovarian cancer is 1.04%. Ovarian Cancer can be called a rare disease but at the same time it is the ninth most common cancer in the USA, with an estimated 22,280 new cases in 2012, and the fifth most deadly, with an estimated 15,500 deaths in 2012.The median age at diagnosis is 63 years. The poor ratio of survival to incidence in EOC results from the high percentage of cases diagnosed at an advanced stage. It is hard to find ovarian cancer early, as it may not cause any symptoms. When symptoms do appear, disease is often advanced and it is well known that the prognosis largely depends on its extent at diagnosis. Less than one-fourth of women present with localized disease. Despite advances in surgery and chemotherapy, survival of patients with EOC stands at about 31-45% at 5 years. Despite the efficacy of platinum-based chemotherapy, over 75% of women with stage III/IV EOC ultimately relapse and die from their disease. Median survival for women whose disease does not respond or in whom duration of response is short is less than 12 months. Although new drugs hold the potential of improved responses in advanced and recurrent EOC, a greater impact could be made by recognition of high-risk patients and by offering the proper advice and risk-reducing surgery when indicated. It is important that health care professionals can recognize women with possible hereditary Ovarian Cancer and have the basic knowledge to inform them of their management options. Details about the Genetics of Breast and Ovarian Cancer are available at the National Cancer Institute site and other relevant sites and publications [1-6].

2. The pathogenesis of ovarian cancer – The role of genes

The pathogenesis of ovarian carcinoma remains unclear and represents a fascinating research area. It is possible that several pathways lead to ovarian cancer. Certain theories have been proposed to explain its epidemiology including the theory of incessant ovulation, gonadotropin stimulation, excess androgenic stimulation, and inflammation. Associated risk factors for ovarian cancer support some or all of these hypotheses. Multiparity, oral contraceptive use, and breastfeeding are associated with a decreased risk of ovarian cancer. Oophorectomy reduces but does not completely eliminate the risk of ovarian cancer. A history of tubal ligation or hysterectomy with ovarian conservation is also associated with a decreased risk of ovarian cancer. Risk is increased in women with a family history of ovarian cancer, with the postmenopausal use of hormone therapy, and among women who have used fertility drugs. Obesity, tall height, and high body mass index have also been associated with increased risk of ovarian cancer. Perineal exposure to talcum powder has been investigated as possible risk factor for ovarian cancer. It is very important to note that some women are at an increased risk due to an inherited susceptibility to ovarian cancer with the magnitude of that risk depending on the affected gene and specific mutation [1-5,7,8].

There is significant heterogeneity within the EOC group. Histologically defined subtypes such as serous, endometrioid, mucinous, and low- and high-grade malignancies all have variable clinical manifestations and underlying molecular signatures. Substantial advances have been made in understanding the genetic alterations and biologic processes in ovarian cancer; however, the etiology remains poorly understood. According to a recent publication by S Vaughan et al the term ovarian cancer is misleading. Ovarian Cancer is not a single disease, and a considerable proportion of tumors do not arise from ovarian tissue. "The unifying clinical feature of all ovarian cancers is frequent loco-regional dissemination to the ovary and related pelvic organs. We considered whether the term ovarian cancer should be replaced with the terms pelvic or peritoneal cancer but we recognized the confusion that might ensue for patients and physicians, as well as in the scientific literature, especially during a transition period. Before the term ovarian cancer is abandoned, the disparate origins of this disease need to be more widely understood by patients, physicians and scientists."[1-5, 7, 8]

While approximately 90% of ovarian cancers occur sporadically, 10% of women with ovarian cancer have inherited genetic changes that predisposed them to ovarian cancer. It is very important to identify these persons and properly manage them. The following information is very useful for the candidates of genetic testing: Genes carry information in the form of DNA within each cell of the human body. There are 30,000 different genes in each cell's chromosomes and there are 23 pairs of chromosomes in each cell. One chromosome of each pair is inherited from the person's father and one from the person's mother. Genes control how a cell functions, including how quickly it grows, how often it divides, and how long it lives. To control these functions, genes produce proteins that perform specific tasks and act as messengers for the cell. Therefore, it is essential that each gene have the correct instructions or "code" for making its protein so that the protein can perform the proper function for the cell [1-5].

Many cancers begin when one or more genes in a cell are mutated creating an abnormal protein or no protein at all. The information provided by an abnormal protein is different from that of a normal protein, which can cause cells to multiply uncontrollably and become cancerous. A person may either be born with the genetic mutation in all of their cells (germline mutation) or acquire a genetic mutation in a single cell during his or her lifetime. An acquired mutation is passed on to all cells that develop from that single cell (somatic mutation). A germline mutation or a hereditary mutation, according to the NCI definition, is a gene change in a body's reproductive cell that becomes incorporated into the DNA of every cell in the body of the offspring. Germline mutations are passed on from parents to offspring. Somatic mutations, according to the NCI, are alterations in DNA that occur after conception. Somatic mutations can occur in any of the cells of the body except the germ cells and therefore are not passed on to children. These alterations can (but do not always) cause cancer or other diseases. If the mutant cell continues to divide, the individual will come to contain a patch of tissue of genotype different from the cells of the rest of the body. So this is a change in the genetic structure that is neither inherited nor passed to offspring. These changes can be caused by environmental factors such as ultraviolet radiation from the sun and cigarette smoke or can occur if a mistake is made as DNA copies itself during cell division. Mutations may also occur in a single cell within an early embryo. As all the cells divide during growth and development, the individual will have some cells with the mutation and some cells without the genetic change. This situation is called mosaicism. Some genetic changes are very rare; others are common in the population. Genetic changes that occur in more than 1 percent of the population are called polymorphisms. They are common enough to be considered a normal variation in the DNA. Polymorphisms are responsible for many of the normal differences between people such as eye color, hair color, and blood type. Although many polymorphisms have no negative effects on a person's health, some of these variations may influence the risk of developing certain disorders [1-5, 9-17].

Most ovarian cancers (about 85% to 90%) are considered sporadic, meaning that the damage to the genes occurs by chance after a person is born and there is no risk of passing on the gene to a person's children. Inherited ovarian cancers are less common (about 10% to 15%) and occur when gene mutations are passed within a family, from one generation to the next. Every cell usually has two copies of each gene: one inherited from a person's mother and one inherited from a person's father. Most types of hereditary ovarian cancer follow an autosomal dominant inheritance pattern, in which a mutation needs to happen in only one copy of the gene for the person to have an increased risk of getting the disease. This means that a parent with a gene mutation may pass on a copy of the normal gene or a copy of the gene with a mutation. Therefore, a child who has a parent with a mutation has a 50% chance of inheriting that mutation. A brother, sister, or parent of a person who has a gene mutation also has a 50% chance of having the same mutation. Autosomal dominant inheritance of breast/ovarian cancer is characterized by transmission of cancer predisposition from generation to generation, through either the mother's or the father's side of the family, with an inheritance risk of 50%. Although the risk of inheriting the predisposition is 50%, not everyone with the predisposition will develop cancer because of incomplete penetrance and/or gender-restricted or gender-related expression. Both males and females can inherit and transmit an autosomal dominant cancer predisposition. A male who inherits a cancer predisposition can still pass the altered gene on to his sons and daughters [1-5, 9-17].

3. The BRCA1 and BRCA2 genes

Breast and ovarian cancer are components of several autosomal syndromes but most strongly associated with both cancers are the BRCA1 or BRCA2 mutation syndromes, which account for about 90% of hereditary cases. The BRCA1 gene is located on chromosome 17q21, while BRCA2 is located on chromosome 13q12. BRCA1 and BRCA2 play major roles in the repair of DNA doublestrand breaks by homologous recombination. Homologus recombination repairs doublestrand breaks that occur in late S and G2 phase of the cell cycle and also has a key role in repairing doublestrand breaks that result from unrepaired single-strand break. BRCA1 signals the presence of doublestrand breaks, while BRCA2 is directly involved in the mechanism of homologous recombination. So the BRCA1 and BRCA2 proteins are considered caretakers of the genome, and play key roles in the signaling of DNA damage, the activation of DNA repair, the induction of apoptosis, and the monitoring of cell cycle checkpoints. Cells that lack functional BRCA have increased aneuploidy, centrosome amplification, and chromosomal aberrations, which make them susceptible to further mutations. BRCA appears to function as a cofactor for a variety of transcription factors, and the associated ovarian cancers are more likely to be high grade and of serous histopathology. In the absence of BRCA1 or BRCA2, alternative DNA repair pathways are used, which result in chromosomal instability and cell death. Normal cell of carriers are usually heterozygote with loss of the second allele occurring during tumorigenesis in the tumor cells of these women. [1-5, 7,8].

There are several genetic conditions linked to an increased risk of ovarian cancer involving mutations in several other genes, including TP53, PTEN, STK11/LKB1, CDH1, CHEK2, ATM, MLH1, and MSH2.Some of the most common hereditary cancer syndromes associated with ovarian cancer risk are the following:

1. **Hereditary breast and ovarian cancer syndrome.** This syndrome is associated with mutations in the BRCA1 or BRCA2 genes (BRCA stands for BReast CAncer) and it is related with an increased risk of breast cancer and ovarian cancer. There have also been reports of a small number of families with an excess of ovarian cancer, but no breast cancer, called site-specific ovarian cancer families. These families have been linked to mutations in BRCA1 and are thought to represent a unique phenotype of the hereditary breast-ovarian syndrome. The majority of hereditary breast cancers can be accounted

for by inherited mutations in BRCA1 and BRCA2. Overall, it has been estimated that inherited BRCA1 and BRCA2 mutations account for 5 to 10 percent of breast cancers and 10 to 15 percent of ovarian cancers among white women in the United States. When examining consecutive series of patients with ovarian cancer who have been unselected for family history, approximately 10% to 15% of patients have a deleterious mutation in either of these genes. When studying patients with ovarian cancer who have a family history of ovarian cancer or early onset breast cancer, the likelihood of finding a BRCA1 or BRCA2 mutation rises considerably. In fact, it is generally stated that the majority of hereditary ovarian cancer is explained by BRCA1 or BRCA2 abnormalities. The Gynecologic Oncology Group conducted a prospective study of women with ovarian cancer and a positive family history. Specifically, they enrolled patients with ovarian cancer who had any of the following features: a first degree relative with ovarian cancer, a second-degree relative with ovarian cancer plus a first-degree relative with early-onset breast cancer (defined as younger than 50 years), or a first- and second-degree relative with early onset breast cancer. Of 26 eligible patients screened for mutations, 12 had deleterious alterations, eight in BRCA1 and four in BRCA2 [1-5, 7, 8]. Although reproductive, demographic, and lifestyle factors affect risk of ovarian cancer, the single most important ovarian cancer risk factor is a family history of the disease. A large meta-analysis of 15 published studies estimated an odds ratio of 3.1 for the risk of ovarian cancer associated with at least one first degree relative with ovarian cancer. The family characteristics that suggest hereditary breast and ovarian cancer predisposition include the following: 1) Multiple cancers within a family. 2) Cancers that are usually diagnosed at an earlier age than in sporadic. 3) History of two or more primary cancers in a single particular individual. The Claus and the Gail models are widely used in research studies and clinical counseling. Both have limitations, and the risk estimates derived from the two models may differ for an individual patient. Several other models, which include more detailed family history information, are also in use. The use of these models requires specific knowledge and expertise. 4) Cases of male breast cancer are definitely indications for genetic testing [1-5, 9-17].

2. **Lynch syndrome or hereditary nonpolyposis colon cancer (HNPCC).** Lynch syndrome increases a woman's risk of ovarian cancer. It is caused by mutations in several different genes and it also increases the risk of colorectal cancer, as well as cancers of the stomach, small intestine, liver, bile duct, urinary tract, endometrium, the brain and central nervous system, and possibly breast cancer. Defects in mismatch repair in patients with Lynch syndrome account for approximately 10% of hereditary ovarian cancers and for 1% to 2% of overall cases. Patients with this syndrome, however, individually carry an approximately 12% risk of developing ovarian cancer. The mechanism of increased risk is through defects in the mismatch-repair machinery and its resulting genetic instability that places cells at risk of multiple mutations; however, carcinogenesis in ovarian cancer has not been well studied beyond a description of mismatch repair defects.

Genetic conditions that are also associated with a small increased risk of ovarian cancer are the following:

1. **Peutz - Jeghers syndrome.** This syndrome is caused by a specific genetic mutation in the STK11 gene and is associated with multiple polyps in the digestive tract that become noncancerous tumors, increased pigmentation on the face and hands and with an increased risk of ovarian, breast, uterine, and lung cancers.

2. **Nevoid basal cell carcinoma syndrome or Gorlin syndrome** is associated with a mutation in PTCH and a 20% life time risk of developing stromal tumors and fibromas of the ovaries. There is a small risk that these fibromas could develop into fibrosarcoma. People with Gorlin syndrome often have multiple basal cell carcinomas and jaw cysts and may develop medulloblastoma in childhood.

3. **Li-Fraumeni syndrome.** The Li-Fraumeni syndrome is a rare condition associated with a specific genetic mutation. People with Li-Fraumeni syndrome have a higher risk of developing osteosarcoma, soft tissue sarcoma, leukemia, breast cancer, brain cancer, and adrenal cortical tumors.

4. **Ataxia telangiectasia.** Ataxia telangiectasia is a rare disorder associated with a specific genetic mutation. It causes progressive neurological problems and an increased risk of leukemia, lymphoma, and possibly sarcoma, breast, ovarian and stomach cancer. Germline mutations in the genes responsible for those syndromes produce different clinical phenotypes of characteristic malignancies and, in some instances, associated nonmalignant abnormalities.

A study of genetic disorders can provide great insight into the etiology and early events in carcinogenesis. Evaluation of BRCA1 and BRCA2 mutant and sporadic tumors with gene expression profiling has demonstrated that the greatest contrast in expression patterns was between that of BRCA1 and BRCA2 mutant tumors and that sporadic tumors shared characteristics of both. This intriguing finding suggests that BRCA1 and BRCA2 tumors may have variable pathways in carcinogenesis and that even sporadic tumors may develop as a result of alterations in either pathway. Ovarian carcinogenesis, as in most cancers, involves multiple genetic alterations. A great deal has been learned about proteins and pathways important in the early stages of malignant transformation and metastasis, as derived from studies of individual tumors, microarray data, animal models, and inherited disorders that confer susceptibility. However, a full understanding of the earliest recognizable events in epithelial ovarian carcinogenesis is limited by the lack of a well-defined premalignant state common to all ovarian subtypes and by the paucity of data from early-stage cancers. Evidence suggests that ovarian cancers can progress both through a stepwise mutation process (low-grade pathway) and through greater genetic instability that leads to rapid metastasis without an identifiable precursor lesion (high-grade pathway). In an interesting review, CN Landen et al. discuss many of the genetic and molecular disorders in each key process that is altered in cancer cells, and present a model of ovarian pathogenesis that incorporates the role of tumor cell mutations and factors in the host microenvironment important to tumor initiation and progression [1-5, 9-17]. Borderline tumors have a much less frequent incidence of BRCA mutations, which also suggests a different molecular origin. Other than in hereditary syndromes, BRCA genes are rarely mutated in sporadic ovarian cancers, although epigenetic changes alternate splicing, and other genetic factors may affect BRCA function in as many as 82% of sporadic occurrences.

An analysis of genomic changes in ovarian cancer has provided the most comprehensive and integrated view of cancer genes for any cancer type to date. Ovarian serous adenocarcinoma tumors from 500 patients were examined by The Cancer Genome Atlas (TCGA) Research Network and analyses were reported in 2011.These findings confirm that mutations in a single gene, TP53, are present in more than 96 percent of all such cancers. TP53 encodes a tumor suppressor protein that normally prevents cancer formation. Mutations in the gene disrupt this protein's function, which contributes to uncontrolled growth of ovarian cells. Several less-frequent mutations in other genes have also been identified and was also established how sets of genes are expressed in a fashion that can predict patient survival, identifying patterns for 108 genes associated with poor survival and 85 genes associated with better survival. Patients whose tumors had a gene-expression signature associated with poor survival lived for a period that was 23 percent shorter than patients whose tumors did not have such a signature. To identify opportunities for targeted treatment, the investigators searched for existing drugs that might inhibit amplified or over-expressed genes that were suggested to play a role in ovarian cancer. Sixty-eight genes have been identified that could be targeted by existing or experimental therapeutic compounds. One type of drug, a PARP (Poly ADP ribose polymerase) inhibitor, might be able to counteract the DNA repair gene observed in half of the ovarian tumors studied. These drugs could be effective against the disease, this study revealed that 50 percent of tumors might be responsive to drugs that exploit the genetic instability of the tumors and induce the cancer cells to die. The results of this study support the existence of four distinct subtypes of the disease, based on the patterns seen in the transcription of RNA from DNA. They also support the existence of four related subtypes based on the patterns of DNA methylation—a chemical reaction in which a small molecule called a methyl group is added to DNA, changing the activity of individual genes. These patterns likely reflect the functional changes associated with ovarian serous adenocarcinoma, but are not strongly associated with survival duration. In this study, approximately 21 percent of the tumors showed mutations in BRCA1 and BRCA2 genes. Analysis of these tumors confirmed observations that patients with mutated BRCA1 and BRCA2 genes have better survival odds than patients without mutations in these genes. If either of the BRCA1 and BRCA2 genes is mutated, there is improved survival duration. However, if BRCA1 activity is instead reduced by methylation, there is no improved survival duration [1-5, 9-17].

4. Genetic testing

Only genetic testing can determine whether a person has a genetic mutation. Most experts strongly recommend that people considering genetic testing first consult a genetic counselor if possible. Genetic counselors are trained to explain the risks and benefits of genetic testing. If a Genetic counselor is not available the clinician treating a patient with Ovarian Cancer has the duty to take its role. He/she must consider if each patient with ovarian cancer is a candidate for genetic testing. Hereditary cancer syndromes have a major ethical, legal and psychological impact on the individual as well as family members and the caring physician. As a result, a careful counseling before, during and after the testing is necessary. There are many issues that one has to know before proceeding with the genetic testing.

Criteria for recommending genetic testing: Currently, there are no standard criteria for recommending or referring someone for BRCA1 orBRCA2 mutation testing American Society of Clinical Oncology (ASCO) has published some guidelines for Genetic Testing of cancer patients and their families. ASCO also encourages Oncologists to assume the responsibility of genetics counseling with patients and their families. ASCO General recommendation as to indications for genetic testing in generally are the following: 1) When a person has a strong family history of cancer or very early age of onset of disease. 2) Test can be adequately interpreted. 3) Result will influence medical management of the patient/family member. In a family with a history of breast and/or ovarian cancer, it may be most informative to first test a family member who has breast or ovarian cancer. If that person is found to have a harmful BRCA1 or BRCA2 mutation, then other family members can be tested to see if they also have the mutation. Women who have a relative with a harmful BRCA1 or BRCA2 mutation and women who appear to be at increased risk of breast and/or ovarian cancer because of their family history should consider genetic counseling to learn more about their potential risks and about BRCA1 and BRCA2 genetic tests.

ASCO Recommendation as to indications for genetic testing for Breast and Ovarian cancers are the following: 1) Family with more than two breast cancer cases and one or more cases of ovarian cancer diagnosed at any age. 2) Family with more than three breast cancer cases diagnosed before age 50. 3) Sister pairs with two of the following cancers diagnosed before age 50: two breast cancers; two ovarian cancers; or a breast and ovarian cancer.4) Relatives of individuals with breast cancer diagnosed before the age of 30.Despite the above recommendations, there are individuals who do not fit any of the above categories and yet like to be tested. Such individuals need to be counseled to determine the appropriateness of genetic testing [1-5, 9-17].

Genetic counseling: Genetic counseling is generally recommended before and after a genetic test. This counseling should be performed by a health care professional experienced in cancer genetics. Genetic counseling usually involves a risk assessment based on the individual's personal and family medical history and discussions about the appropriateness of genetic testing, the specific test(s) that might be used and the technical accuracy of the test(s), the medical implications of a positive or a negative test result, the possibility that a test result might not be informative (an ambiguous result), the psychological risks and benefits of genetic test results, and the risk of passing a mutation to children. In case genetic testing turns positive health care professional must explain to her that a positive test result indicates that a person has inherited a known harmful mutation in BRCA1 or BRCA2 and, therefore, has an increased risk of developing cancer. Women considering genetic testing must know in advance certain facts about the risk to develop Ovarian Cancer if the tests are positive as well as the available prevention options. The lifetime risk for women who are BRCA1 carriers is about 40-50% and for BRCA2 carriers about 10-20%. The following information must be provided to genetic testing candidates according to the NCI. Women must know that in addition to family history, other environmental and lifestyle factors may increase their risk of ovarian cancer. Discussing their family history and personal risk factors with a doctor helps them to better understand their risk. People with a higher than average risk may benefit from genetic counseling, and the implementation of early detection and prevention strategies.

There can be benefits to genetic testing, whether a person receives a positive or a negative result. The potential benefits of a negative result include a sense of relief and the possibility that special preventive checkups, tests, or surgeries may not be needed. A positive test result can bring relief from uncertainty and allow people to make informed decisions about their future, including taking steps to reduce their cancer risk. In addition, many people who have a positive test result may be able to participate in medical research that could, in the long run, help reduce deaths from breast cancer. The direct medical risks, or harms, of genetic testing are very small, but test results may have an effect on a person's emotions, social relationships, finances, and medical choices. People who receive a positive test result may feel anxious, depressed, or angry. They may choose to undergo preventive measures, such as prophylactic surgery, that have serious long-term implications and whose effectiveness is uncertain. People who receive a negative test result may experience "survivor guilt," caused by the knowledge that they likely do not have an increased risk of developing a disease that affects one or more loved ones. Because genetic testing can reveal information about more than one family member, the emotions caused by test results can create tension within families. Test results can also affect personal choices, such as marriage and childbearing. Issues surrounding the privacy and confidentiality of genetic test results are additional potential risks.

Ovarian cancer may run in the family if first-degree relatives (mother, sisters, daughters) or many other family members (grandmothers, aunts, nieces, granddaughters) have had ovarian cancer. If a woman's first-degree relatives developed ovarian cancer, her risk of ovarian cancer is about three times higher than the average woman's risk of ovarian cancer. The risk increases if other close relatives have had ovarian cancer. When using family history to assess risk, the accuracy and completeness of family history data must be taken into account. A reported family history may be erroneous, or a person may be unaware of relatives affected with cancer. In addition, small family sizes, premature deaths, immigration and poor medical records may limit the information obtained from a family history. Breast or ovarian cancer on the paternal side of the family usually involves more distant relatives than on the maternal side and thus may be more difficult to obtain. When comparing self-reported information with independently verified cases, the sensitivity of a history of breast cancer is relatively high, at 83% to 97%, but lower for ovarian cancer, at 60%. [1-5, 10,11]

However, **a positive test** result provides information only about a person's risk of developing cancer. It cannot tell whether an individual will actually develop cancer or when. It must be stressed that not all women who inherit a harmful BRCA1 or BRCA2 mutation will develop breast or ovarian cancer. A positive genetic test result may have important health and social implications for family members, including future generations. Unlike most other medical tests, genetic tests can reveal information not only about the person being tested but also about that person's relatives. Both men and women who inherit harmful BRCA1 or BRCA2 mutations, whether they develop cancer themselves or not, may pass the mutations on to their sons and daughters. However, not all children of people who have a harmful mutation will inherit the mutation. How a **negative test** result will be interpreted depends on whether or not someone in the tested person's family is known to carry a harmful BRCA1 or BRCA2 mutation. If someone in the family has a known mutation, testing other family members for the same mutation can provide information about their cancer risk. If a person tests negative for a known mutation in his or her family, it is unlikely that they have an inherited susceptibility to cancer associated with BRCA1 orBRCA2. Such a test result is called **a "true negative."** On the other hand having a true negative test result does not mean that a person will not develop cancer; it means that the person's risk of cancer is probably the same as that of people in the general population. In cases in which a family has a history of breast and/or ovarian cancer and no known mutation in BRCA1 or BRCA2 has been previously identified, a negative test result is not informative. It is not possible to tell whether an individual has a harmful BRCA1 or BRCA2 mutation that was not detected by testing and this is called a **"false negative test"** or whether the result is a true negative. In addition, it is possible for people to have a mutation in a gene other than BRCA1 or BRCA2 that increases their cancer risk but is not detectable by the test(s) used. If genetic testing shows a change in BRCA1 or BRCA2 that has not been previously associated with cancer in other people, the person's test result may be interpreted as **"ambiguous"** and the result is considered as uncertain. It is estimated that 10 percent of women who underwent BRCA1 and BRCA2 mutation testing had this type of ambiguous result. Because everyone has genetic differences that are not associated with an increased risk of disease, it is sometimes not known whether a specific DNA change affects a person's risk of developing cancer. As more research is conducted and more people are tested for BRCA1 or BRCA2 changes, we expect to learn more about these changes and cancer risk [1-5, 9-17].

Genetic tests: Several methods are available to test for BRCA1 and BRCA2 mutations. Most of these methods look for changes in BRCA1 and BRCA2 DNA. At least one method looks for changes in the proteins produced by these genes. Frequently, a combination of methods is used. A blood sample is needed for these tests. The blood is drawn in a laboratory, doctor's office, hospital, or clinic and then sent to a laboratory that specializes in the tests. It usually takes several weeks or longer to get the test results. Genetic tests are expensive and this represents a major problem in every day practice.

5. Management of women with mutated genes

The options available today for women who have tested positive can be divided into secondary and primary prevention. Methods of secondary prevention, such as surveillance, attempt to diagnose cancers at an early stage, while primary prevention prevents cancer development. Chemoprevention and prophylactic oophorectomy are examples of primary prevention. Not all methods are appropriate for all patients, and potential adverse effects, complications, cost, and efficacy of these interventions must be considered and reviewed with patients before implementation. It must be stressed that having a particular genetic mutation linked to ovarian cancer cannot predict that a person will develop cancer. [1-5, 18-29].

Cancer prevention is action taken to lower the chance of getting cancer. By preventing cancer, the number of new cases of cancer in a group or population is lowered. Hopefully, this will lower the number of deaths caused by cancer. To prevent new cancers from starting, we must consider risk and protective factors. Anything that increases one person's chance of developing cancer is called a cancer risk factor; anything that decreases the chance of developing cancer is called a cancer protective factor. Some risk factors for cancer can be avoided, but many cannot. For example, both smoking and inheriting certain genes are risk factors for some types of cancer, but only smoking can be avoided. Regular exercise and a healthy diet may be protective factors for some types of cancer. Avoiding risk factors and increasing protective factors may lower the risk but it does not mean that cancer will be avoided. Different ways to prevent cancer are being studied, including: Changing lifestyle or eating habits, avoiding things known to cause cancer or taking medicines to treat a precancerous condition or to keep cancer from starting[1-5,18-29]. According to the NCI's PDQ cancer information about **Ovarian cancer prevention** the following risk factors may **increase** the risk of ovarian cancer: Family history of ovarian cancer, inherited risk, hormone replacement therapy, fertility drugs, talc and obesity. Factors associated with a **decreased** risk of ovarian cancer include: (a) using oral contraceptives, (b) having and breastfeeding children, (c) having a bilateral tubal ligation or hysterectomy, and (d) having a prophylactic oophorectomy. Multiple studies have consistently demonstrated a decrease in ovarian cancer risk in women who take oral contraceptives. The protective association increases with the duration of oral contraceptive use and persists up to 25 years after discontinuing oral contraceptives. A review of the literature demonstrated a 10% to 12% decrease in risk associated with use for 1 year and an approximate 50% decrease after 5 years of use. This reduced risk was present among both nulliparous and parous women. A protective association between oral contraceptives and risk of ovarian cancer has been observed in most studies among women who carry a mutation in BRCA1 and BRCA2 genes but a population-based study did not observe an association between oral contraceptives and ovarian cancer, while parity was protective. There may be a slight increase in a woman's risk of breast cancer during the time she is taking oral contraceptives. This risk decreases over time. Pregnancy and breastfeeding are linked to a decreased risk of ovarian cancer. Ovulation stops or occurs less often in women who are pregnant or breastfeeding and women who ovulate less often have a decreased risk of ovarian cancer. Factors that increase risk for ovarian cancer include increasing age and nulliparity, while those that decrease risk include surgical history and use of Oral contraceptives. Relatively few studies have addressed the effect of these risk factors in women who are genetically susceptible to ovarian cancer. Ovarian cancer incidence rises in a linear fashion from age 30 years to age 50 years and continues to increase, though at a slower rate, thereafter. Before age 30 years, the risk of developing epithelial ovarian cancer is remote, even in hereditary cancer families. Nulliparity is consistently associated with an increased risk of ovarian cancer, including among BRCA1/BRCA2mutation carriers. Risk may also be increased among women who have used fertility drugs, especially those who remain nulligravid. Evidence is growing that the use of menopausal HRT is associated with an increased risk of ovarian cancer, particularly in long-time users and users of sequential estrogen-progesterone schedules [1-5].

Surveillance means cancer **screening**, or a way of detecting the disease early. Screening does not, however, change the risk of developing cancer. The goal is to find cancer early, when it may be most treatable. **Screening**, looking for cancer before a person has any symptoms, can help find cancer at an early stage and increase the chances for cure or prolong survival. By the time symptoms appear, the disease may have begun to spread and treatment results are usually disappointing. Before recommending screening it is important to estimate women who have increased risk to develop ovarian cancer in order to suggest the proper screening tests, when to start screening and how often to repeat it. If screening tests are abnormal then the physician has to proceed to diagnostic tests. There are unfortunately no satisfactory standard screening tests for ovarian cancer. Family members of ovarian cancer patients must be informed that tests that may detect ovarian cancer are the following: Pelvic examination, transvaginal ultrasound and CA-125 assay. Although screening for ovarian cancer has not been proven to decrease the death rate from the disease, this approach is the only available screening today for the possible early diagnosis for Ovarian Cancer and this is what we must follow. Several biomarkers with potential application to ovarian cancer screening are under development but have not yet been validated or evaluated for efficacy in early detection and mortality reduction. The Pap test, which is considered by many women as the "screening for Gynecological Cancer", may occasionally detect malignant ovarian cells, but it is not sensitive, the reported sensitivity is about 10%–30%, and has not been evaluated for the early detection of ovarian cancer. Other methods of detection, including cytologic examination of peritoneal lavage obtained by culdocentesis and proteomics used to identify patterns or specific serum markers that may be used in place of, or in conjunction with, CA 125 measurements remain under study. Given the low incidence of ovarian cancer in the general population, the use of these modalities has not been adopted for screening purposes in the general population. To be cost effective and avoid unnecessary surgical interventions, the use of transvaginal ultrasound and CA-125 would need to be nearly 100% specific and sensitive. Premenopausal women in particular have a high incidence of benign ovarian cysts. Although CA-125 can be a reliable marker for recurrence in women with a previous diagnosis of ovarian cancer, only 50% of early-stage ovarian cancers are associated with an abnormal CA-125. It must be noted that CA-125 can also show spurious elevations in association with any process, which irritates the peritoneal or pleural cavity, such as endometriosis, pneumonia, pulmonary embolism, or even normal menses. Prospective screening trials, using ultrasound and CA-125, in women in the general population have resulted in approximately 30 surgeries for every cancer diagnosed and have failed to detect disease at an early stage. Given the higher prevalence of ovarian cancer in patients with BRCA mutations, there has been speculation that pelvic ultrasound and CA-125 may be useful screening strategies for these patients. In fact, annual or semiannual screening with pelvic examination, transvaginal ultrasonography, and serum CA-125 was recommended as appropriate interventions for women at high risk of ovarian cancer in a National Institutes of Health consensus conference although they did concede that there was no evidence of efficacy. Indeed, multiple investigations have been performed that cast doubt on the efficacy of these interventions. For example, a recent study prospectively screened 1,110 women with increased risk of ovarian cancer with pelvic ultrasound and CA-125 measurements. About half of patients were at moderate risk of developing ovarian cancer, with a 4% to 10% lifetime risk and half were at high risk with more than 10% lifetime risk. Invasive ovarian cancer was diagnosed in 12 patients. Two patients had stage I disease, one had stage II, four had stage III, and one had stage IV. These screening techniques missed an additional two patients with stage III disease and one patient with stage IV ovarian cancer. Based on abnormal ultrasound findings, 29 additional women underwent surgery for what turned out to be benign processes. The positive predictive value was 17%, and the sensitivity was less than 50%. These screening techniques are especially problematic for premenopausal women (the cohort with BRCA mutations is of highest interest) in which the false-positive rate was 79%. The conclusion is that the use of pelvic ultrasound and CA-125 does not meet World Health Organization screening standards for women with an increased risk for ovarian cancer. The advantages of surveillance include avoidance of premature menopause and the fact that there is no intervention for those without disease. It allows management with other techniques, which may be available in the future. However, surveillance does not prevent disease, and an objective assessment of the data on screening for ovarian cancer does not support the use of these modalities, even in patients at elevated risk. For women who have not finished childbearing or are deferring prophylactic oophorectomy for other reasons, current practice guidelines from the National Comprehensive Cancer Network recommends concurrent transvaginal ultrasound and CA-125 every 6 months starting at age 35 or 5 to 10 years earlier than the earliest ovarian cancer diagnosis in the family (and preferably days 1 to 10 of cycle for premenopausal women). If initiated, it is important for these women to understand the shortcomings of surveillance. They should be aware of the high likelihood of an abnormal scan in ovulating women, and also understand that a normal scan does not guarantee absence of disease, even in the advanced stages [1-5, 18-29].

Chemoprevention involves the use of natural or synthetic substances to reduce the risk of developing cancer or to reduce the chance that cancer will come back. It has been postulated that incessant ovulation may be one mechanism by which ovarian cancer develops. Consistent with this theory is the observation that parity is associated with a reduction in risk. **The use of oral contraceptives** has also been shown to reduce ovarian cancer risk by as much as 50% in the general population. However, there have been relatively few investigations studying the effect of oral contraceptive use on ovarian cancer risk in women with BRCA mutations. Unfortunately, the available data are conflicting. In one retrospective investigation of 451 patients with BRCA mutations, women who used oral contraceptives for 6 or more years had an odds ratio of ovarian cancer of 0.62 (95% confidence interval [CI], 0.35–1.09). Although not a statistically significant reduction in risk, this study suggests that oral contraceptives may be an effective form of chemoprevention in carriers. In contrast, Modan et al performed a case-control study of 1,591 Jewish women, 257 of whom underwent genetic testing and were found to have a BRCA mutation. They did not find clear evidence of a protective effect with oral contraceptive use in BRCA carriers. Given the low incidence of adverse effects, before more definitive investigations are available, the use of oral contraceptives as a chemopreventive strategy would appear to be a reasonable approach for the patient who declines prophylactic salpingo-oophorectomy and for whom prevention of pregnancy is acceptable. However, the conflicting data should be reviewed with the patient before initiation [1-5, 18-29].

Prophylactic salpingo-oophorectomy. The use of oral contraceptives, having and breast-feeding children do not certainly offer enough protection for BRCA1/BRCA2 carriers. The removal of the "at-risk" tissue is the most important step to prevent Ovarian Cancer. Women who have a high risk of ovarian cancer must be informed about the possibility of a prophylactic oophorectomy. This includes women who have inherited certain changes in the BRCA1 and BRCA2 genes or in the genes linked to hereditary nonpolyposis colon cancer (HNPCC). It is very important to have a cancer risk assessment and counseling before making this decision. These and other factors should be discussed: Early menopause: 90% reduction in risk of ovarian cancer observed among women with a BRCA1 or BRCA2 mutation. BRCA1 or BRCA2 mutations occur in 0.1–0.8% of the general population and are inherited in an autosomal dominant manner. They are well recognized to have a higher incidence in certain ethnic groups, such as women of Ashkenazi Jewish descent. S Vaughan Given the newly appreciated importance of the fallopian tube in the genesis of high-grade serous ovarian cancer, it is recommended that the complete removal of the fallopian tube should become standard of care in any woman undergoing hysterectomy and/or removal of the ovaries (oophorectomy). Oophorectomy in premenopausal women induces early menopause. As a consequence, and with the changed view of the role of the fallopian tube in ovarian cancer, some clinicians have recommended that only the fallopian tubes should be removed (salpingectomy) in women with germline BRCA1 or BRCA2 mutations, or in women with a strong family history of breast and/or ovarian cancer34. However, until comprehensive comparative data are available, it is premature to recommend that only the fallopian tubes are removed in high-risk women [1-5, 30-43].

Women who have completed childbearing are candidates for surgery. For the majority of women, this surgery can be performed laparoscopically as an outpatient procedure. In contrast to surveillance and chemoprevention, this intervention is very effective in reducing the risk of ovarian cancer. Bilateral tubal ligation and hysterectomy are associated with reduced ovarian cancer risk, including in BRCA1/BRCA2 mutation carriers. Ovarian cancer risk is reduced more than 90% in women with documented BRCA1 or BRCA2 mutations who chose risk-reducing salpingo-oophorectomy. In this same population, prophylactic removal of the ovaries also resulted in a nearly 50% reduction in the risk of subsequent breast cancer. In a retrospective analysis of 551 patients, Rebbeck et al showed that women who had undergone prophylactic salpingo-oophorectomy had an odds ratio of 0.04 for ovarian cancer, compared with carriers without prophylactic salpingo-oophorectomy. Over a median follow-up of 8.8 years, two primary peritoneal cancers were diagnosed in the 259 women who underwent prophylactic salpingo-oophorectomy compared with 58 ovarian/peritoneal cancers in the 292 women who did not have prophylactic salpingo-oophorectomy. An added benefit was a 47% reduction in the risk of breast cancer in premenopausal women who had prophylactic salpingo-oophorectomy. The effectiveness of prophylactic salpingo-oophorectomy in reduction of ovarian cancer risk has also been demonstrated in prospective studies. Prophylactic salpingo-oophorectomy failures may be divided into groups of those patients who are found to harbor an occult malignancy at the time of surgery and those who go on to develop carcinoma at a later time. The existence of occult ovarian cancer in BRCA carriers with apparently healthy ovaries has been documented in small samples for a number of years. In a recent investigation that included 555 women who underwent prophylactic salpingo-oophorectomy, the rate of occult fallopian tube or ovarian cancer was 2.2%, consistent with prior reports. Although a low incidence, this risk should routinely be discussed with patients before surgery and highlights the need for an extensive pathologic assessment of the entire adnexa, including the fallopian tubes [30-43]. Development of primary peritoneal carcinoma (PPC) represents the vast majority of failures after prophylactic salpingo-oophorectomy. In a multicenter investigation of 1,828 carriers, the cumulative risk of PPC was 4.3% at 20 years after prophylactic salpingo-oophorectomy.24 It is hypothesized that PPC arises from the peritoneal coelomic epithelium, derived from the same embryonic tissue that gives rise to the epithelial covering of the ovaries. Ovarian and peritoneal epithelium share common embryonal origin, originating both from the coelomic epithelium (mesodermal origin). Coelomic epithelium is thought to be of mesonephric origin. With the overall point being that normal ovarian and peritoneal tissue is derived from the mesonephros. On the contrary, fallopian tube epithelium, endometrium and endocervix are related to paramesonephros (Müllerian duct). Surprisingly, epithelial ovarian cancer and primary peritoneal cancer are histologically similar to the Mullerian epithelium; not their embryonal origin, the mesonephros. Either a metaplasia has occurred or Mullerian remnants have been left behind in coelemic epithelium, which have turned oncogenic. Although the precise causes are not known, a link with certain variants of BRCA1/2 has been described. Furthermore, women with BRCA1/2 mutation have a 5% risk of developing primary peritoneal cancer even after prophylactic oophorectomy. Primary peritoneal carcinoma shows similar rates of tumor suppressor gene dysfunction (p53, BRCA, WT1) as ovarian cancer and can also show an increased expression of HER-2/neu. An association with vascular endothelial growth factor has been observed. Although the absolute risk of fallopian tube cancer is unknown in patients with BRCA mutations, it is agreed that it is substantially elevated, with a relative risk of 120 in one study. It remains unknown if the 4.3% failure rate found by Finch et al consists entirely of PPC or if a proportion is in fact peritoneal recurrences of a fallopian tube carcinoma missed at the time of prophylactic salpingo-oophorectomy. Regardless, it is widely accepted that removal of the fallopian tubes is essential at the time of prophylactic surgery. There is an abundance of evidence supporting the efficacy of prophylactic salpingo-oophorectomy, but less information exists to counsel the clinician as to the optimal timing of prophylactic surgery. Reasonable guidelines can be inferred from existing data regarding the onset of ovarian cancer in BRCA carriers. The cumulative incidence of breast cancer is 11.6% by age 40 for women with BRCA1 mutations. In contrast, the rate is only 2.3% for ovarian cancer by age 40. By age 45, 6.5% of BRCA1 carriers will be diagnosed with ovarian cancer; 13.2% by age 50. As a result, for BRCA1 carriers, most physicians recommend prophylactic salpingo-oophorectomy between ages 35 to 40 years. However, performing prophylactic salpingo-oophorectomy before age 45 must be considered in the context of the potential morbidity of estrogen deprivation at an early age. Oophorectomy before age 45 has been associated with a hazard ratio of 1.96 for death from all causes (p 0.002). However, administration of estrogen replacement eliminated this risk. Many physicians consider estrogen therapy for women without a personal history of breast cancer who undergo prophylactic salpingo-oophorectomy before the age of 45.29 It should be noted that early prophylactic salpingo-oophorectomy is less important for BRCA2 carriers who are known to develop ovarian cancer at approximately the same age as patients with sporadic cancer. Only 1.2% of BRCA2 carriers will have ovarian cancer by the age of 50, so prophylactic salpingo-oophorectomy may safely be delayed until these patients are closer to menopause. The disadvantages of prophylactic salpingo-oophorectomy include the fact that it is an invasive surgical intervention, there is loss of ovarian tissue with accompanying hormone deprivation, and it is an irreversible decision. However, in contrast to surveillance and chemoprevention, prophylactic salpingo-oophorectomy has proven efficacy over an extended time period. Cost analyses comparing surveillance, oral contraceptives, and prophylactic salpingo-oophorectomy have shown that although any primary prevention strategy was cost effective, prophylactic salpingo-oophorectomy dominated all other strategies in women with BRCA mutations. Consequently, prophylactic salpingo-oophorectomy is recommended for all BRCA carriers, with timing dependent on the type of BRCA1 or BRCA2 mutation, childbearing status, and the age of onset of ovarian cancer within the family. The resultant physical and emotional outcomes of repeated gynecological screening or prophylactic oophorectomy must be discussed before and after genetic testing. A study of 315 women with documented HNPCC–associated germline mutations found no ovarian cancer among 47 women who had bilateral salpingo-oophorectomy and 12 cases (5%) among women with mutations who had not had surgery for a prevented fraction of 100% (95% CI, 62%–100%).

The degree of risk of ovarian cancer, potential morbidity and mortality of surgery, and the risks associated with early menopause, should be taken into account when considering prophylactic oophorectomy for high-risk women. Adverse effects of bilateral oophorectomy and premature menopause include infertility, vasomotor symptoms, decline in sexual interest and activity, cardiovascular disease, and osteoporosis. Among women who have not taken hormone therapy, women undergoing bilateral oophorecotmy were twice as likely to have moderate or severe hot flashes than women who underwent natural menopause (odds ratio [OR] = 2.44; 95% CI, 1.03–5.77). Women at increased hereditary risk of ovarian cancer who underwent oophorectomy without hormone therapy reported statistically significantly more vasomotor symptoms than women choosing screening or those using hormone replacement therapy (HRT). These women also reported lower sexual function scores but the difference was not statistically significant. A meta-analysis of early menopause as a risk factor for cardiovascular disease observed a pooled risk of 4.55 (95% CI, 2.56–8.01) among women with bilateral oophorectomy and early menopause (defined as younger than 50 years). Early menopause is also associated with an increased risk of fracture (OR = 1.5; 95% CI, 1.2–1.8).

6. Treatment

Over the past ten years, the focus of management for BRCA1/2mutation carriers has been on cancer prevention and early cancer detection. However, despite prophylactic measures to reduce risk of EOC, many BRCA1/2 carriers have cancer at the time their mutation is diagnosed and more will develop in the future. The treatment of patients with BRCA associated EOC is so far identical to those with sporadic disease. Data suggested that cancers associated with BRCA mutations responded differently to chemotherapy. Tan et al. compared 22 BRCA-positive patients with EOC to 44 nonhereditary EOC controls in a matched case-control study. They found that BRCA-positive patients have higher response rates to first line platinum-based treatment (81.8%versus 43.2%, P =.004) as well as to subsequent lines of platinum-based treatments (second line, 91.7% versus 40.9%, P =.004), third line, 100% v 14,3% (P<. 002) and time of first relapse (5v 1.6 years; P<. 001). They conclude that BRCA-positive EOC patients have better outcomes than nonhereditary EOC cases. There exists a clinical syndrome of BRCAness that includes serous histology, high response rates to first and subsequent lines of platinum-based treatment, longer tumor free interval between relapses and improved overall survival [44].

Over recent years the investigation of DNA repair in cancer cells has been a very active area of translational research. All cells have a number of overlapping pathways to protect the genome from DNA damage, which occurs as a result of normal cell cycling, environmental insults, or cytotoxic chemotherapy. It is well recognized that when mutations occur within these DNA repair pathways there is an increased risk of malignant transformation and chemotherapy resistance. Much research has focused on protecting cells from DNA damage and/or restoring DNA repair function. However, emerging data suggest that the concept of "synthetic lethality," that is, exploiting the vulnerability of cancer cells, which have lost one mechanism of DNA repair by targeting a second pathway, may be a particularly attractive therapeutic approach.. Targeting the nuclear enzyme PARP-1 represents a new and novel approach to the treatment of EOC and appears to be particularly promising for those carrying mutations in the BRCA1 and 2 genes. Poly(ADPribose) polymerase (PARP) is an enzyme, which plays an important role in the recognition and repair of single-strand DNA breaks via the base excision repair pathway. Over the last few years it has become apparent that in cells, which have lost BRCA1 or BRCA2, components of a second DNA repair pathway, homologous recombination, are particularly sensitive to PARP inhibition. These data suggest that PARP inhibitors may be particularly useful for the treatment of women with hereditary BRCA1/2-associated EOC. Targeted therapy using PARP inhibitors has become an important novel strategy for treating those with hereditary ovarian cancer. Furthermore the identification of other subpopulations of women with EOC who may benefit from this approach is an active area of research. There are currently 17 members of the PARP superfamily identified. PARP-1 is the most studied enzyme. In the preclinical setting, PARP-1 inhibitors enhance the cytotoxic effects of ionizing radiation and cytotoxic chemotherapy. Additionally, in the preclinical setting, the use of PARP-1 inhibitors as single agents did not cause any measurable toxicity, but the combination of PARP-1 inhibitor with temozolomide in the tumor bearing mice caused significant toxicity. There did not seem to be a correlation, however, between the antitumor activity and the toxicity of the PARP inhibitor-temozolomide combinations, suggesting that toxicity and chemosensitization were by different mechanisms. In 2005, two preclinical papers demonstrated the sensitivity of BRCA1- and BRCA2-deficient cell lines to PARP inhibition. The first paper by Bryant et al. demonstrated reduced survival of BRCA2-deficient cell lines with four PARP inhibitors. They concluded that BRCA2- deficient cells were sensitive to PARP inhibition, and that monotherapy with one of these agents could selectively kill cancer cells. In the same year, Farmer et al. demonstrated how both BRCA1- and BRCA2-deficient cells lines were sensitive to inhibition of PARP-1, and that BRCA2 deficient cells were more than 1000 times more sensitive to nanomolar concentrations of PARP inhibitor. Both of these papers demonstrated how homozygotes (tumor cells) are sensitive to the mechanism of PARP inhibition, whereas heterozygotes (the rest of the patient's cells) are insensitive to this mechanism and should not exhibit toxicity. These findings from two independent groups using different chemical classes of PARP inhibitors on different BRCA deficient cell lines were the first to suggest the potent effect of PARP inhibition. A number of PARP inhibitors have entered the clinic in both intravenous and oral formulations. The four, which are furthest along in terms of development, are AGO14699 (Pfizer), AZD2281 (AstraZeneca), ABT-888 (Abbott), and BSI-201 (BI Par), and all four of these compounds demonstrate profound inhibition of PARP-1.Olaparib (AZD2281, KU-0059436, AstraZeneca) is an oral small-molecule PARP inhibitor. Yap et al. presented the first clinical evidence demonstrating the sensitivity of BRCA-mutated cancers to PARP inhibitor monotherapy in a study in 2007. This phase I trial included 44 patients, of which 11 patients had a BRCA mutation associated cancer. Dose escalation was guided by toxicity, pharmacokinetic and pharmacodynamic data. Based on the encouraging antitumor activity, many in whom had BRCA1/2 mutations, the trial was subsequently expanded to concentrate on cancers in patients with BRCA mutations. The drug was well tolerated in both BRCA mutated and normal populations. Most toxicities were grade 1-2 (≥95%), consisting of fatigue (28%), nausea (28%), vomiting (18%), loss of taste (13%), and anorexia (12%). Grade 3-4 toxicities were rare, consisting of myelosuppression (≤5%), nausea and vomiting (2-3%), and dizziness or mood changes (2- 3%) [27]. Of the 60 patients that were enrolled and treated, 19 of 23 BRCA-positive carriers were evaluable. 12 of the 19 (63%) had a clinical benefit from olaparib, with radiologic or tumor marker responses, or stable disease for 4 months or more. Patient response was seen in those receiving a minimum of 100 mg twice daily up to 400 mg twice daily. Response was the greatest in patients with platinum-sensitive disease, although duration of response was the same regardless of the platinum-free interval. Recently data was presented from a phase II study of olaparib in women with advanced EOC with known mutations in BRCA1/2. Two patient cohorts received continuous oral olaparib in 28-day cycles; 33 patients received 400 mg orally twice daily, while 24 patients received 100 mg twice daily. The choice of dosing and schedule was based on the phase I trial above. The objective response rate measured by RECIST criteria was 33% at the 400 mg dose, and 12.5% at the 100 mg dose, suggesting that there may be a dose response effect. The toxicity profile was mainly mild, consisting of grade 1 or 2 nausea (44%) and fatigue (35%), with few grade 3 or 4 toxicities. Interestingly, although numbers were low, in this study there appeared to be a higher response rate in platinum resistant patients (38% versus 14%), which was opposite to that observed in the earlier phase I study, where response was the greatest in platinum-sensitive patients. Laboratory studies have previously suggested that platinum resistant patients may reacquire BRCA function thus potentially making them resistant to the effects of PARP inhibition. Taken together, the clinical data suggest that we still have a lot to learn with regard to target populations and the role of PARP inhibition. Furthermore, data from the phase II study appears to give an early indication that response (both RECIST and CA125) may be greater in those patients with BRCA2 mutations. This would be in line with the known mechanism of action of the two BRCA proteins as BRCA2 plays a key role in the repair pathway; whereas BRCA1 functions as a signaling molecule. This phase II study concluded that oral olaparib is well-tolerated and highly active in advanced, chemotherapy refractory BRCA-deficient EOC, with greater activity seen at a higher dose of 400 mg twice daily. The optimal patient group with respect to platinum sensitivity has not been defined. Reassuringly in the clinical studies there does not appear to be an increase in toxicity between BRCA mutation carriers compared to noncarriers, supporting the theory that PARP inhibitors should not result in increased toxicity to heterozygote cells. These recent phase I and phase II trials are particularly promising for patients with BRCA-associated EOC. Further phase II trials are currently underway which will help further elucidate the role and potential for this new targeted therapy. Loss of BRCA1/2 function is not exclusive to inheriting a mutation in the BRCA1/2 genes. The results seen in known BRCA1 and 2 mutation carriers may also be relevant to the sporadic EOC patient population. Epigenetic gene inactivation is a well-recognized phenomenon with 31% of EOC exhibiting aberrant methylation of the BRCA1 promoter. Furthermore, genetic or epigenetic events occurring in other components of the HR pathway can be found in sporadic EOC. These tumors seem to be similar to BRCA1- or BRCA2-mutated tumors, even though they do not have mutations to either of these genes, a concept called "BRCAness." One molecular characterization study suggested that over 50% of patients with high-grade EOC had loss of BRCA function, either by genetic or epigenetic events [34]. Studies have shown that the loss of functional proteins in the HR pathway may lead these cells to be sensitive to PARP inhibition. Identification of "BRCA-like" EOC populations who may benefit from this new therapy through the identification and validation of biomarkers is an active area of ongoing research. Several PARP inhibitors are under investigation either as single agents and/or in combination with other agents or treatment modalities. Phase II studies in women with advanced EOC in both BRCA1/2 mutation carriers and high-grade EOC of unknown BRCA status are ongoing. Currently, olaparib is being evaluated in a randomized phase II trial comparing this agent with pegylated liposomal doxorubicin in patients with BRCA-mutated EOC with a platinum-free interval of 0–12 months. More combination studies in women with both hereditary and sporadic EOC are expected in the future. Further defining the role of PARP inhibitors in the clinic is ongoing. Olaparib is being evaluated in a randomized placebo-controlled trial as a maintenance therapy in patients with sporadic EOC at high risk of early recurrence. Furthermore, some suggest that PARP inhibitors could be used to prevent cancers in patients who are BRCA mutation carriers. This approach, however, requires careful consideration and some caution with the potential for the development of drug resistance in long-term use of PARP inhibitors. Investigation of the PARP inhibitors in the nonhereditary EOC population is very active with both the impact of treatment on patients without BRCA defects and the search for populations of women who have lost functional proteins in the HR pathway. Investigation of PARP inhibitor resistance and ways to overcome this resistance are emerging fields. The emerging data regarding the use of PARP inhibitors in patients with BRCA-associated EOC are encouraging. Identification of further patient groups who will benefit from this approach is also indicated. Clinical trials underway will hopefully improve the prognosis of women with Epithelial Ovarian Cancer [45-53].

7. Conclusions

Genetic testing can identify women with a hereditary increased risk to develop Ovarian Cancer. This information is extremely useful if the candidate for genetic testing is willing to accept prophylactic surgery. For patients who already have Ovarian Cancer Genetic testing will offer useful information for the relatives but it can also help plan their own treatment. Published data regarding the use of PARP inhibitors in patients with BRCA-associated EOC are encouraging. Studies in combination with chemotherapy are also producing encouraging results and there are several ongoing studies in patients with hereditary and sporadic cancer as well. These studies will clarify the mechanisms of DNA repair and how this can be exploited to improve treatment results. The development of diagnostic tests in order to select patients likely to be sensitive to PARP inhibitors will also be very useful. The combination of prevention, early diagnosis and more effective disease management will hopefully improve EOC prognosis in the near future.

Author details

Constantine Gennatas

2nd Department Of Surgery, Areteion Hospital, University of Athens, Athens, Greece

References

[1] National Cancer Institute: PDQ® Ovarian Epithelial Cancer Treatment. Bethesda, MD: National Cancer Institute. Date last modified 06/22/2012. Available at: http://cancer.gov/cancertopics/pdq/treatment/ovarianepithelial /Health Professional. Accessed 09/16/2012.

[2] National Cancer Institute: PDQ® Ovarian Cancer Prevention. Bethesda, MD: National Cancer Institute. Date last modified 02/06/2012. Available at: http://cancer.gov/cancertopics/pdq/prevention/ovarian/HealthProfessional. Accessed 08/08/2012.

[3] National Cancer Institute: PDQ® Ovarian Cancer Screening. Bethesda, MD: National Cancer Institute. Date last modified 01/26/2012. Available at:http://cancer.gov/cancertopics/pdq/screening/ovarian/HealthProfessional. Accessed 09/16/2012.

[4] National Cancer Institute: PDQ® Ovarian Cancer Screening. Bethesda, MD: National Cancer Institute. Date last modified 09/30/2011. Available athttp://cancer.gov/cancertopics/pdq/screening/ovarian/Patient version. Accessed 09/16/2012.

[5] Genetics of Breast and Ovarian Cancer (PDQ) Health Professional Version Last modified 08/08/2012. Available at: http://cancertopics/pdq/genetics/breast-and-ovarian Health Professional. Accessed 09/01/2012.

[6] American Cancer Society: Cancer Facts and Figures 2012. Atlanta, Ga: American Cancer Society, 2012. Available online http://www.cancer.gov/global/web/policies/ page 8. Last accessed July 31, 2012.

[7] Landen Jr, CN,Birrer MJ and Sood AK. Early Events in the Pathogenesis of Epithelial Ovarian Cancer. Doi: 10.1200/JCO.2006.07.9970 JCO 2008; 26(6) 995-100.

[8] Vaughan S et al. Rethinking ovarian cancer: recommendations for improving outcomes. Nature Reviews Cancer 2011; 11 719-725.

[9] Spellman, et al. Integrated Genomic Analyses of Ovarian Carcinoma. Nature 2011;DOI: 10.1038/nature 10166.

[10] BRCA1 and BRCA2: Cancer Risk and Genetic Testing. National Cancer Institute. Available on-line. Reviewed: 05/29/2009 accessed 9/22/2012.

[11] Dowdy SC and Hartmann LC. Management of Hereditary Ovarian Cancer by American Society of Clinical Oncology 2007 Educational book.

[12] Greene MH, Kohlmann W, Popik WC and Offit K. Cancer Genetics in Practice: Current Guidelines and Emerging Issues. ASCO Educational Book 2004.

[13] Risch HA, McLaughlin JR, Cole DE, et al. Prevalence and penetrance of germline BRCA1 and BRCA2 mutations in a population series of 649 women with ovarian cancer. Am J Hum Genet 2001; 68:700-710.

[14] Garber JE, Offit K. Hereditary cancer predisposition syndromes. J Clin Oncol 2005; 23 276-292.

[15] King MC, Marks JH, Mandell JB. Breast and ovarian cancer risks due to inherited mutations in BRCA1 and BRCA2. Science 2003; 302 643-646.

[16] Reedy M, Gallion H, Fowler JM, et al. Contribution of BRCA1 and BRCA2 to familial ovarian cancer: A gynecologic oncology group study. Gynecol Oncol 2002; 85 255-259.

[17] Guillem JG, Wood WC, Moley JF, et al. ASCO/SSO review of current role of risk-reducing surgery in common hereditary cancer syndromes. J Clin Oncol 2006; 24 4642-4660.

[18] NIH Consensus Conference. Ovarian cancer: Screening, treatment, and follow-up: NIH Consensus Development Panel on Ovarian Cancer. JAMA. 1995; 273 491-497.

[19] National Comprehensive Cancer Network. Hereditary breast and/or ovarian cancer: NCCN Practice Guidelines in Oncology - v. 1.2006. National Comprehensive Cancer Network, 2006.

[20] Buys SS, Partridge E, Greene MH, et al. Ovarian cancer screening in the Prostate, Lung, Colorectal and Ovarian (PLCO) cancer screening trial: findings from the initial screen of a randomized trial. Am J Obstet Gynecol 2005;193 (5) 1630-9.

[21] Partridge E, Kreimer AR, Greenlee RT, et al. Results from four rounds of ovarian cancer screening in a randomized trial. Obstet Gynecol 2009; 113 (4) 775-82.

[22] Menon U, Gentry-Maharaj A, Hallett R, et al. Sensitivity and specificity of multimodal and ultrasound screening for ovarian cancer, and stage distribution of detected cancers: results of the prevalence screen of the UK Collaborative Trial of Ovarian Cancer Screening (UKCTOCS). Lancet Oncol 2009; 10 (4) 327-40.

[23] Kobayashi H, Yamada Y, Sado T, et al. A randomized study of screening for ovarian cancer: a multicenter study in Japan. Int J Gynecol Cancer 2008; 18 (3) 414-20.

[24] Einhorn N, Bast R, Knapp R, et al. Long-term follow-up of the Stockholm screening study on ovarian cancer. Gynecol Oncol 2000; 79 (3) 466-70.

[25] Vasen HF, Tesfay E, Boonstra H, et al. Early detection of breast and ovarian cancer in families with BRCA mutations. Eur J Cancer 2005; 41 (4): 549-54.

[26] Olivier RI, Lubsen-Brandsma MA, Verhoef S, et al. CA125 and transvaginal ultrasound monitoring in high-risk women cannot prevent the diagnosis of advanced ovarian cancer. Gynecol Oncol 2006; 100 (1) 20-6.

[27] Buys SS, Partridge E, Black A, et al.: Effect of screening on ovarian cancer mortality: the Prostate, Lung, Colorectal and Ovarian (PLCO) Cancer Screening Randomized Controlled Trial. JAMA2011; 305 (22) 2295-303.

[28] Zhang Z, Bast RC Jr, Yu Y, et al.: Three biomarkers identified from serum proteomic analysis for the detection of early stage ovarian cancer. Cancer Res 2004; 64 (16) 5882-90.

[29] Petricoin EF, Ardekani AM, Hitt BA, et al.: Use of proteomic patterns in serum to identify ovarian cancer. Lancet 2002; 359 (9306): 572-7.

[30] Rebbeck TR, Lynch HT, Neuhausen SL, et al. Prophylactic oophorectomy in carrier 21 of BRCA1 or BRCA2 mutations. N Engl J Med 2002;346 1616-1622.

[31] Kauff ND, Satagopan JM, Robson ME, et al. Risk-reducing salpingooophorectomy in women with a BRCA1 or BRCA2 mutation. N Engl J Med 2002;346 1609-1615.

[32] Finch A, Beiner M, Lubinski J, et al. Salpingo-oophorectomy and the risk of ovarian, fallopian tube, and peritoneal cancers in women with a BRCA1 or BRCA2 Mutation. JAMA 2006; 296 185-192.

[33] Colgan TJ, Murphy J, Cole DE, et al. Occult carcinoma in prophylactic oophorectomy specimens: Prevalence and association with BRCA germline mutation status. Am J Surg Pathol 2001; 25 1283-1289.

[34] Lu KH, Garber JE, Cramer DW, et al. Occult ovarian tumors in women with BRCA1 or BRCA2 mutations undergoing prophylactic oophorectomy. J Clin Oncol 2000; 18 2728-2732.

[35] Hankinson SE, Hunter DJ, Colditz GA, et al.: Tubal ligation, hysterectomy, and risk of ovarian cancer. A prospective study. JAMA 1993; 270 (23) 2813-8.

[36] Rebbeck TR, Lynch HT, Neuhausen SL, et al. Prophylactic oophorectomy in carriers of BRCA1 or BRCA2 mutations. N Engl J Med 2002;346 (21) 1616-22.

[37] Tobacman JK, Greene MH, Tucker MA, et al. Intra-abdominal carcinomatosis after prophylactic oophorectomy in ovarian-cancer-prone families. Lancet 1982; 2 (8302) 795-7.

[38] Piver MS, Jishi MF, Tsukada Y, et al.: Primary peritoneal carcinoma after prophylactic oophorectomy in women with a family history of ovarian cancer. A report of the Gilda Radner Familial Ovarian Cancer Registry. Cancer 1993; 71 (9) 2751-5.

[39] Casey MJ, Synder C, Bewtra C, et al. Intra-abdominal carcinomatosis after prophylactic oophorectomy in women of hereditary breast ovarian cancer syndrome kindreds associated with BRCA1 and BRCA2 mutations. Gynecol Oncol 2005; 97 (2) 457-67.

[40] Madalinska JB, van Beurden M, Bleiker EM, et al. The impact of hormone replacement therapy on menopausal symptoms in younger high-risk women after prophylactic salpingo-oophorectomy. J Clin Oncol 2006; 24 (22) 3576-82. 47.

[41] Schmeler KM, Lynch HT, Chen LM, et al. Prophylactic surgery to reduce the risk of gynecologic cancers in the Lynch

[42] Offit K, Kauff ND: Reducing the risk of gynecologic cancer in the Lynch syndrome. N Engl J Med 2006; 354 (3) 293-5. syndrome. N Engl J Med 2006;354 (3) 261-9.

[43] Rebbeck TR, Lynch HT, Neuhausen SL, et al. Prophylactic oophorectomy in carriers of BRCA1 or BRCA2 mutations. N Engl J Med 2002; 346 (21)1616-22.

[44] Tan DS, Rothermundt C, Thomas K, Bancroft E, Eeles R, Shanley S, Ardern-Jones A, Norman A, Kaye SB, Gore ME. "BRCAness" syndrome in ovarian cancer: a case-control study describing the clinical features and outcome of patients with epithelial ovarian cancer associated with BRCA1 and BRCA2 mutations. J Clin Oncol 2008; 1; 26(34):5530-6. Epub 2008 Oct 27.

[45] Roux R. Zwifel M,Gordon JS and Rustin GJS. Biologicals in the Up front Treatment of Ovarian Cancer: Focus on Bevacizumab and Poly(ADP-Ribose) Polymerase Inhibitors. Journal of Oncology 2010; Article ID 151750, 6 pages doi:10.1155/2010/151750

[46] Gien LT and Mackay HJ. Review Article The Emerging Role of PARP Inhibitors in the Treatment of Epithelial Ovarian Cancer. Journal of Oncology 2010; Article ID 151750, 6 pages doi:10.1155/2010/151750

[47] Huehls AM, Wagner JM, Huntoon CJ, Karnitz LM. Identification of DNA Repair Pathways that Affect the Survival of Ovarian Cancer Cells Treated with a PARP Inhibitor in a Novel Drug Combination. Mol Pharmacol 2012; July 25. [Epub ahead of print]

[48] Marchetti C, Imperiale L, Gasparri ML, Palaia I, Pignata S, Boni T, Bellati F, Benedetti Panici P. Olaparib, PARP1 inhibitor in ovarian cancer.Expert Opin Investig Drugs 2012; 21(10):1575-84. Epub 2012 Jul 13.PMID:22788971

[49] Maxwell KN, Domchek SM. Cancer treatment according to BRCA1 and BRCA2 mutations.Nat Rev Clin Oncol 2012; 14;9(9):520-8. doi: 10.1038/nrclinonc.2012.123. Epub 2012 Jul 24.PMID: 22825375

[50] Marchetti C, Imperiale L, Gasparri ML, Palaia I, Pignata S, Boni T, Bellati F, Benedetti Panici P. Olaparib, PARP1 inhibitor in ovarian cancer.Expert Opin Investig Drugs 2012; 21(10) 1575-84. Epub 2012 Jul 13.PMID22788971Ratner ES, Sartorelli AC, Lin ZP Poly (ADP-ribose) polymerase inhibitors: on the horizon of tailored and personalized therapies for epithelial ovarian cancer. Curr Opin Oncol 2012; 24(5) 564-71. PMID: 22759740.

[51] Westin SN, Herzog TJ, Coleman RL. Investigational agents in development for the treatment of ovarian cancer.Invest New Drugs 2012; June 4. [Epub ahead of print] PMID: 22661305.

[52] Shigetomi H, Higashiura Y, Kajihara H, Kobayashi H.Targeted molecular therapies for ovarian cancer: an update and future perspectives (Review).Oncol Rep 2012; 28(2) 395-408. doi: 10.3892/or.2012.1833. Epub 2012 May 25.PMID: 22641286

[53] Tinker AV, Gelmon K. The Role of PARP Inhibitors in the Treatment of Ovarian Carcinomas. Curr Pharm Des. 2012;18 (25):3770-4. PMID: 22591423

Section 3

Ovarian Cancer Therapeutics

Chapter 8

Surgical Treatment of Ovarian Cancer

Lucas Minig, M. Guadalupe Patrono,
Rafael Alvarez Gallego,
Javier Valero de Bernabé and Ivan Diaz-Padilla

Additional information is available at the end of the chapter

http://dx.doi.org/10.5772/53972

1. Introduction

Despite great efforts in developing novel screening, diagnosis and therapeutic strategies, the incidence and mortality of ovarian cancer have not significantly changed in the last 30 years. [1] It remains the leading cause of death from gynecologic malignancy with a lifetime probability of developing the disease of 1 in 59.[1] Worldwide, approximately 200.000 women are annually diagnosed with ovarian cancer,[2] and almost 70% of them will be diagnosed at advanced stage disease.[3] With current treatment modalities, the 5-year survival rate ranges from 80–95% for those with organ-confined or early stage disease (International Federation of Gynecology and Obstetrics (FIGO) stage I-II); to 30 – 40% for those women with advanced disease, FIGO stage III-IV. Thus, ovarian cancer is a challenging and complex malignancy.[4]

Surgical management of ovarian cancer remains as the cornerstone treatment of this disease. [5] An adequate full surgical staging in women with early stage disease has demonstrated to improve oncologic outcome.[6] On the other hand, complete surgical cytoreduction is the only modifiable prognosis factor for patients with advanced disease. This chapter will describe the rationale and surgical steps for an adequate surgical staging for women with early stage ovarian cancer, and for obtaining the maximal surgical cytoreduction in women affected by advanced stage and relapsed disease.

2. Surgical treatment of early stage epithelial ovarian cancer

Approximately 25% of newly diagnosed ovarian cancer will be early stage disease. Prognosis is good with survival rates ranging from 80 % to 95 % when recommended treatment is followed.[5] These patients are initially managed by comprehensive surgical staging, which is relevant not only for identifying women with truly early stage disease, but also to select patients who will be candidates for adjuvant chemotherapy.

3. Rationale for surgical staging

Adequate surgical staging procedures include: exploration of abdomen/pelvis, peritoneal washings, bilateral salpingo-oophorectomy, hysterectomy, peritoneal biopsies of Cul-de-sac, pelvic walls, paracolic gutters, diaphragm, suspicious areas, omentectomy, appendectomy, as well as pelvic and para-aortic node dissection up to the renal veins. (TABLE 1)[7],[8] These procedures are needed to find hidden disease in nearly 18% of women[8], which has implications in the prognosis and subsequent patient treatment.[9] Surgeon expertise is crucial given that it was correlated with under-staged ovarian cancer. Several studies demonstrated that over 30% of patients operated by general gynecologists or general surgeons were upstaged by gynecologist oncologists by finding disease on pelvic-aortic lymph nodes, diaphragm biopsies and omentum.[6, 10] Moreover, as it has been demonstrated, inadequate initial surgical staging leads to a higher risk of developing recurrent disease despite receiving adjuvant chemotherapy.[6] Thus, if the operative risk is not too high, all patients should be routinely re-staged before starting chemotherapy.

• Peritoneal cytology/ascites drainage
• Careful and systematic abdominal exploration – inspect and palpate all peritoneal surface
• Infracolicomentectomy
• Total abdominal hysterectomy and bilateral salpingo-oophorectomy
• Pelvic and aortic lymphadenectomy
• Random and directed peritoneal biopsies – posterior cul-de-sac, bladder reflection, both pelvic sidewalls and both paracolic spaces
• Biopsy or scrapings from the undersurface of both diaphragms
• Appendectomy (for mucinous histology)

Table 1. Surgical staging procedures for early stage ovarian cancer

4. Surgical staging procedures

Midline vertical incision is the recommended surgical approach for initial management of suspected early stage ovarian cancer. The incision is firstly made from the pubis to the umbilicus and then progressed to xifoid appendix, if surgical staging is indicated following the frozen section diagnosis. The abdominal-pelvic cavity is opened and visualized. If free fluid is present, a minimum sample of 100 cc[3] should be obtained for cytological examination.

Peritoneal washing from paracolic gutters, pelvis and abdominal cavity should be done in the absence of ascites. It is estimated that over 30% of patients with stage I disease have tumoral cells on cytological examination.[11] Careful inspection and palpation is preformed to detect extra-ovarian implants in a systematic way: starting by right paracolic space, advancing the hand to the right kidney, suprahepatic space, the right diaphragm, right hepatic lobe, gallbladder, Morrison´s pouch, left hemi-diaphragm, left hepatic lobe, spleen, stomach, transverse colon, left kidney and left paracolic space. The lesser sac is entered on the left side of the gastrocolic ligament. Both surfaces of the mesentery should be examined and retroperitoneal vascular areas should be palpated as well. The result of this comprehensive procedure should be properly described.

The ovaries need to be examined for capsule rupture or external excrescences. The affected ovary must then be removed for frozen section. Although the influence on the prognosis of the intraoperative rupture of malignant ovarian tumors is controversial,[12] adnexal masses should be removed intact. If malignancy is confirmed in the frozen section, full surgical staging, as previously described, must be performed by the extension of the incision up to xifoid appendix. Contralateral oophorectomy and total hysterectomy is completed due to the possibility of synchronous cancer.

Even though controversial, random peritoneal biopsies are indicated in early-stage disease. A retrospective study demonstrated that less than 4% of patients with ovarian cancer were upstaged due to positive peritoneal biopsies. No patient, however, had a change in treatment recommendations based on these biopsies.[13] Infracolic omentectomy should be performed from the hepatic to splenic flexure. During dissection, the lesser sac is developed dissecting the posterior and anterior layer of the transverse mesocolon, while preserving the middle colic artery. The omentum is removed and the pedicles are sequentially sutured – ligated. Appendectomy is only reserved for mucinous histology.

5. Retropetitoneal lymph node dissection

The incidence of lymph-node involvement in patients with disease confined to the ovary is 5% in only pelvic nodes, 9% in aortic nodes and 6% in both pelvic and aortic nodes.[14] Systematic lymphadenectomy as part of surgical staging of apparent early stage ovarian cancer is associated with a statistically significant increase in median operative time, median blood loss, and the proportion of patients undergoing blood transfusions.[15] Systematic lymphadenectomy, however, significantly improves progression-free survival (PFS) rates, without a statistically significant impact on overall survival (OS). [14, 15] Lymphatic drainage of the ovaries is known to follow the gonadal blood supply that reaches the renal vein, on the left side, and the inferior vena cava, on the right side. Pelvic lymphadenectomy should include removal of nodes from paravesical and pararectal spaces, including bilateral common iliac nodes. Aortic nodes should be removed from aortic bifurcation to the renal veins.[14]

6. Minimally invasive surgery for surgical staging ovarian cancer

Over the last years, laparoscopy has gained an important role for the management of suspected adnexal masses. High-volume centers have reported their experience in performing a comprehensive surgical staging by using minimally invasive surgery.[16],[17] Nezhat et al. [16] reported a case series of 36 patients with early stage invasive ovarian carcinoma managed by laparoscopy. They showed 100% OS rate with a mean duration of follow-up of 55.9 months. Chi et al. [17] conducted a case control study by staging 20 patients with early ovarian cancer with laparoscopy compared with 30 patients staged with laparotomy. There were no differences in the omental specimen size or number of lymph nodes removed. Blood loss and hospital stay were lower for the laparoscopy group, with longer operating time. There were no conversions to laparotomy or other intraoperative complications in the laparoscopy group.

Despite laparoscopic staging of early ovarian cancer seems to be a safe and feasible procedure performed by expert surgeons, the possibility of cyst rupture or port-site metastases remain controversial. The immediate effect of tumor rupture is that a patient with a potentially curable disease will require additional adjuvant chemotherapy. Preoperative evaluation is essential, as well as the surgical experience and the quality of laparoscopic instruments.[18] Even though there are no specific recommendations, adnexal masses up to 5-6 cm could be reasonably managed by laparoscopy.

The etiology of port-site metastases is uncertain. Several hypotheses include tumor cell entrapment, direct spread from the trocar in which instruments are exchanged, and the "chimney effect," which suggests that tumor cells travel along the sheath of the trocars with the leaking gas. Port-site metastases have been reported in 1% to 2% of patients with ovarian cancer. However, <5% of port metastases are clinically detected and these sites are likely to respond to chemotherapy.[9]

Robotic surgery has emerged as an innovative minimally invasive approach in the field of gynecology. The da Vinci Surgical System (Intuitive Surgical, Inc, Sunnyvale, California, USA) offers several advantages over conventional laparoscopy including three-dimensional view, greater dexterity, and tremor filtration. Most of the data regarding the application of robotic technology for ovarian cancer staging are included in the literature used in the assessment for its implementation in other gynecologic malignancies, such as cervical and endometrial cancer.[19] Data are still scarce but promising.

7. Treatment of advanced stage disease: Surgical cytoreduction

Advanced-stage disease means that the disease is extended to pelvic/ aortic lymph nodes, peritoneum, intra-abdominal organs or disease outside the abdominal cavity.[20] In 1975, a landmark study quantified residual disease and demonstrated for the first time an inverse relationship between residual tumor and oncologic outcome. [21] The goal of surgery is to resect as much tumor as possible obtaining, ideally, a complete resection. The standard

http://dx.doi.org/10.5772/53972

worldwide recommendation consists of primary maximal surgical cytoreduction followed by 6 cycles of intravenous carboplatin plus paclitaxel. [5,7] An alternative strategy is reserved for selected patients and it includes surgical cytoreduction in between chemotherapy courses, usually after three or four cycles. This strategy is called neoadjuvant chemotherapy followed by interval debulking surgery. (fig 1) The appropriate selection of patients for each modality of treatment will be described below.

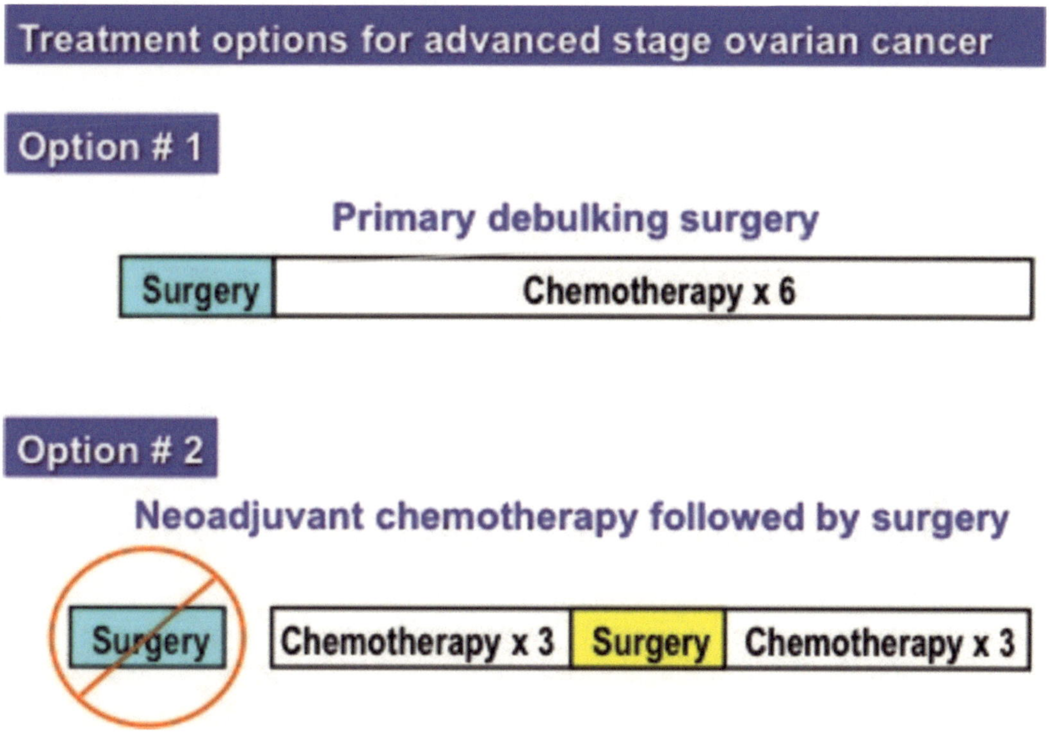

Figure 1. Treatment options for advanced stage ovarian cancer

8. Prognostic factors

Prognostic factors in women with advanced stage EOC was described in literature based on retrospective data.[22] Recently, Du Buois et al., [23] did a combined exploratory analysis of three prospective randomized phase III multicenter trials, which enrolled 3388 patients with advanced EOC between 1995 and 2002. Univariate and multivariate analysis revealed non-modifiable significant prognostic factors for OS and PFS such as: age, performance status (ECOG 2 versus 0-1), FIGO stage (IIIC-IV versus IIB-IIIB), subtype histology (Mucinous versus serous), histology grade (grade 2-3 versus 1), presence of large volume ascites (> 500 mL). The only significant modifiable prognosis factor was postoperative residual tumor (0 versus >1 mm). (Table 2) This study highlighted the importance of an adequate surgical management of women affected by ovarian cancer as the key-point for improving oncologic outcomes given that the quality of surgical cytoreduction was the only modifiable prognosis factor for survival.

Non-modifiable
• Patient performance status
• FIGO stage
• Hystology subtype
• Hystology grade
• Large volume of ascites
Modifiable
• Post-surgical residual tumor

Table 2. Prognosis factors of overall survival and progression free survival in patients with advanced stage epithelial ovarian cancer

9. Rationale for primary surgical cytoreduction

1. **Improvement of oncologic outcomes:** a large body of retrospective and non-randomized prospective studies consistently show an inverse correlation between survival and the amount of postoperative residual disease [22]. Results of two meta-analysis[22],[24] evaluated women affected by advanced stage EOC that were treated with primary surgical cytoreduction and platinum-based neoadjuvant chemotherapy and demonstrated a mean weighted median survival of 29 and 24 months respectively.

2. **Surgical reduction of tumor burden prior to chemotherapy:** it has been postulated that the proportion of tumor cells destroyed with each cycle of chemotherapy is constant. Thus, in cases of tumor cells not resistant to chemotherapy, fewer cycles would be necessary to eradicate them if the absolute number were less.[25] In addition, tumor size is correlated with an increased spontaneous mutation rate of malignant cells.[26] Animal models have also demonstrated that drug exposure allows the resistant cells to outgrow the sensitive tumor cells population.[27] Primary surgical cytoreduction, thus, reduces the number of cancer cells decreasing the chance of inducing drug resistance.

3. **Improved drug diffusion:** large bulky tumors may have hypoperfused areas where concentration of chemotherapy agents can be suboptimal, increasing the possibility of drug resistance.[28]

4. **Increased tumor cells growth rate:** During initial tumor growth, cancer cell division is almost exponential. But then, cell growth reaches a plateau. Thus, the great majority of cells in large tumoral masses are not dividing, being in G_0 phase of the cell cycle, which

are essentially resistant to chemotherapy.[29] Primary surgical cytoreduction may stimulate G_0 residual tumor cells to re-enter in the normal cell cycle, increasing the chemotherapy efficacy.[29]

10. Residual tumor disease: Definition and relevance

Residual tumor disease is commonly described as the diameter, in millimeters, of the biggest nodule left after surgical debulking. Griffiths *et al.*, first described the importance of residual disease after surgery in women with ovarian cancer.[21] They demonstrated an inverse relationship between residual disease and patient survival. In 1994, the Gynecology Oncology Group (GOG) published a sub-analysis of two retrospective series (GOG protocol 52 & 97) of patients affected by advanced stage EOC who underwent primary cytoreduction followed by chemotherapy. The study showed significant differences in OS in women with microscopic disease or less than 2 cm in comparison with of residual disease of more than 2 cm diameter. The maximum diameter of residual disease was firstly found to be an independent predictor of OS after controlling other variables. Thus, surgery with residual disease of less than 2 cm was defined as "optimal" cytoreduction; while more than 2 cm was called "suboptimal".[30]

In 2002, a meta-analysis of 6885 patients with stage III or IV ovarian cancer was reported. [22]The study analyzed 81 cohorts of patients treated in the platinum era to evaluate the effect of maximal cytoreductive surgery and other prognostic factors on survival. The investigators demonstrated that each 10% increase in the proportion of patients undergoing maximal cytoreduction was associated with a concomitant 5.5% increase in median cohort survival time. The mean weighted median survival time was 29 months. Thus, for all clinical trials that followed, the GOG established ≤ 1 cm residual disease as the criterion for optimal cytoreduction.

Winter III et al. [31] reported the GOG collective experience analyzing the data of seven trials (GOG 11, 114, 132, 152, 158, 162 and 172) that studied the efficacy of chemotherapy in 1895 stage III and 360 stage IV ovarian cancer patients. All patients underwent primary debulking surgery followed by 6 courses of cisplatin and paclitaxel. Residual disease after surgery was an independent prognostic factor. The median OS reported was 79.1, 42.4 and 35 months in patients with microscopic, 1-10 mm and > 10 mm of residual disease, respectively. The authors suggested a modification of the term "optimal residual disease" from < 1 cm to microscopic.

These results were confirmed when 3 large phase III randomized trials conducted by the AGO (AGO-OVAR 3, 5 and 7) of patients with stage IIB-IV ovarian cancer receiving platinum/taxanes chemotherapy following primary cytoreduction surgery were analyzed. [23] Patients with microscopic residual disease had significantly longer median OS than those with any residual disease, 99.1 months versus less than 36 months, respectively. Thus the current goal of the surgery in ovarian cancer is to obtain a complete cytoreduction. (Fig 2)

The goal of the surgery in ovarian cancer is to obtain a complete cytoreduction

Figure 2. Goal of the surgery in ovarian cancer

Chang and Bristow in 2012, reported a single institution series and cooperative group trials since 2003 of patients who underwent primary debulking surgery followed by adjuvant chemotherapy. Over 14000 patients in 15 studies were analyzed.[32] A marked inverse correlation between the maximal diameter of residual tumor and OS was noted. The weighted median OS for 3593 patients with no gross residual disease was 77.8 months compared to 39.0 months for the 4780 patients with 0.1–1 cm residual disease and 31.1 months for the 3518 patients with residual tumor >1 cm in maximal diameter. The magnitude of the incremental improvement in OS strongly suggests that complete resection should be the surgical objective whenever feasible.

11. Feasibility of complete primary cytoreduction

In the presence of a preoperative suspected adnexal mass whit ascites and peritoneal carcinomatosis are present, the feasibility of complete cytoreduction should be determined by exclusion of multiple liver or pulmonary metastases by imaging studies such as computed tomography (CT). In the absence of extra-peritoneal lesions and surgical contraindications, patients should undergo primary debulking surgery. The feasibility of optimal cytoreduction depends on the disease distribution, the patient´s overall medical condition and the surgeon's expertise. However, obtaining an optimal cytoreduction ≤ 1 cm of residual disease is not an easy task. In highly specialized centers, the rate with optimal primary cytoreduction is over 75 %. (Fig 3) But this rate falls down to 25% when low-volume ovarian cancer surgeries centers are included in the analysis. (Fig 4) Nevertheless, as it was previously mentioned, according with collecting data of the latter,[23],[31] primary debulking surgery is beneficial if complete cytoreduction is achieved. According with the literature, this is achievable in only 30% of patients when a gynecologist oncologist performs the surgery, a higher rate when compared with general gynecologists or general surgeons.[33]-[38]

12. Neoadjuvant chemotherapy followed by interval debulking surgery

Despite upfront primary debulking surgery (PDS) for newly diagnosed patients with advanced stage ovarian cancer is considered the standard of care,[5] limitations to this strategy have been postulated.[39],[40] For instance, patients with incomplete primary cytoreduction seem to have no meaningful impact on OS.[23],[31] Furthermore, only experienced surgeons

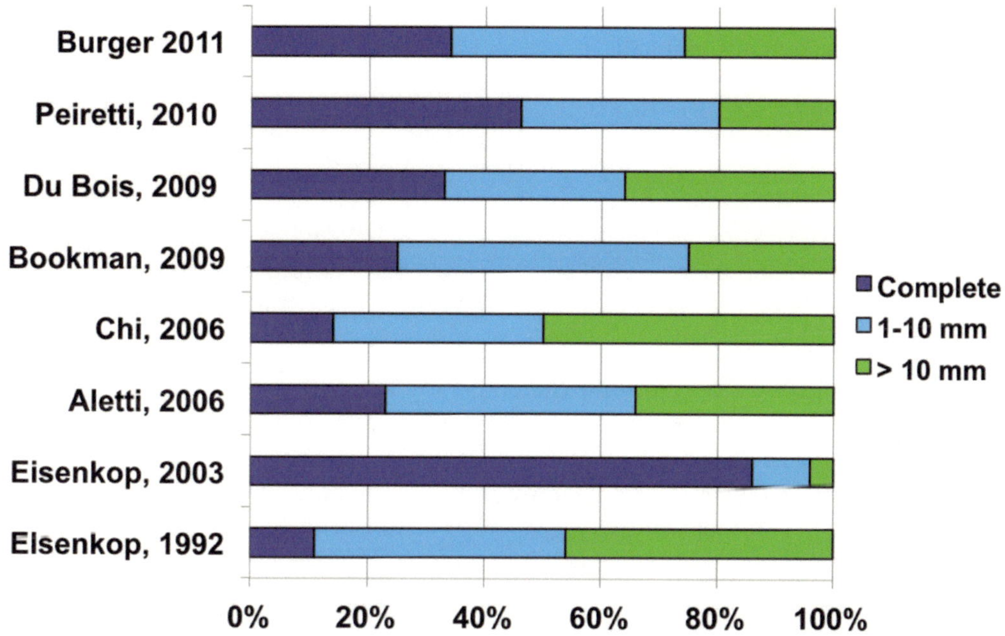

Figure 3. Stratified residual tumor on expert series/international traits

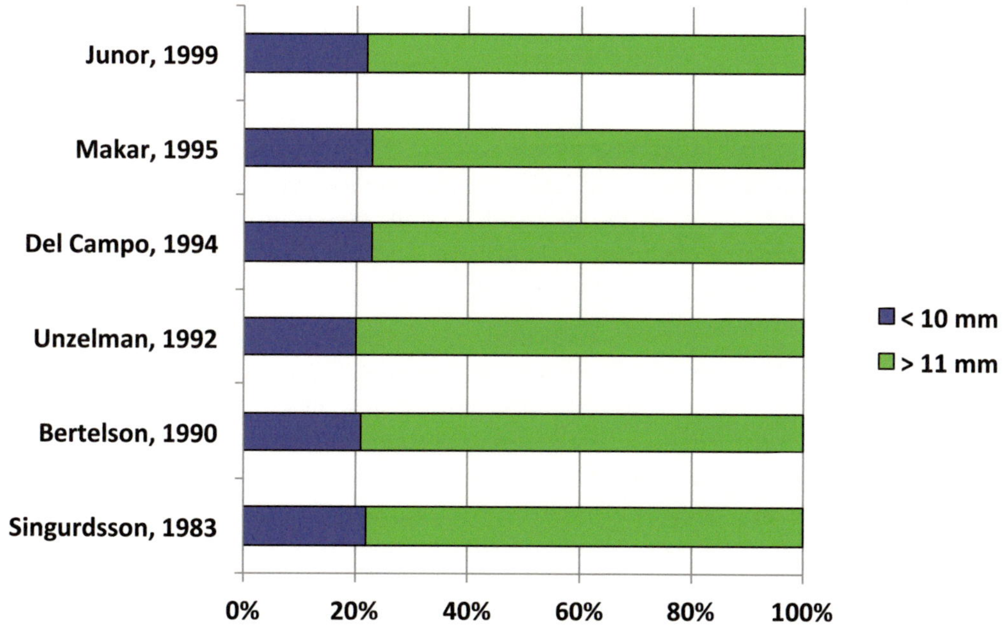

Figure 4. Stratified residual tumor on less experienced centers

with extended formal training in cytoreductive techniques obtain an acceptable complete primary cytoreduction rate.[41]-[43]

Consequently, an alternative approach such as neoadjuvant chemotherapy (NACT) has been proposed by several authors.[39],[40] This strategy of treatment consists in the administration of at least 3 courses of platinum-taxanes chemotherapy followed by an interval debulking surgery (IDS) and further adjuvant treatment in patients responsive to chemotherapy. [44] (Figure 1) The goal of this modality is to reduce the extension of the disease and, by performing a less radical surgical procedure, to improve the complete cytoreduction rate reducing the surgical time and complication rate, while improving the PFS and OS rate.

Objective indications for neoadjuvant chemotherapy are patients with poor performance status and with significant medical co-morbidities making them unsuitable for an aggressive debulking surgery. These indications include, however, the smallest proportion of patients who underwent neoadjuvant chemotherapy in the series published in the literature. [39],[40],[45],[46] The majority of women receive either NACT or PDS based on tumor extension and on estimated tumor resectability.[47] The latter is a subjective and highly surgeon-dependent indication. [24] Although several criteria have been tested for predicting the surgical resectability of ovarian tumors, its accuracy and clinical applicability is still controversial. [48] Some of these criteria include ascites volume, serum CA 125 values[48] and computer tomography scan parameters.[49] For example, terms like "dense adhesion between bowel and omentum", "large diaphragm disease", and "large tumor nodules adherent to abdominal structures" have been postulated by some authors as criteria of unresectability.[50] These terms show how subjective is the definition of a patient as debulkable or not. These criteria are mostly based on CT scan findings but, sometimes, a direct laparoscopic assessment of is recommended.[51] (Fig. 5)

On the other hand it is a common belief to associate NACT with less complex surgical procedures, shorter surgical time, and lower incidence of complications after IDS.[44],[46] However, this strategy does not exclude the necessity of performing complex surgical procedures at the time of IDS in order to obtain an optimal cytoreduction. Thus, referring these patients to a specialized gynecologist is mandatory as well.

Recently, the results of a randomized, controlled, prospective trial conducted by the European Organization for Research and Treatment of Cancer (EORTC) were published.[52] Six hundred and seventy patients with stage IIIC and IV ovarian cancer were randomly assigned to primary cytoreductive surgery group or neoadjuvant chemotherapy group. There were no significant differences in OS (29 months for primary cytoreductive surgery group versus 30 months for neoadjuvant chemotherapy group) between the two groups. Complete cytoreduction with no gross residual disease was possible in 20% of patients who underwent primary cytoreduction and 52% of those who had neoadjuvant chemotherapy. On multivariate analysis, the strongest independent predictor factor of prolonged survival was the absence of residual tumor after surgery ($p < 0.001$). The authors concluded that neoadjuvant chemotherapy followed by interval debulking surgery has similar efficacy compared with primary debulking surgery followed by chemotherapy for patients with stage IIIC or

IV ovarian cancer and complete resection of all gross lesions remains the objective of the cytoreductive surgery whether performed as primary or after neoadjuvant chemotherapy. However, optimal cytoreduction (<1 cm residual disease) was achieved in only 41.6% of patients in the PDS arm, a substantially lower rate than the published by expert series.[31],[42],[43] The PFS and OS for patients randomized to the PDS arm were substantially lower than those reported in previous studies, including prospective trials of the Gynecologic Oncology Group (GOG) as well.[30],[31],[43]

A recent report from the Memorial Sloan-Kettering Cancer Center contradicts the findings of the EORTC study and suggests that the strategy of neoadjuvant chemotherapy requires further investigation. A total of 316 stage IIIC–IV ovarian cancer patients were treated at the institution during the same period in which the EORTC-NCIC trial were evaluated, using identical inclusion criteria.[53] The optimal cytoreduction rate was 71% and the median OS time was 50 months. This study suggested that primary cytoreductive surgery should be considered as t he preferred initial management strategy for patients with this disease.

It seems, therefore, that neoadjuvant chemotherapy should not be performed routinely in patients with advanced ovarian cancer and be done in selected patients who are at risk of morbidity associated with primary surgery and less likely to have a complete cytoreduction. (Fig. 5)

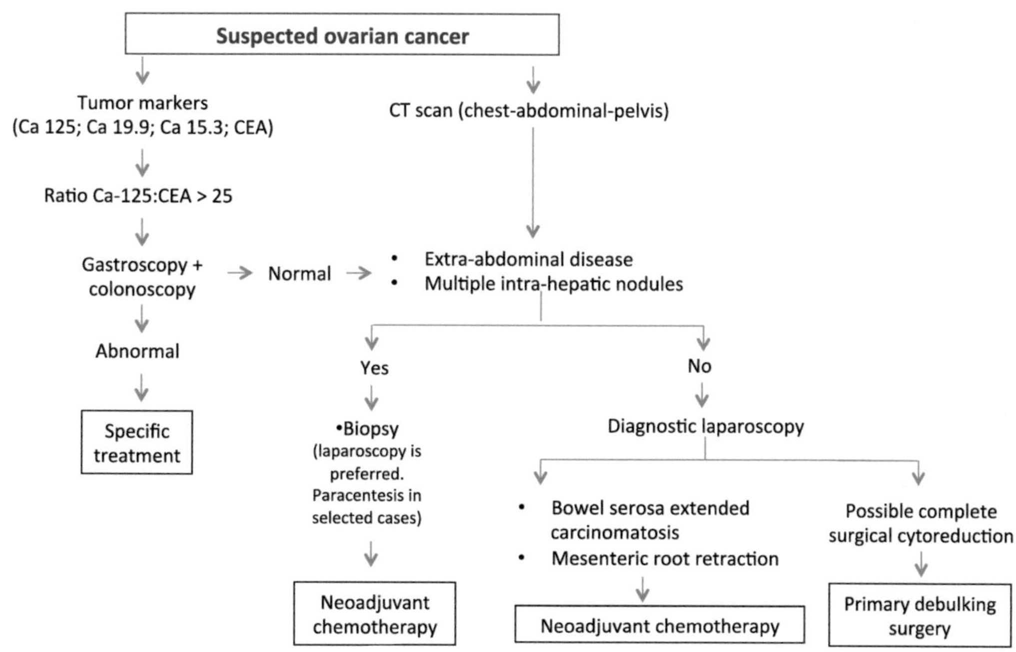

Figure 5. Initial approach of suspected advanced ovarian cáncer

13. Surgical cytoreduction technique

Women should be placed on supine position with legs spread apart. Vertical midline incision is recommended in order to access to the entire abdominal cavity. Ascites is evacuated and sent for cytological evaluation. As described above, a careful inspection and palpation of the entire peritoneal cavity and retroperitoneum is carried out in order to assess the extent of the primary and metastatic disease. The localization and diameter of the primary tumor and its extension into surrounding organs is described as the diameter of the larger metastases. Sometimes, there are regions that cannot be accessed before larger tumor masses are removed. This careful inspection and palpation is essential in order to establish the feasibility and extension of surgical cytoreduction. Complete cytoreduction may by difficult in cases of bulky suprarenal nodes, extensive disease in the liver parenchyma, along the root of the small bowel mesentery and in the bowel serosa, close to the origin of the superior mesenteric artery, or in the porta hepatis. If complete surgical cytoreduction is not feasible, neoadjuvant chemotherapy is preferred. (Figure 5)

Radical omentectomy use to be the first surgical step because it is the first tumor encountered upon entering the peritoneal cavity. The infracolic omentum is separated from the transverse colon and resected. If the omental metastases involve the gastrocolic omentum, it is resected as well. The next step is to remove the primary tumor in the pelvis with the other adnexa and the uterus in the usual fashion if no extension to other pelvic organs is present. However, advanced ovarian cancer often involves the uterus, rectosigmoid, cecum, ileum and bladder. Metastases of the pelvic peritoneum sometimes completely obliterate the anterior and posterior cul-de-sac. In this case, the retroperitoneal approach is the most reasonable way for removing *in block* the entire tumor. This procedure is accompanied by performing a rectosigmoid resection with an end-to end mechanical anastomosis.[54] Tumor spread to the hilum of the spleen may be carefully inspected as well. Splenectomy may be sometimes indicated to achieve maximal tumor debulking. Any peritoneal implants should be removed, particularly if there are large, isolated masses and their removal will render the patient optimally cytoreduced. Diaphragm peritoneum should be visualized and resected if the disease is present. Sometimes, it can involve muscle resection that can be sutured with non-reabsorbed monofilament continuous suture. Pelvic and /or aortic lymph node involvement is seen is approximately 60% of patient with advanced stage disease. Despite controversial, pelvic and aortic lymphadenectomy should be completed starting form aortic bifurcation up to the renal veins. The incidence of complications and morbidity of this approach should be also taken into consideration for patient selection. The most common complications include: infections, cardiac morbidity, pulmonary thromboembolism, coagulopathy, gastrointestinal, renal failure, re-laparotomy and death.

14. Surgical treatment of relapsed ovarian cancer: Secondary cytoreduction

Once recurrence is confirmed, the next step is to determine the best treatment approach for each individual case. Recurrent epithelial ovarian carcinoma is, however, a therapeutic dilemma for physicians. To date, there is no consensus for optimal treatment strategies. Three essential options are proposed: surgical resection followed by chemotherapy, chemotherapy only or enrollment into clinical trials. This dilemma will be fundamentally responded by the localization of the disease, by the disease free interval (DFI) between the end of standard front-line chemotherapy (platinum/taxanes-based) and the date of documented disease recurrence. This period will divide patients in three groups: *platinum sensible* with a DFI more than 6 months; *platinum resistant:* patients with a DFI less than 6 months; and the group of *platinum refractory:* patients who will never respond to front line therapy or who will experience progression of disease. The latter represents 20-30% of the patients with FIGO stage III-IV who underwent surgical cytoreduction followed by carboplatin /paclitaxel.[55],[56] DFI has been established as the most important predictor factor for response to treatment of the relapsed disease.[55],[57],[58]

15. Secondary cytoreduction

Surgical resection for ovarian cancer recurrence means secondary cytoreduction. Although primary cytoreductive surgery is well accepted as the cornerstone of initial management, the use of cytoreductive surgery in the setting of recurrent disease is defined less clearly. Benefits of secondary cytoreduction are encountered in several studies.[59] No randomized studies exist regarding the benefits of surgical resection over chemotherapy in patients with recurrent disease. The available data is controversial and biased by the decision whether or not to expose patients to a surgical treatment. In general, studies included patients with more favorable characteristics such as younger age, fewer medical comorbidity, scarce number of lesions, better performance status, absence of ascites at recurrence, early stage at diagnosis, DFI more than 12 months, and optimal primary cytoreduction.[60]-[64] All of the previous characteristics are favorable prognostic factors and constitute the standard indications for secondary surgical resection.[60] A recent meta-analysis studied 2.019 patients enrolled in 40 retrospective and prospective trials who underwent secondary cytoreduction due to recurrent ovarian cancer. The mean weighted median OS time after recurrence was 30.3 months. Complete cytoreduction was identified as an independent factor for the improving OS after secondary cytoreduction. In addition, the multivariate analysis showed that the survival time is increased 3.0 months each 10 % increase in the proportion of patients undergoing complete cytoreductive surgery.[65]

The objective of secondary cytoreduction should be to achieve complete debulking. In patients who are able to tolerate a major surgical procedure, secondary cytoreduction should be offered to those with a single site disease regardless of DFI, as well as to all patients with a DFI of greater than 30 months regardless the amount of disease sites. Patients with carcinomatosis and a DFI of less than 12 months should not be considered for secondary cytoreduction. The decisions must be, however, individualized based on each patient's goals, performance status, operative risk, and available therapeutic options.[66] (Table 3)

Disease-Free Interval	Single site of recurrence	Multiple site od recurrence – but no carcinomatosis	Carcinomatosis
6 – 12 months	Offer SC	Consider SC	No SC
12 – 30 months	Offer SC	Offer SC	Consider SC
> 30 months	Offer SC	Offer SC	Offer SC

Table 3. Recommendations for secondary cytoreduction (SC)

16. Specialized gynecologists

Surgical evaluation of a pelvic mass is one of the most common indications for gynecologic surgery and, therefore, it is unlikely that all patients with adnexal masses will be referred to a gynecologic oncologist. To assist in the referral process, the Society of Gynecologic Oncology established a guideline for patient referral with suspected ovarian cancer.[67]

It has been demonstrated that patients operated on by gynecologic oncologists are more likely to undergo an adequate staging procedure in early stage disease[34],[36],[37],[68] and a better percentage of optimal primary cytoreduction in advanced stage disease can be achieved in comparison to general gynecologists or general surgeons.[33]-[38] Moreover, many studies from several countries around the world have shown over 10 months increased OS when ovarian cancer patients were initially operated by a gynecological oncologist rather than general gynecologist [33],[34],[69]-[71] or general surgeons.[68],[72] Thus, optimal primary cytoreductive surgery performed by a surgeon with extended formal training in cytoreductive techniques followed by an appropriate chemotherapy combination is among the most powerful clinician-driven determinants of survival for women with ovarian cancer.[24]

17. Multidisciplinary team and centralization of treatment

Ovarian cancer is a challenging, complex and multidisciplinary disease. It is not only important how well trained physicians are, but also how many physicians of different specialties are involved in the management of this malignancy. The holistic conception of patient care and the intrinsic complexity of ovarian cancer require the involvement of different specialties to optimize the quality of care. The concept of multidisciplinary team approach in ovarian cancer is not restricted to the operating room settings. Multidisciplinary approach is crucial from the diagnosis to the demise of disease.

Results of different studies consistently show that patients with ovarian cancer treated at referral teaching high-volume hospitals receive better quality of care as accomplished by better surgical staging, better optimal cytoreduction[35],[39],[69],[73]-[75] and better chemotherapy administration rate and schemes.[69],[75]-[78] Treating patients at referral hospitals was independently associated with 10%-20% increased probability of survival at 5 years after first treatment.[69],[72],[73],[75],[79] In absolute numbers, this translates in an extension of survival of more than 10 months.[79]

Despite the consensus and the advantages explained above, population-based studies indicate that access to specialist care in gynecologic oncology for women with suspected ovarian cancer has been less than universal.[35],[36],[70] Reports from countries such as USA,[80] and UK[35],[81] have consistently shown that the majority of patients were treated in low-volume hospitals by low-volume surgeons. For example, the accessibility of patients with ovarian cancer to a specialized center was reported in 18% of patients in The Netherlands[74], 35% in Canada[72] and 40% in Maryland, USA.[82]

In summary, the configuration of health-care delivery systems to facilitate quick and consistent centralized referral will be necessary to ensure widespread access for women with suspected ovarian cancer to such health-care providers. Only through such efforts will contemporary patterns of surgical practice conform to the definition of high-quality cancer care.[83]

Author details

Lucas Minig[1*], M. Guadalupe Patrono[1], Rafael Alvarez Gallego[2],
Javier Valero de Bernabé[1] and Ivan Diaz-Padilla[2]

*Address all correspondence to: lucasminig@yahoo.com

1 Gynecologic Oncology Division, Department of Obstetrics and Gynecology. HM Universitario Sanchinarro, Centro Integral Oncológico Clara Campal, Madrid, Spain

2 Medical Oncology Division, Gynecologic Oncology Program, Medical Oncology Division, HM Universitario Sanchinarro, Centro Integral Oncológico Clara Campal, Madrid, Spain

References

[1] Jema A, Siegel R, Ward E, Hao Y, Xu J, Murray T, Thun M. Cancer Statistics, 2008. CA Cancer J Clin 2008;58;71-96.

[2] Siegel R, Desantis C, Virgo K, Stein K, Mariotto A, Smith T, Cooper D, Gansler T, Lerro C, Fedewa S, Lin C, Leach C, Cannady RS, Cho H, Scoppa S, Hachey M, Kirch R, Jemal A, Ward E.Cancer treatment and survivorship statistics, 2012.CA Cancer J Clin. 2012 Jul;62(4):220-41.

[3] Pecorelli S, Creasman WT, Petterson F, Benedet JL, Shepard JH. FIGO annual report on the results of treatment in gynaecological cancer. J Epidemiol Biostat. 1998;3:75–102.

[4] Bookman MA, Brady MF, McGuire WP, Harper PG, Alberts DS, Friedlander M, Colombo N, Fowler JM, Argenta PA, De Geest K, Mutch DG, Burger RA, Swart AM, Trimble EL, Accario-Winslow C, Roth LM. Evaluation of new platinum-based treatment regimens in advanced-stage ovarian cancer: a Phase III Trial of the Gynecologic Cancer Intergroup. J Clin Oncol. 2009 Mar 20;27(9):1419-25.

[5] GCIG-Consensous. Stuart GC, Kitchener H, Bacon M, duBois A, Friedlander M, Ledermann J, Marth C, Thigpen T, Trimble E; participants of 4th Ovarian Cancer Consensus Conference (OCCC); Gynecologic Cancer Intergroup.2010 Gynecologic Cancer InterGroup (GCIG) consensus statement on clinical trials in ovarian cancer: report from the Fourth Ovarian Cancer Consensus Conference.Int J Gynecol Cancer. 2011 May;21(4):750-5

[6] Le T, Adolph A, Krepart GV, Lotocki R, Heywood MS. The benefits of comprehensive surgical staging in the management of early-stage epithelial ovarian carcinoma. Gynecol Oncol. 2002 May;85(2):351-5.

[7] NIH consensus conference. Ovarian cancer. Screening, treatment, and follow-up. NIH Consensus Development Panel on Ovarian Cancer. JAMA. 1995 Feb 8;273(6): 491-7

[8] Buchsbaum HJ, Brady MF, Delgado G, Miller A, Hoskins WJ, Manetta A, Sutton G. Surgical staging of carcinoma of the ovaries. Surg Gynecol Obstet. 1989;169(3):226-32.

[9] Salani R, Bristow RE. Surgical management of epithelial ovarian cancer. Clin Obstet Gynecol. 2012;55(1):75-95.

[10] Bagley CM Jr, Young RC, Schein PS, Chabner BA, DeVita VT. Ovarian carcinoma metastatic to the diaphragm--frequently undiagnosed at laparotomy. A preliminary report. Am J Obstet Gynecol. 1973 Jun 1;116(3):397-400.

[11] Zuna RE, Behrens A. Peritoneal washing cytology in gynecologic cancers: long-term follow-up of 355 patients. J Natl Cancer Inst. 1996 17;88(14):980-7.

[12] Sigurdsson K, Alm P, Gullberg B. Prognostic factors in malignant epithelial ovarian tumors. Gynecol Oncol. 1983;15(3):370-80.

[13] Powless CA, Bakkum-Gamez JN, Aletti GD, Cliby WA. Random peritoneal biopsies have limited value in staging of apparent early stage epithelial ovarian cancer after thorough exploration. Gynecol Oncol. 2009;115(1):86-9.

[14] Angioli R, Plotti F, Palaia I, Calcagno M, Montera R, Cafà EV, Sereni MI, Panici PB. Update on lymphadenectomy in early and advanced ovarian cancer. Curr Opin Obstet Gynecol. 2008;20(1):34-9.

[15] Panici PB, Maggioni A, Hacker N, Landoni F, Ackermann S, Campagnutta E, Tamussino K, Winter R, Pellegrino A, Greggi S, Angioli R, Manci N, Scambia G, Dell'Anna T, Fossati R, Floriani I, Rossi RS, Grassi R, Favalli G, Raspagliesi F, Giannarelli D, Martella L, Mangioni C. Systematic aortic and pelvic lymphadenectomy versus resec-

tion of bulky nodes only in optimally debulked advanced ovarian cancer: a randomized clinical trial. J Natl Cancer Inst. 2005 Apr 20;97(8):560-6.

[16] Nezhat FR, Ezzati M, Chuang L, Shamshirsaz AA, Rahaman J, Gretz H. Laparoscopic management of early ovarian and fallopian tube cancers: surgical and survival outcome. Am J Obstet Gynecol. 2009;200(1):83.e1-6.

[17] Chi DS, Abu-Rustum NR, Sonoda Y, Ivy J, Rhee E, Moore K, Levine DA, Barakat RR. The safety and efficacy of laparoscopic surgical staging of apparent stage I ovarian and fallopian tube cancers. Am J Obstet Gynecol. 2005 May;192(5):1614-9.

[18] Tozzi R, Schneider A. Laparoscopic treatment of early ovarian cancer. Curr Opin Obstet Gynecol. 2005;17(4):354-8.

[19] Magrina JF, Zanagnolo V, Noble BN, Kho RM, Magtibay P. Robotic approach for ovarian cancer: perioperative and survival results and comparison with laparoscopy and laparotomy. Gynecol Oncol. 2011 Apr;121(1):100-5.

[20] FIGO. The new FIGO staging system for cancers of the vulva, cervix, endometrium and sarcomas. Gynecologic Oncology 115 (2009) 325–328

[21] Griffiths CT. Surgical resection of tumor bulk in the primary treatment of ovarian carcinoma. Natl Cancer Inst Mongr 1975;421:1014.

[22] Bristow RE, Tomacruz RS, Armstrong DK, Trimble EL, Montz FJ.Survival effect of maximal cytoreductive surgery for advanced ovarian carcinoma during the platinum era: a meta-analysis.J Clin Oncol. 2002 Mar 1;20(5):1248-59.

[23] du Bois A, Reuss A, Pujade-Lauraine E, Harter P, Ray-Coquard I, Pfisterer J. Role of surgical outcome as prognostic factor in advanced epithelial ovarian cancer: a combined exploratory analysis of 3 prospectively randomized phase 3 multicenter trials: by the Arbeitsgemeinschaft Gynaekologische Onkologie Studiengruppe Ovarialkarzinom (AGO-OVAR) and the Groupe d'Investigateurs Nationaux Pour les Etudes des Cancers de l'Ovaire (GINECO).Cancer. 2009 Mar 15;115(6):1234-44.

[24] Bristow RE, Chi DS.Platinum-based neoadjuvant chemotherapy and interval surgical cytoreduction for advanced ovarian cancer: a meta-analysis.Gynecol Oncol. 2006 Dec;103(3):1070-6.

[25] Skipper HE.Adjuvant chemotherapy.Cancer. 1978 Mar;41(3):936-40.

[26] Goldie JH, Coldman AJ. A mathematic model for relating the drug sensitivity of tumors to their spontaneous mutation rate. Cancer Treat Rep. 1979 Nov-Dec;63(11-12): 1727-33.

[27] Curt GA, Clendeninn NJ, Chabner BA. Drug resistance in cancer. Cancer Treat Rep. 1984 Jan;68(1):87-99.

[28] Skipper HE.Thoughts on cancer chemotherapy and combination modality therapy.JAMA. 1974;18;230(7):1033-5.

[29] Gunduz N, Fisher B, Saffer EA. Effect of surgical removal on the growth and kinetics of residual tumor. Cancer Res. 1979 Oct;39(10):3861-5.

[30] Hoskins WJ, McGuire WP, Brady MF, et al.: The effect of diameter of largest residual disease on survival after primary cytoreductive surgery in patients with suboptimal residual epithelial ovarian carcinoma. Am J Obstet Gynecol 1994, 170:974–980.

[31] Winter WE 3rd, Maxwell GL, Tian C, Carlson JW, Ozols RF, Rose PG, Markman M, Armstrong DK, Muggia F, McGuire WP; Gynecologic Oncology Group Study. Prognostic factors for stage III epithelial ovarian cancer: a Gynecologic Oncology Group Study. J Clin Oncol. 2007 Aug 20;25(24):3621-7.

[32] Chang SJ, Bristow RE. Evolution of surgical treatment paradigms for advanced-stage ovarian cancer: redefining 'optimal' residual disease. Gynecol Oncol. 2012 May; 125(2):483-92.

[33] Junor EJ, Hole DJ, McNulty L, Mason M, Young J. Specialist gynaecologists and survival outcome in ovarian cancer: a Scottish national study of 1866 patients. Br J Obstet Gynaecol 1999;106:1130– 6.

[34] Engelen MJA, Kos HE, Willemse PHB, et al. Surgery by consultant gynecologic oncologists improves survival in patients with ovarian carcinoma. Cancer 2006; 106: 589–98.

[35] Olaitan A, Weeks J, Mocroft A, Smith J, Howe K, Murdoch J. The surgical management of women with ovarian cancer in the south west of England. Br J Cancer. 2001;85:1824-30.

[36] Grossi M, Quinn MA, Thursfield VJ, Francis PA, Rome RM, Planner RS, Giles GG. Ovarian cancer: patterns of care in Victoria during 1993-1995. Med J Aust. 2002 Jul 1;177(1):11-6.

[37] Kumpulainen S, Kuoppala T, Leminen A, Penttinen J, Puistola U, Pukkala E, et al. Surgical treatment of ovarian cancer in different hospital categories—A prospective nation-wide study in Finland. Eur J Cancer 2006;43:388–95.

[38] Vernooij F, Heintz P, Witteveen E, van der Graaf Y. The outcomes of ovarian cancer treatment are better when provided by gynecologic oncologists and in specialized hospitals: a systematic review. Gynecol Oncol. 2007;105:801-12.

[39] Vergote I, DeWever I, TjalmaW, Van Gramberen M, Decloedt J, van Dam P. Neoadjuvant chemotherapy or primary debulking surgery in advanced ovarian carcinoma: a retrospective analysis of 285 patients. Gynecol Oncol 1998;71:431–6.

[40] Schwartz PE, Rutherford TJ, Chambers JT, Kohorn EI, Thiel PR. Neoadjuvant chemotherapy for advanced ovarian cancer: long-term survival. Gynecol Oncol 1999;72:93–9.

[41] Eisenkop SM, Spirtos NM, Friedman RL, et al. Relative influences of tumor volume before surgery and the cytoreductive outcome on survival for patients with advanced ovarian cancer: a prospective study. Gynecol Oncol 2003;90:390–6.

[42] Aletti GD, Gostout BS, Podratz KC, Cliby WA. Ovarian cancer surgical resectability: relative impact of disease, patient status, and surgeon. Gynecol Oncol 2006;100:33–7.

[43] Chi DS, Eisenhauer EL, Lang J, Huh J, Haddad L, Abu-Rustum NR, et al. What is theoptimal goal of primary cytoreductive surgery for bulky stage IIIC epitelialovarian carcinoma (EOC)? Gynecol Oncol 2006;103:559–64.

[44] Pecorelli S, Odicino F, Favalli G. Interval debulking surgery in advanced epithelial ovarian cancer. Best Prac Res, Clin Obstet Gynaecol 2002;16:573–83.

[45] Hegazy MA, Hegazi RA, Elshafei MA, Setit AE, Elshamy MR, Eltatoongy M, Halim AA. Neoadjuvant chemotherapy versus primary surgery in advanced ovarian carci noma. World J Surg Oncol. 2005 Aug 31;3:57.

[46] Hou JY, Kelly MG, Yu H, McAlpine JN, Azodi M, Rutherford TJ, Schwartz PE. Neoadjuvant chemotherapy lessens surgical morbidity in advanced ovarian cancer and leads to improved survival in stage IV disease. Gynecol Oncol. 2007;105:211-7.

[47] Chi DS, Schwartz PE. Cytoreduction vs. neoadjuvant chemotherapy for ovarian cancer. Gynecol Oncol. 2008;111:391-9.

[48] Eltabbakh GH, Mount SL, Beatty B, Simmons-Arnold L, Cooper K, Morgan A. Factors associated with cytoreducibility among women with ovarian carcinoma. Gynecol Oncol 2004;95:377–83.

[49] Nelson BE, Rosenfield AT, Schwartz PE. Preoperative abdominopelvic computed tomographic prediction of optimal cytoreduction in epithelial ovarian carcinoma. J Clin Oncol 1993;11(1):166–72.

[50] Bristow RE, Santillan A, Diaz-Montes TP, Gardner GJ, Giuntoli RL, Meisner BC, et al. Centralization of care for patients with advanced-stage ovarian cancer: a costeffectiveness analysis. Cancer 2007;109:1513–22.

[51] Fagotti A, Ferrandina G, Fanfani F, Ercoli A, Lorusso D, Rossi M, Scambia G. A laparoscopy-based score to predict surgical outcome in patients with advanced ovarian carcinoma: a pilot study. Ann Surg Oncol. 2006 Aug;13(8):1156-61

[52] Vergote I, Tropé CG, Amant F, Kristensen GB, Ehlen T, Johnson N, et al. European Organization for Research and Treatment of Cancer — Gynaecological Cancer Group; NCIC Clinical Trials Group. Neoadjuvant chemotherapy or primary surgery in stage IIIC or IV ovarian cancer. N Engl J Med 2010;363:943–53.

[53] Chi DS, Musa F, Dao F, Zivanovic O, Sonoda Y, Leitao MM. An analysis of patients with bulky advanced stage ovarian, tubal, and peritoneal carcinoma treated with primary debulking surgery (PDS) during an identical time period as the random- ized

EORTC-NCIC trial of PDS vs neoadjuvant chemotherapy (NACT). Gynecol Oncol 2012;124:10–4.

[54] Hudson CN, Chir M. Surgical treatment of ovarian cáncer. Gynecol Oncol 1973;1:370-8.

[55] Markman M, Reichman B, Hakes T, Jones W, Lewis JL Jr, Rubin S, et al. Responses to second-line cisplatin-based intraperitoneal therapy in ovarian cancer: influence of a prior response to intravenous cisplatin. J Clin Oncol. 1991;9:1801-5.

[56] McGuire WP, Markman M. Primary ovarian cancer: current standards of care. BJC 2003; 89 Suppl. 3: S3-8

[57] Gore ME, Fryatt I, Wiltshaw E, Dawson T. Treatment of relapsed carcinoma of the ovary with cisplatin or carboplatin following initial treatment with these compounds. Gynecol Oncol. 1990;36:207-11.

[58] Hoskins PJ, O'Reilly SE, Swenerton KD. The 'failure free interval' defines the likelihood of resistance to carboplatin in patients with advanced epithelial ovarian cancer previously treated with cisplatin: relevance to therapy and new drug testing. Int J Gynecol Cancer 1991; 1: 205-8.

[59] Munkarah AR, Coleman RL. Critical evaluation of secondary cytoreduction in recurrent ovarian cancer. Gynecol Oncol. 2004;95:273-280.

[60] Chi DS, McCaughty K, Diaz JP, Huh J, Schwabenbauer S, Hummer AJ, Venkatraman ES, Aghajanian C, Sonoda Y, Abu-Rustum NR, Barakat RR.Guidelines and selection criteria for secondary cytoreductive surgery in patients with recurrent, platinum-sensitive epithelial ovarian carcinoma.Cancer. 2006 May 1;106(9):1933-9.

[61] Eisenkop SM, Friedman RL, Spirtos NM. The role of secondary cytoreductive surgery in the treatment of pa- tients with recurrent epithelial ovarian carcinoma. Cancer. 2000;88:144-53.

[62] Harter P, du Bois A, Hahmann M, Burges A, Loibl S,Gropp M, et al. Surgery in recurrent ovarian cancer: the Arbeitsgemeinschaft Gynaekologische Onkologie (AGO) DESKTOP OVAR trial. Ann Surg Oncol. 2006;13:1702-10.

[63] Scarabelli C, Gallo A, Carbone A. Secondary cytoreduc- tive surgery for patients with recurrent epithelial ovarian carcinoma. Gynecol Oncol. 2001;83:504-12.

[64] Zang RY, Zhang ZY, Li ZT, Chen J, Tang MQ, Liu Q, et al. Effect of cytoreductive surgery on survival of patients with recurrent epithelial ovarian cancer. J Surg Oncol. 2000;75:24-30.

[65] Bristow RE, Puri I, Chi DS. Cytoreductive surgery for recurrent ovarian cancer: a meta-analysis. Gynecol Oncol. 2009;112(1):265-74.

[66] Leitao MM Jr, Chi DS.Surgical management of recurrent ovarian cancer.Semin Oncol. 2009 Apr;36(2):106-11.

[67] SGO. Guidelines for referral to a gynecologic oncologist: rationale and benefits. The Society of Gynecologic Oncologists.Gynecol Oncol. 2000 Sep;78(3 Pt 2):S1-13.

[68] Earle CC, Schrag D, Neville BA, Yabroff KR, Topor M, Fahey A, et al. Effect of surgeon specialty on processes of care and outcomes for ovarian cancer patients. J Natl Cancer Inst 2006;98(3): 172–80.

[69] Paulsen T, Kjaerheim K, Kaern J, Tretli S, Trope C. Improved short-term survival for advanced ovarian, tubal, and peritoneal cancer patients operated at teaching hospitals. Int J Gynecol Cancer 2006;16(Suppl 1):11–7.

[70] Carney ME, Lancaster JM, Ford C, Tsodikov A, Wiggins CL. A population-based study of patterns of care for ovarian cancer: who is seen by a gynecologic oncologist and who is not? Gynecol Oncol 2002; 84: 36–42.

[71] Eisenkop SM, Spirtos NM, Montag TW, Nalick RH, Wang HJ. The impact of subspecialty training on the management of advanced ovarian cancer. Gynecol Oncol 1992;47:203– 9.

[72] Elit L, Bondy SJ, Paszat L, Przybysz R, Levine M. Outcomes in surgery for ovarian cancer. Gynecol Oncol 2002;87(3):260–7.

[73] Vernooij F, Heintz A, Coebergh J, Massuger L, Witteveen P, van der Graaf Y. Specialized and high-volume care leads to better outcomes of ovarian cancer treatment in the Netherlands. Gynecol Oncol 2009;112:455–461.

[74] Vernooij F, Heintz APM, Witteveen E, et al. Specialized care and survival of ovarian cancer patients in The Netherlands: nationwide cohort study. J Natl Cancer Inst 2008;100:399–406.

[75] Tingulstad S, Skjeldestad FE, Hagen B. The effect of centralization of primary surgery on survival in ovarian cancer patients. Obstet Gynecol. 2003;102:499-505.

[76] Cress RD, O'Malley CD, Leiserowitz GS, Campleman SL. Patterns of chemotherapy use for women with ovarian cancer: a population-based study. J Clin Oncol. 2003;21:1530-5.

[77] Schrag D, Earle C, Xu F, Panageas KS, Yabroff KR, Bristow RE, et al. Associations between hospital and surgeon procedure volumes and patient outcomes after ovarian cancer resection. J Natl Cancer Inst 2006;98 (3):163–71.

[78] Harlan LC, Clegg LX, Trimble EL. Trends in surgery and chemotherapy for women diagnosed with ovarian cancer in the United States. J Clin Oncol 2003;21(18):3488–94.

[79] Wolfe CD, Tilling K, Raju KS. Management and survival of ovarian cancer patients in south east England. Eur J Cancer 1997;33(11):1835–40.

[80] Goff BA, Matthews BJ, Wynn M, Muntz HG, Lishner DM, Baldwin LM. Ovarian cancer: patterns of surgical care across the United States. Gynecol Oncol. 2006 Nov; 103(2):383-90.

[81] Jolly K, Parry J, Rouse A, Stevens A. Volumes of cancer surgery for breast, colorectal and ovarian cancer 1992– 97: is there evidence of increasing sub-specialization by surgeons? Br J Cancer 2001;84:1308– 13.

[82] Diaz-Montes TP, Zahurak ML, Giuntoli II RL, Gardner GJ, Gordon TA, Armstrong DK, et al. Surgical care of elderly women with ovarian cancer: a population-based perspective. Gynecol Oncol 2005;99(2):352–7.

[83] Bristow RE, Berek JS. Surgery for ovarian cancer: how to improve survival. Lancet. 2006;367:1558-60.

Chapter 9

The Role of Chemotherapy in Recurrent Ovarian Cancer

Miguel Angel Alonso Bermejo, Ana Fernandez Montes, Eva Perez Lopez, Miguel Angel Nuñez Viejo, Jesus Garcia Gomez and Jesus Garcia Mata

Additional information is available at the end of the chapter

http://dx.doi.org/10.5772/54171

1. Introduction

Epithelial ovarian cancer causes more deaths than any other cancer of the female reproductive system and it is the leading cause of death from gynecologic cancer. There is no universally accepted consensus on the surveillance of ovarian cancer, but if we review the main clinical guidelines, we can find similar recommendations for follow-up for patients with ovarian cancer after chemotherapy treatment.

Approximately 60% of patients will experience a relapse after the standard first-line treatment including cytoreductive surgery and adjuvant chemotherapy [1]. At this time, when relapse occurs, the chance of cure decreases drastically and treatment is solely palliative. This makes the increase in overall survival and the quality of life the primary endpoints. Surgery is not sufficiently validated due to the lack of phase III clinical trials, and there are no approved targeted therapies in relapsed ovarian cancer. Therefore, chemotherapy is the only option to achieve these objectives. We will review the role of chemotherapy in recurrent ovarian cancer in this chapter.

2. Diagnosis of epithelial ovarian cancer relapse

In stages I, II, III and IV complete responders, American guidelines recommend that, after completing primary surgery and adjuvant chemotherapy, follow-up visits should include a physical examination with a pelvic exam every 2 to 4 months for the first two years, then every 3 to 6 months until the fifth year, and then annually after the fifth year. Periodic monitoring of CA 125 and other tumor markers (e.g., CA 19.9, CEA) are also recommended if the markers were elevated previously. The rest of the examination, which ranges from performing

Computerized Tomography (CT), Magnetic Resonance Imaging (MRI) or Positron Emission Tomography/Computerized Tomography (PET/CT), will be performed as clinically indicated such as weight loss, fatigue, bloating, pelvic pain or bowel occlusion [2].

European clinical guidelines recommend a physical exam and routine measurement of CA 125 every 3 months for 2 years, every 4 months during the third year and every 6 months during years 4 and 5. CT scan will be performed if the CA 125 is elevated or if there is clinical evidence of relapse [3].

A physical examination to detect recurrent ovarian cancer has limited value and detects abnormalities that indicate a recurrence only in 3.8 to 4.6% of patients [4, 5]. CT has a sensitivity of 40 - 93%, depending on the presence of peritoneal disease, tumor location and the presence of ascites. The sensitivity of MRI ranges from 62 to 91%, depending on the location of the tumor and tumor size. MRI facilitates the detection of disease on the peritoneal and intestinal surface [6].

We can define the relapse of ovarian cancer with the RECIST (Response Evaluation Criteria in Solid Tumors) criteria. However, relapse can also be defined as a doubling from the upper limit of normal value of CA 125 (30 U/mL) in patients who normalized their value after finishing their treatment, or doubling this value from the nadir (minimum value) in patients who never had normalized values [7-9]. It is estimated that this rise in the CA 125 level precedes the clinical detection of recurrence by about three months [10], and this may have implications at the beginning of the second-line treatment.

3. Classification of relapse

There are several classifications of patients with relapsed ovarian cancer based on the platinum-free interval (Table 1).

Markman suggested that the probability of response in the re-treatment with platinum-based chemotherapy depends on the platinum-free interval. In a retrospective analysis conducted at the Memorial Sloan-Kettering Cancer Center (New York, United States of America), these authors found a subgroup of patients with a higher likelihood of response to platinum salts. They selected 82 patients who received initial chemotherapeutic treatment with a cisplatin-based regimen and second-line treatment with a cisplatin- or carboplatin-based regimen, with a platinum-free interval of more than 4 months. The response rate to second-line treatment in the three groups according to the platinum-free interval at 5 to 12 months, 13 to 24 months and more than 24 months, was 27%, 33% and 59%, respectively [11]. They proposed to classify patients into different groups according to their previous response to platinum-based treatment and platinum-free interval: primary platinum-resistant (patients who progressed before the completion of the planned treatment), secondary platinum-resistant (patients who responded to a platinum regimen and did not respond to a second platinum-based treatment), and potentially platinum-sensitive (all patients who respond to a platinum-based treatment, subdivided into patients with platinum-free intervals of less than 6, 6 to 12 months and more than 12 months) [12].

http://dx.doi.org/10.5772/54171

In 1993, Thigpen defined two subgroups of patients with relapsed ovarian carcinoma based on the volume of relapse and the time to relapse after the end of treatment with platinum. Patients with small-volume disease confined to the peritoneal cavity have a far better chance of achieving a response to second-line chemotherapy with subsequent prolonged survival than those with bulky disease or disease outside the abdomen. Thus, we can classify the patients into those who are still "clinically sensitive" to the platinum-based regimens (initial response to platinum-based therapy and relapse more than 6 months after cessation of treatment) and those with "clinically resistant" disease (defined as progression disease during or within 6 months of first-line treatment platinum-based therapy). We should choose a platinum-containing regimen for relapse for those patients classified as clinically sensitive and an alternative treatment without platinum salts for those with clinically resistant disease [13]. Until recently, this was the most utilized and simplest classification.

Author	Best response to platinum	Platinum Free Interval	Classification
Markman [11,12]	Progression	-----	Primary Platinum-resistant
	No response	Any	Primary Platinum-resistant
	Response	< 6 months	Potentially platinum-sensitive
	Response	> 6 months	Potentially platinum-sensitive
Thigpen [13]	Progression	----	Platinum-resistant
	No response	Any	Platinum-resistant
	Response	< 6 months	Platinum-resistant
	Response	> 6 months	Platinum-sensitive
1998 International Workshop Consensus [14]	Progression	----	Platinum-refractory
	No response	Any	Platinum-refractory
	Response	< 4 months	Platinum-refractory
	Response	> 4 - 12 months	Intermediate platinum-sensitive
	Response	> 12 months	Platinum-sensitive
NICE 2005 [15]	Progression	----	Platinum-refractory
	No response	Any	Platinum-refractory
2010 GCIG Consensus [16]	Response	< 6 months	Platinum-resistant
	Response	> 6 - 12 months	Partially platinum-sensitive
	Response	> 12 months	Platinum-sensitive

Table 1. Classification of relapsed ovarian cancer

The International Workshop Consensus established a different classification in 1998 and stratified patients into platinum-refractory (progression during or within 4 months), intermediate platinum-sensitive (initial response but relapse 4 -12 months) and platinum-sensitive (relapse after 12 months) [14].

More recently, the National Institute for Health and Clinical Excellence (NICE) in 2005 [15] and the Gynecologic Cancer InterGroup (GCIG) in 2010 [16] have developed new classifications, including partially platinum-sensitive patients (those who relapse between 6 and 12 months after completion of initial platinum-based chemotherapy).

4. Treatment of platinum-sensitive disease

Until the early 2000s, monotherapy with platinum salts was the standard treatment for patients with platinum-sensitive disease because clinical trials attempting to prove the superiority of polychemotherapy were negative.

More recent clinical trials have demonstrated the superiority of polychemotherapy versus monotherapy, making this strategy the standard treatment in patients with platinum-sensitive disease. We discuss the main previous studies in this section.

4.1. Carboplatin versus carboplatin/paclitaxel (ICON4/AGO-OVAR 2.2)

In parallel, two pragmatic clinical trials were designed to determine whether the combination of carboplatin and paclitaxel should be used at first relapse after platinum-based chemotherapy [the International Collaborative Ovarian Neoplasm 4 (ICON4), coordinated by the Instituto Mario Negri, Milan, Italy (IRFMN) and the Medical Research Council's Clinical Trials Unit, London, United Kingdom (MRC CTU), and Arbeitsgemeinschaft Gynaekologische Onkologie (AGO) OVAR 2.2 coordinated by AGO, Karlsruhe, Germany] [17].

They randomized 802 patients with relapsed epithelial ovarian cancer who previously received platinum-based chemotherapy and had a platinum-free interval of more than 6 months (more than 12 months in the ICON4 group) to receive a conventional platinum-based chemotherapy (the majority of patients (71%) received carboplatin alone) or a combined treatment with paclitaxel 175 mg/m^2 plus cisplatin 50 mg/m^2 or carboplatin AUC 5 – 6 every 3 weeks for at least 6 cycles. The primary endpoint was overall survival (OS), and secondary endpoints were progression-free survival (PFS) and quality of life. The platinum-free interval was greater than 12 months in 75% of patients.

Patients in the AGO protocol must have previously received cisplatin or carboplatin plus paclitaxel, patients in the MRC CTU protocol trial were permitted to have had more than one line of previous chemotherapy and patients randomized into the Italian protocol required measurable disease.

With a median follow-up of 42 months, OS was increased by 5 months (24 versus 29 months), with an absolute difference in 2-year survival of 7% in favor of paclitaxel plus platinum-based chemotherapy (57% versus 50%; Hazard Ratio (HR): 0.82; 95% CI 0.69 - 0.97; p = 0.02). For PFS, there was a HR: 0.76 (95% CI 0.66 - 0.89; p = 0.0004) in favor of paclitaxel plus platinum-based chemotherapy, which translates into an absolute difference in median PFS of 3 months in favor of the combination regimen (9 versus 12 months). The response rate (RR) seemed to be higher in the combination arm (66%) compared to the conventional chemotherapy arm (p = 0.06). There were no differences between the quality of life measures in both groups. The results showed no difference between different subgroups (randomization group, time to relapse, number of previous lines of chemotherapy, type of prior chemotherapy, age and performance status).

Paclitaxel plus platinum-based chemotherapy was generally more toxic than conventional platinum-based chemotherapy, causing more alopecia and neurotoxicity (20% of patients), while conventional platinum-based chemotherapy was associated with more hematological toxic effects than paclitaxel plus platinum chemotherapy.

The ICON4/AGO-OVAR 2.2 trial was the first large clinical trial that showed the superiority of polychemotherapy versus monotherapy in platinum-sensitive ovarian cancer.

Similar results were found in a Spanish randomized phase II clinical trial conducted by GEICO (Grupo Español de Investigación en Cáncer de Ovario) [18]. In this trial, 81 patients with platinum-sensitive recurrent ovarian carcinoma were randomized to carboplatin or carboplatin plus paclitaxel. The primary endpoint was objective response and secondary endpoints were time to progression, overall survival, tolerability and quality of life. The platinum-free interval was greater than 12 months in 57.7% of patients. In the intent-to-treat analysis, they reported a higher response rate in the group treated with carboplatin plus paclitaxel than in the carboplatin group (75.6% versus 50%; p = 0.017). The median time to progression (49.1 versus 33.7 weeks; p = 0.021) and overall survival (not reached versus 72.7 weeks; p = 0.0021) were also better in the group treated with the combination therapy. There were no differences in the quality of life. As in the ICON4/AGO-OVAR 2.2 trial, alopecia (86.8%) and neurotoxicity (23.7%) were more frequent in patients treated with paclitaxel. Stomatitis (18.4%) and myalgias/arthralgias (36.8%) were also more frequent in this group. In the ICON4/AGO OVAR 2.2 trial, only 40% of patients received paclitaxel as part of a previous treatment, which could affect the superiority of the paclitaxel arm following the relapse. In the Spanish trial, 87.2% of patients received paclitaxel previously, so it was suggested that carboplatin plus paclitaxel could be administered at relapse in patients who received this treatment as first-line therapy.

4.2. Carboplatin versus carboplatin/gemcitabine (AGO-OVAR 2.5)

Neurotoxicity is the main drawback for the re-treatment with carboplatin plus paclitaxel because, among other factors, co-administration of paclitaxel and platinum compounds can increase the development of neurotoxicity [19]. Neurotoxicity is a cumulative dose-dependent toxicity; 715 mg/m^2 is the mean cumulative dose to onset of grade 2 or greater neurotoxicity [20].

In the ICON4-AGO OVAR 2.2 study, moderate or severe neurological effects were observed in 20% of patients in the combination arm, and the majority of patients experienced grades 1 to 4 neurotoxicity (75% to 83%) with the combination of carboplatin–paclitaxel and cisplatin-paclitaxel.

For these reasons, an alternative combination with carboplatin and gemcitabine was designed to avoid toxic effects, such as neurotoxicity, derived from the combination of carboplatin or cisplatin and paclitaxel.

In the AGO-OVAR 2.5 [21] clinical trial, the AGO-OVAR investigators, in collaboration with the National Cancer Institute of Canada Clinical Trials Group (NCIC CTG) and the European Organization for Research and Treatment of Cancer Gynecological Cancer Group (EORTC GCG), randomized 356 patients with platinum-sensitive recurrent ovarian cancer to receive either carboplatin alone (AUC 5) every 21 days or carboplatin AUC 4 on day 1 plus gemcitabine 1000 mg/m^2 on days 1 and 8, every 21 days. Patients could receive 6 to 10 cycles in both arms. The primary objective was progression-free survival, and secondary objectives included the response rate, duration of response, overall survival, quality of life and toxicity. Both groups were well balanced: 70.8% of patients had received platinum-based plus taxane as first-line therapy, and 59.8% of patients had a platinum-free interval greater than 12 months. The study was not powered to detect differences in OS.

With a median follow-up of 17 months, the median PFS in the combination arm and the single-agent arm were 8.6 months (95% CI, 7.9 - 9.7) and 5.8 months (95% CI, 5.2 - 7.1), respectively, with a 28% reduction in the progression-free event rate (HR: 0.72; 95% CI, 0.58 - 0.90; p = 0.0031). On the other hand, the RR was significantly higher in the gemcitabine plus carboplatin arm than in the carboplatin arm (47.2% versus 30.9%; p = 0.0016). The HR for overall survival was 0.96 (95% CI, 0.75 - 1.23; p = 0.7349). There was no difference in OS, which was 18 months for patients treated with carboplatin and gemcitabine versus 17.3 for patients treated with carboplatin alone. Furthermore, there was no difference in the quality of life between treatment arms.

A significant increase in serious (grade 3 to 4) hematologic adverse events was documented in both arms, including neutropenia (71% versus 12%), thrombocytopenia (35% versus 11%) and anemia (27% versus 8%). These adverse events appeared more commonly in the combination arm. The use of granulocyte colony-stimulating factor was more frequent in patients treated with carboplatin and gemcitabine (24% versus 10%).

The results of the AGO-OVAR 2.5 trial confirmed the superiority of platinum-based polychemotherapy over platinum salts in monotherapy.

The results of this clinical trial provide a treatment alternative to carboplatin/paclitaxel, with a different profile of toxicity, including less alopecia and neurotoxicity, which can affect the quality of life for women with ovarian cancer.

4.3. Carboplatin/paclitaxel versus carboplatin/Pegylated Liposomal Doxorubicin (PLD) (CALYPSO)

In an attempt to establish a new second-line treatment with improved tolerance and equal or greater efficacy than the standard treatment with carboplatin and paclitaxel, the CALYPSO clinical trial was designed [22].

In this trial, a total of 976 patients with histologically confirmed ovarian cancer with recurrence more than 6 months after first- or second-line platinum- and taxane-based therapies were randomly assigned to receive carboplatin AUC 5 on day 1 plus pegylated liposomal doxorubicin (PLD) 30 mg/m^2 on day 1, every 28 days, or carboplatin AUC 5 on day 1 plus paclitaxel 175 mg/m2 on day 1 at 3-week intervals for at least 6 cycles (in case of stabilization of disease or if partial response was achieved after 6 courses, the patients were allowed to receive therapy until progression). The platinum-free interval was greater than 12 months in 63.9% of patients.

The study was designed as a non-inferiority trial. The primary endpoint was progression-free survival, and secondary endpoints were toxicity, quality of life, and overall survival.

With a median follow-up of 22 months, PFS was statistically superior for patients treated with carboplatin/PLD than patients in the carboplatin/paclitaxel arm (11.3 versus 9.4 months with HR: 0.821; 95% CI, 0.72 to 0.94; p = 0.005).

Severe non-hematologic toxicity (grades 3 to 4) was more frequent in patients in the carboplatin/paclitaxel arm than in patients treated with carboplatin/PLD (36.8% versus 28.4%; p = 0.001). Grade 2 or greater palmar-plantar erythrodisestesia (12% versus 2.2%), nausea (35.2% versus 24.2%), vomiting (22.5% versus 15.6%) and mucositis (13.9% versus 7%) occurred more commonly in the carboplatin/PLD arm. Grade 2 or greater neurotoxicity (4.9% versus 26.9%), complete hair loss (7% versus 83.6%) and allergic/hypersensitivity reactions (5.6% versus 18.8%) were more frequent in patients treated with carboplatin and paclitaxel. The allergic/hypersensitivity reactions were mainly secondary to carboplatin administration and was the reason for significantly lower rates of early discontinuation of one or both drugs in the paclitaxel arm compared with the PLD arm (1% versus 6%; p > 0.001). Fewer patients discontinued treatment early for toxicity in the carboplatin/PLD arm (6% versus 15%; p < 0.001).

Regarding hematologic toxicities, they were generally similar between the treatment groups, although grades 3 to 4 neutropenia was more frequent in patients treated with carboplatin/paclitaxel (35.2% versus 45.7%) and grades 3 to 4 thrombocytopenia was more frequent in patients treated with carboplatin/PLD (15.9% versus 6.2%). There were no differences in febrile neutropenia or the use of supportive treatment (e.g., transfusion, granulocyte colony-stimulating factor).

Recently, data on the final OS were reported. With a median follow-up of 49 months, no statistically significant difference in OS was observed between the two arms (HR: 0.99; 95% CI: 0.85 - 1.16; p = 0.94). The median OS was 30.7 months in patients treated with carboplatin and PLD and 33.0 months for patients treated with carboplatin and paclitaxel. The authors rationalize this fact with an imbalanced post-study cross-over between arms, with a greater proportion of patients randomized to carboplatin/paclitaxel receiving post-study PLD (68%) than patients in the carboplatin/PLD arm receiving post-study paclitaxel (43%; p < 0.001) [23].

The improved disease-related outcomes achieved with carboplatin/PLD treatment were not at the expense of quality of life [24].

This study provides an optional scheme of treatment for patients with platinum-sensitive ovarian cancer, with a reduction in severe toxicities, including carboplatin hypersensitivity reactions and peripheral neurotoxicity, both of which can be a reason for limiting the dose. Carboplatin/PLD also induced far less alopecia, one of the most feared adverse effects of chemotherapy for the majority of women.

4.4. Carboplatin/gemcitabine versus carboplatin/gemcitabine/bevacizumab (OCEANS)

In ovarian cancer, as in other tumors, the addition of new treatments is required for improved outcomes.

In a phase III clinical trial, 484 patients with relapsed platinum-sensitive ovarian cancer were randomly assigned to receive Carboplatin AUC 4 on day 1 and Gemcitabine 1000 mg/m^2 on days 1 and 8, every 21 days with placebo, or bevacizumab 15 mg/kg on day 1, every 21 days [25]. After 6 to 10 cycles of chemotherapy, bevacizumab or placebo were continued until toxicity or progression. The primary endpoint was progression-free survival, and secondary endpoints were overall response rate, overall survival and the duration of response.

With a median follow-up of 24 months, the analysis showed an increase in PFS (12.4 versus 8.4 months with a HR of 0.484; 95% CI 0.388 to 0.605; $p < 0.0001$) and in the RR (78.5% versus 57.4%, $p < 0.0001$) for bevacizumab. The duration of response was also significantly increased with the addition of bevacizumab (10.4 versus 7.4 months; HR: 0.534; 95% CI: 0.408 - 0.698). With the number of events for the final analysis not yet reached, the OS was 35.2 months in the placebo arm versus 33.3 months in the bevacizumab arm. This could be related to subsequent therapy, including patients receiving bevacizumab in the placebo arm (31%).

The bevacizumab arm had a higher incidence of grade 3 or higher hypertension (17.4% versus 1%) and proteinuria (8.5% versus < 1%). There was no gastrointestinal perforation in any group.

This is the first positive phase III trial evaluating the addition of a targeting therapy to a standard platinum-based chemotherapy regimen for recurrent ovarian cancer.

4.5. New perspectives in the treatment of platinum-sensitive disease

The poly (adenosine diphosphate [ADP]-ribose) polymerases (PARPs) are a family of enzymes that play a role in the repair of DNA damage by repairing base excisions. The tumor-suppressor proteins BRCA1 and BRCA2 are components of the DNA repair pathway, and it is known that a germ-line mutation in BRCA1 or BRCA2 is associated with a high risk of the development of some cancers, including breast, prostate and ovarian cancer. Olaparib (AZD2281) is an oral PARP inhibitor that has shown activity in cancers associated with BRCA1 or BRCA2 mutations with an acceptable side-effect profile [26].

A randomized phase II clinical trial was designed to compare the efficacy of olaparib and PLD in patients with confirmed germ-line BRCA1 or BRCA2 mutations and recurrent or progressed ovarian cancer within 12 months of the most recent platinum-based chemotherapy regimen [27]. The primary endpoint was the progression-free survival by RECIST criteria, and secondary endpoints included the overall response rate, duration of treatment response, overall survival, safety and tolerability, and health-related quality of life. Ninety-seven patients were randomly assigned (1:1:1 ratio) to receive olaparib 200 mg twice per day, 400 mg twice per day continuously or PLD 50 mg/m^2 every 28 days. Patients were stratified by BRCA1 or BRCA2 status and platinum sensitivity (sensitive or resistant). There was no statistically significant difference in PFS between the olaparib 200 mg, olaparib 400 mg and PLD groups (6.5 months, 8.8 months and 7.1 months, respectively). The overall response rate was 25%, 31% and 18%, respectively, with no statistically significant difference. A similar duration of response was also observed (6.0, 6.8 and 5.5 months). There was no difference among groups in the OS or the health-related quality of life. Nausea, vomiting, fatigue and anemia were the most common adverse events related to olaparib; the adverse events related to PLD were stomatitis and palmo-plantar erythrodysesthesia.

In a second randomized phase II study, olaparib was evaluated in the maintenance treatment for patients with platinum-sensitive relapsed high-grade (grades 2 or 3) ovarian cancer who responded to their most recent platinum-based chemotherapy [28]. A total of 265 patients were randomized to receive olaparib 400 mg twice daily or placebo after completion of their last dose of platinum-based chemotherapy. The primary endpoint was progression-free survival; it was significantly longer in the olaparib group (8.4 months) than in the placebo group (4.8 months), with a hazard ratio for progression or death of 0.35 (95% CI 0.25 to 0.49; $p < 0.001$). Secondary efficacy endpoints were time to progression, objective response rate and overall survival. The time to progression was also significantly longer in patients treated with olaparib (8.3 versus 3.7 months; HR: 0.35; 95% CI 0.25 to 0.47; $p < 0.001$). According to the RECIST criteria, there was no difference in the response rate (12% versus 4%; $p = 0.12$) or in the overall survival in the interim analysis at 38% maturity (29.7 versus 29.9 months; $p = 0.75$). Nausea, vomiting, fatigue and anemia were the adverse events, with an incidence of at least 10% or higher in the olaparib group; the majority of them were grade 1 or 2.

The results of these two trials underline the necessity of further exploring the role of olaparib and other PARP inhibitors in the treatment of women with recurrent ovarian cancer. It may well be that their use has to be restricted to BRCA mutated patients, but a better definition of BRCAness should then be standardized. [29]

5. Treatment of platinum-resistant disease

Patients with platinum-resistant disease have a worse prognosis than patients with platinum-sensitive disease and a poorer response rate to cytostatic treatment. Although there is no clear recommendation for the standard treatment in these patients, there is a long list of drugs that have shown activity in phase II clinical trials in this situation: pegylated liposomal doxorubicin, topotecan, gemcitabine, paclitaxel, docetaxel, trabectedin, vinorelbine, ifosfamide, etoposide, and pemetrexed (Table 2).

Drug	Response rate	Main toxicity
Pegylated liposomal doxorubicin	20%	Hand-foot syndrome, mucositis
Topotecan	6 - 20%	Hematologic, alopecia
Gemcitabine	9 - 16%	Hematologic
Paclitaxel	13 - 17%	Neurotoxicity, alopecia
Docetaxel	23%	Hematologic
Trabectedin	6%	Hematologic
Vinorelbine	3 - 21%	Neutropenia
Ifosfamide	12%	Hematologic, central nervous toxicity
Etoposide	27%	Neutropenia
Pemetrexed	9 - 21%	Neutropenia, asthenia

Table 2. Response rate and toxicity for platinum-resistant disease

The comparisons between some of these drugs in phase III clinical trials do not yield superior results for any of the drugs in terms of overall or progression-free survival.

As explained, the response rate to platinum compounds is too low in patients with platinum-resistant disease, so monotherapy with a non-platinum drug is usually preferred because studies with doublets have not demonstrated superiority in platinum-resistant patients or either have presented greater toxicity [30 - 37].

Despite its frequent use in clinical practice, endocrine treatment (e.g., Tamoxifen, Letrozole) is not approved, and there is no good evidence supporting its use. Data on tamoxifen were obtained from observational studies, not comparative ones, and do not allow us to make any evidence-based recommendations [38]. In a phase II trial with letrozol carried out in 44 patients (half of them with platinum-resistant disease) who had primary tumors that expressed the estrogen receptor, a 9% overall response and 42% stabilization at 12 weeks was obtained in 33 patients with radiologically measurable disease, with a minimal toxicity [39]. In any case, there are worse data in the literature on the impact of endocrine therapy versus chemotherapy on progression-free survival [40]. Unfortunately, there are no phase III trials to make any recommendations about the use of hormone treatment in relapsed ovarian cancer.

The main phase III clinical trials comparing different agents in platinum-resistant relapsed ovarian cancer are shown below.

5.1. Topotecan versus paclitaxel

Topotecan and paclitaxel are active in platinum-resistant relapsed ovarian cancer. To compare the activity of these two drugs in this setting, a phase III clinical trial was conducted in patients who had progressed during or after platinum-based therapy [41, 42]. A total of 226 patients were randomized to receive chemotherapy with topotecan 1.5 mg/m^2/24 h on 5 consecutive days, every 21 days (112 patients), or paclitaxel 175 mg/m^2, every 21 days (114 patients). The duration of treatment was dependent on response. Patients with a complete or partial response continued treatment until progression or for 6 months past the maximal response. Patients who progressed were removed from the study and patients with stable disease after six courses were removed from the study or switched to the alternate regimen (the study allowed crossover of the arms). None of the patients had previously received topotecan or paclitaxel (not included in standard first-line therapy as of now). Patients were stratified as platinum-resistant or as early, interim and late relapse groups. In the study, 53% of the patients did not respond to platinum-based treatment or had progression within 6 months; they had platinum-resistant disease (55% in the topotecan group and 52% in the paclitaxel group).

The primary efficacy parameters were the response rate, duration of response and time to progression. The secondary criteria for efficacy were the time to response and survival.

In the whole group of patients in the study, no differences in the response rates (topotecan 20.5% versus paclitaxel 13.2%; p = 0.138) or in the median survival (63 weeks for topotecan versus 53 weeks for paclitaxel, p = 0.44) were achieved. The duration of response was 32.1 weeks in patients treated with topotecan and 19.7 weeks in patients treated with paclitaxel (p = 0.222). There was no statistically significant difference in the time to progression after therapy (18.9 weeks for topotecan versus 14.7 weeks for paclitaxel; p = 0.08). The median time to documented radiologic response was inferior in the paclitaxel group (6 weeks) than in the topotecan group (9 weeks; p = 0.041).

Among platinum-resistant patients, the response rates were superior in the topotecan group than in the paclitaxel group (13.1 versus 6.7%, p = 0.303), and the median overall survival was 28.4 weeks in the topotecan group and 39.7 weeks in patients treated with paclitaxel.

Patients who had no ascites, better performance status and a smaller tumor burden had higher response rates.

The results of questionnaires on the quality of life, including pain, anorexia, diarrhea, fatigue, nausea and vomiting, dyspnea, constipation and insomnia, were similar in both groups.

Different toxicities were observed in the two groups. Hematologic toxicity was more frequent in the topotecan group, including grade 4 neutropenia (79% versus 23% in paclitaxel group; p < 0.01) and grade 4 thrombocytopenia (25% versus 2% in paclitaxel group; p < 0.01). Other toxicities more frequent in patients treated with topotecan were fatigue, nausea and vomiting (generally grades 1 – 2). Patients in the paclitaxel group experienced more alopecia, arthralgia, myalgia and neurotoxicity.

Patients who received topotecan after paclitaxel in their third-line treatment had an overall response rate of 13%, compared to 10% (p = 0.638) in patients who received paclitaxel after topotecan. The data analysis for those patients receiving the other drug (paclitaxel or topotecan) in the third-line therapy showed that there was a degree of non-cross-resistance between them [43]. Therefore, the use of paclitaxel in first-line therapy does not prevent the administration of topotecan in relapsed epithelial ovarian cancer.

5.2. Paclitaxel versus pegylated liposomal doxorubicin

One study compared PLD 50 mg/m^2 every 4 weeks versus paclitaxel 175 mg/m^2 every 3 weeks in 214 patients with relapsed epithelial ovarian cancer [44].

There were no differences in the response rates among patients who received pegylated liposomal doxorubicin and patients who received paclitaxel (17.8% versus 22.4%; p = 0.034). There was also no difference in the PFS (21.7 weeks versus 22.4 weeks; p = 0.15) or OS (45.7 weeks versus 56.1 weeks; p = 0.44).

There were no observed differences in the PFS or OS in platinum-resistant or platinum-sensitive patients.

In the PLD group, hand-foot syndrome, stomatitis, nausea, and vomiting were more frequent. Conversely, alopecia, myalgia, arthralgia, and paresthesia were more frequent in the paclitaxel group.

5.3. Pegylated liposomal doxorubicin versus topotecan

To compare the efficacy and safety of PLD and topotecan in relapsed ovarian cancer after chemotherapy with platinum and taxanes, a phase III clinical trial was carried out in 474 patients [45, 46].

Patients were randomized to receive treatment with PLD 50 mg/m^2 every 28 days (239 patients), or topotecan 1.5 mg/m^2/24 h on 5 consecutive days, every 21 days (235 patients). The primary endpoint was time to progression, and the secondary endpoints included overall survival, response rate, time to response, duration of response and toxicity. The trial included 54% of the platinum-resistant patients in the PLD group and 53% of such patients in the topotecan group.

There was no difference in the rate of response between the two groups (19.7% in patients treated with PLD versus 17% in patients treated with topotecan; p = 0.390). A reduction in the risk of death by 18% was achieved in the group of patients treated with PLD compared to topotecan (HR = 1.216: 95% CI 1.000 to 1.478, p = 0.050). The median survival was 62.7 weeks in the PLD group versus 59.7 weeks in the topotecan group.

In the platinum-sensitive population, there were benefits in survival among patients treated with PLD, with a reduced risk of death by 30% (HR 1.432, 95% CI 1.066 to 1.923, p = 0.017) and a median survival of 107.9 weeks in the PLD group compared to 70.1 weeks in the topotecan group. The progression-free survival was 28.9 weeks for the PLD group and 23.3 weeks for the topotecan group (p =0.037), although the response rate was similar between the two groups (28.4% in the PLD group versus 28.8% in the topotecan group, p = 0.964).

http://dx.doi.org/10.5772/54171

In the subgroup of platinum-resistant patients, (54% of the population of the study; 255 patients) there were no statistically significant differences in the response rate (12.3% for PLD and 6.5% for topotecan, p = 0.118), the PFS (9.1 weeks in patients who received PLD compared to 13.6 weeks in the topotecan group, p = 0.733), or OS (35.6 weeks for the PLD group and 41.3 for the topotecan group, p = 0.455, with a HR = 1.069, 95% CI 0.823 to 1.387, p = 0.618).

The toxicity profiles of the two drugs were different. The main toxicities in patients treated with PLD were hand-foot syndrome (49%) and stomatitis (40%). The main toxicities in patients treated with topotecan were hematological toxicity, so they were more likely to receive granulocyte colony-stimulating factor (29.1%), erythropoietin (23.1%) and transfusions (57.8%). Moreover, the toxicity caused by PLD was usually mild to moderate, while the toxicity caused by topotecan was more severe. Despite this difference, there was no difference in the health-related quality of life questionnaire at 12 weeks.

5.4. Gemcitabine versus pegylated liposomal doxorubicin

Two randomized phase III trials compared gemcitabine with PLD in patients with platinum-resistant disease.

The first trial [47] was carried out in 195 patients with platinum-resistant ovarian cancer who were randomly assigned to receive gemcitabine 1000 mg/m^2 on days 1 and 8, every 21 days, or PLD 50 mg/m^2 every 28 days until the progression of disease or unacceptable toxicity. Cross-over treatment was administered at progression. The primary endpoint was progression-free survival, and secondary endpoints were response rate, time to treatment failure, survival and quality of life.

The response rate was similar in both groups (9.2% for gemcitabine versus 11.7% for PLD, p = 0.772). There was no difference in the progression-free survival between patients treated with gemcitabine and patients treated with PLD (3.6 months versus 3.1 months, p = 0.870). The overall survival was similar in patients treated with gemcitabine followed by PLD and patients who received the inverse sequence (12.7 months versus 13.5 months, p = 0.997).

The toxicity profiles were different, with more hand-foot syndrome and stomatitis in the PLD arm and increased constipation, nausea and vomiting, fatigue and neutropenia in the gemcitabine arm. During the cross-over treatment, toxicity was similar to those observed during the initial treatment phase.

In a second study [48], 153 patients previously treated with platinum/paclitaxel who had relapsed or progressed within 12 months (53% within 6 months) were randomized to receive gemcitabine 1000 mg/m^2 on days 1, 8 and 15, every 28 days, or PLD 40 mg/m^2 every 28 days.

There were no differences in the response rate (29% for gemcitabine versus 16% for PLD, p = 0.066) or time to progression (20 weeks in gemcitabine group versus 16 weeks in PLD group, p = 0.411). Although the overall survival was higher in the PLD arm (51 weeks versus 56 weeks, p = 0.048), this difference was not detected in the platinum-resistant subgroup (relapse or progression < 6 months). The toxicity profile was similar to the previous study. Health-related quality of life favored the PLD arm.

5.5. Canfosfamide versus pegylated liposomal doxorubicin or topotecan

A phase III clinical trial (ASSIST-1) was designed to attempt to demonstrate superiority in the overall survival (primary endpoint) and progression-free survival (secondary endpoint) with canfosfamide versus PLD or topotecan in patients who progressed despite second-line treatment with either topotecan or PLD in platinum-refractory or -resistant patients [49].

The study included 461 patients randomized to an active control arm (PLD 50 mg/m^2 every 28 days or topotecan 1.5 mg/m^2 on days 1 – 5, every 21 days, based on the prior therapy) or canfosfamide 1000 mg/m^2 every 21 days.

The median overall survival was 8.5 months with canfosfamide and 13.5 months in the control arm ($p < 0.01$). The median OS was similar between PLD and topotecan (14.2 versus 10.8 months; $p = 0.1695$). The progression-free survival was longer for patients treated in the control group than for patients in the canfosfamide group (4.3 versus 2.3 months; $p < 0.01$). Hematologic adverse events were more frequent in the control arm, and non-hematologic adverse events were similar in both arms.

6. Extending the platinum-free interval

The cells of ovarian cancer could have intrinsic or acquired resistance to platinum compounds, which is a large clinical obstacle in the treatment of women with relapsed ovarian cancer. There are several mechanisms by which tumor cells can develop resistance to platinum, including increased efflux, enhanced DNA repair of damage caused by chemotherapy and defective cell death pathways. Some of these mechanisms may be reversible with time. It has been hypothesized that artificially extending the platinum-free interval with non-cross-resistant chemotherapy may improve the likelihood of responding to platinum salts subsequently administered and prolong the overall survival [35, 50, 51].

Recently, the OVA-301 trial [35] randomized 672 women with recurrent ovarian cancer to receive trabectedin 1.1 mg/m^2 plus PLD 30 mg/m^2 every 21 days, or PLD 50 mg/m^2 every 28 days. The primary endpoint was progression-free survival, and secondary endpoints included overall survival and safety. The PFS was higher in the combination group in the overall population of the study (7.3 versus 5.8 months; $HR = 0.79$, $p = 0.0190$) and in the platinum-sensitive patients (9.2 versus 7.5 months; $HR = 0.73$, $p = 0.0170$). The most common adverse effects were hand-foot syndrome in the PLD group and neutropenia and a transient ALT increase in the PLD/trabectedin group. After a median follow-up of 47.4 months, no difference in overall survival was observed (22.2 months in the combination group versus 18.9 months in the PLD group; $HR = 0.86$, $p = 0.0835$). Despite stratification based on platinum sensitivity, the authors detected an imbalance in the mean platinum-free interval, which favored the PLD group (13.3 versus 10.6 months; $p = 0.009$) [36].

Furthermore, the data reported in patients with a platinum-free interval of 6 - 12 months are especially interesting. These are the patients who can obtain the most benefit from an extension in the platinum-free interval. In this population, the median PFS was 7.4 months in the PLD/ trabectedin group versus 5.5 months in the PLD group (HR = 0.65; p = 0.0152) [52]. The median OS was 22.4 months in the PLD/trabectedin group versus 16.4 months in the monotherapy arm (HR = 0.64; p = 0.0027) [36].

In the OVA-301 study, similar proportions of patients received subsequent therapy in each arm (77% and 76%), with 56% and 57% receiving platinum-based therapies in the 6 - 12 months subgroup. In this subgroup, the time from randomization to subsequent platinum-based therapy was significantly longer for patients treated with PLD/trabectedin (9.8 versus 7.9 months; p = 0.0167). Patients randomized to the combination group experienced significantly longer survival after the initiation of subsequent platinum-based therapy (13.3 versus 9.8 months; HR = 0.63, p = 0.0357) [52]. These data support the hypothesis that the enhanced survival benefits may be due to an artificial extension of the platinum-free interval. In any case, this hypothesis should be confirmed in prospective randomized trials.

When the data on patients who received platinum-based therapy as the first subsequent treatment after PLD/trabectedin or PLD in the 6 - 12 months subset were analyzed, platinum was delayed 4 months (11.5 versus 7.5 months; HR: 0.61, p = 0.0203) and the overall survival from the first platinum treatment was significantly extended by a median of 8.7 months (18.6 versus 9.9 months; HR = 0.54, p = 0.0169) [53].

The delay in platinum re-treatment could promote the recovery from toxicities, such as polyneuropathy or alopecia.

7. Discussion

As previously shown, a longer platinum-free interval is the most important factor associated with a higher likelihood of response and prolongation of progression-free survival. Therefore, patients who relapse after six months of completion of chemotherapy and are responders are candidates for re-treatment with platinum salts.

The considerations in the choice of a second and subsequent line of chemotherapy in recurrent ovarian cancer may also include assessment of efficacy, cumulative toxicities and the optimal sequencing of available agents.

Currently, in patients with platinum-sensitive disease, it is preferred to administer a combination regimen including a platinum compound and a second active drug (Table 3). The platinum compound most commonly used is carboplatin, due to its better toxicity profile. These treatments provide a high response rate and significant improvements in the quality of life and progression-free survival compared to platinum monotherapy. However, the ideal platinum combination is unknown, and several regimens are available. Recently, schemes without platinum, such as PLD/trabectedin, have been developed and can be useful. Nevertheless, there are no data comparing these regimens to platinum-based schemes, so we must be prudent.

Clinical Trial	Scheme	Patients	RR	PFS	OS
ICON4/AGO-OVAR 2.2 [20]	C vs. C/P	n = 802	54% vs. 66%	9 vs. 12 m	24 vs. 29 m
AGO-OVAR 2.5 [24]	C vs. C/Gem	n = 356	30.9 vs. 47.2%	5.8 vs. 8.6 m	18 vs. 17.3 m
CALYPSO [25]	C/P vs. C/PLD	n = 976	Not achieved	9.4 vs. 11.3 m	33 vs. 30.7 m
OCEANS [28]	C/Gem/Pl vs. C/Gem/Bev	n = 484	57.4% vs. 78.5%	8.4 vs. 12.4 m	35.2 vs. 33.3 m

Abbreviations: RR: response rate. PFS: progression-free survival. OS: overall survival. C: carboplatin. P: paclitaxel. Gem: gemcitabine. PLD: pegylated liposomal doxorubicin, m: months.

Table 3. Main phase III clinical trials in platinum-sensitive relapsed ovarian cancer

The ICON4/AGO-OVAR 2.2 trial was the first clinical trial that showed the superiority of polychemotherapy to monotherapy in patients with platinum-sensitive relapsed ovarian cancer. The combination of carboplatin and paclitaxel may be used in patients who have no residual neurotoxicity, especially if the platinum-free interval is greater than one year.

A valid alternative is the administration of carboplatin plus PLD (CALYPSO), which has demonstrated similar efficacy to carboplatin/paclitaxel and a more favorable toxicity profile, with less alopecia, neurotoxicity and allergic/hypersensitivity reactions. Perhaps this is the most commonly used scheme by oncologists worldwide, now conditioned by a globally limited availability of PLD.

Although no survival benefit was achieved in the AGO-OVAR 2.5 trial with carboplatin and gemcitabine, the results of this clinical trial allow us to recommend this chemotherapy scheme as an alternative to carboplatin/paclitaxel, due to its different, and perhaps more favorable, toxicity profile. This scheme is especially useful for patients with risk factors for neurotoxicity development. The addition of an anti-angiogenic drug, such as bevacizumab (OCEANS), can improve outcomes without a significant increase in toxicity.

The incorporation of new active drugs into the treatment of patients with platinum-sensitive ovarian cancer is also important. Thus, we must be aware of the results of the phase III clinical trial, HECTOR (ClinicalTrials.gov Identifier: NCT00437307), which compares the combination of carboplatin plus topotecan with the current standard of care (carboplatin/paclitaxel, carboplatin/gemcitabine or carboplatin/PLD). The trial may be completed in 2013.

Because the response rate to platinum salts is too low in patients with platinum-resistant disease, monotherapy with a non-platinum drug is usually the choice in this setting. Comparisons of the efficacy of different active drugs in phase III clinical trials show no superiority of any of them, and there is no clear recommendation for the standard treatment in these patients. Therefore, the selection of treatment for platinum-resistant patients will be based on other criteria, such as toxicity, patient preferences and physician experience. Whenever possible, patients with platinum-resistant disease should be considered for treatment in clinical trials.

Recurrent platinum-resistant ovarian cancer has limited treatment options and is generally treated sequentially with multiple single-agent regimens consisting of non-platinum and non-taxane chemotherapy.

The most common options are PLD, topotecan and gemcitabine. These options have been compared in several phase III clinical trials (Table 4), but none of the options have proven superior. PLD and gemcitabine could be used in patients who do not desire alopecia. Additionally, PLD is dosed less frequently than topotecan and gemcitabine, which results in improved convenience for the patient and a reduction in the use of resources.

Subsequent lines of treatment will be made with available drugs.

Author, year	Drugs	Patients	RR	PFS	OS
ten Bokkel Huinink W, 2004	Topotecan vs. Paclitaxel	n = 226	13.1% vs. 6.7%**	23.1 vs. 14 w*	28.4 vs. 39.7 w**
O'Byrne KJ, 2002	Paclitaxel vs. PLD	n = 214	22.4% vs. 17.8%*	22.4 vs. 21.7 w*	56.1 vs. 45.7 w*
Gordon AN, 2004	PLD vs. Topotecan	n = 474	12.3% vs. 6.5%**	9.1 vs. 13.6 w**	35.6 vs. 41.3 w**
Mutch DG, 2007	Gemcitabine vs. PLD	n = 195	9.2% vs. 11.7%**	3.6 vs. 3.1 m**	12.7 vs. 13.5 m**
Ferrandina G, 2008	Gemcitabine vs. PLD	n = 153	29% vs. 16%*	20 vs. 16 w*	51 vs. 56 w*

*Data from the whole group

**Data from platinum-resistant patients

Abbreviations: RR: response rate, PFS: progression-free survival, OS: overall survival, PLD: pegylated liposomal doxorubicin, w: weeks, m: months.

Table 4. Main phase III clinical trials including platinum-resistant relapsed ovarian cancer

Recently, the use of non-platinum agents in relapsed ovarian cancer to extend the platinum-free interval has gained interest. The answer to the question of whether the prolongation of the platinum-free interval increases overall survival after the reintroduction of platinum should be revealed by two phase III trials currently in progress. The MITO-8 (ClinicalTrials.gov Identifier: NCT00657878) trial compares carboplatin/paclitaxel followed by PLD versus the reverse sequence (PLD followed by carboplatin/paclitaxel), and the INOVATYON trial (ClinicalTrial.gov identifier: NCT01379989) compares the administration of carboplatin/PLD followed by treatment at the discretion of the investigator versus PLD/trabectedin followed by a platinum-based.

Author details

Miguel Angel Alonso Bermejo[1], Ana Fernandez Montes[1*], Eva Perez Lopez[1], Miguel Angel Nuñez Viejo[2], Jesus Garcia Gomez[1] and Jesus Garcia Mata[1]

*Address all correspondence to: afm1003@hotmail.com

1 Medical Oncology Service at the University Hospital Ourense, Ourense, Spain

2 Palliative Care Department at the University Hospital Ourense, Ourense, Spain

References

[1] Díaz-montes, T. P, & Bristow, R. E. Secondary cytoreduction for patients with recurrent ovarian cancer. Curr Oncol Rep (2005). , 7(6), 451-8.

[2] National Comprehensive Cancer NetworkNCCN Guidelines for Treatment of Cancer by Site. Ovarian Cancer ~ (2012). Available at: http://www.nccn.org/professionals/physician_gls/pdf/ovarian.pdfAccessed Aug 15, 2012)., 3

[3] Colombo, N, Peiretti, M, Parma, G, et al. Newly diagnosed and relapsed epithelial ovarian carcinoma: ESMO Clinical Practice Guidelines for diagnosis, treatment and follow-up. Ann Oncol (2010). Suppl 5:, 23-30

[4] Chan, K. K, Tam, K. F, Tse, K. Y, et al. The role of regular physical examination in the detection of ovarian cancer recurrence. Gynecol Oncol (2008). , 110(2), 158-61.

[5] Menczer, J, Chetrit, A, Sadetzki, S, et al. Follow-up of ovarian and primary peritoneal carcinoma: the value of physical examination in patients with pretreatment elevated CA 125 levels. Gynecol Oncol (2006). , 103(1), 137-40.

[6] Gadducci, A, & Cosio, S. Surveillance of patients after initial treatment of ovarian cancer. Crit Rev Oncol Hematol (2009). , 71(1), 43-52.

[7] Rustin, G. J, Nelstrop, A. E, Tuxen, M. K, et al. Defining progression of ovarian carcinoma during follow-up according to CA 125: a North Thames Ovary Group Study. Ann Oncol (1996). , 7(4), 361-4.

[8] Rustin, G. J, Marples, M, Nelstrop, A. E, et al. Use of CA-125 to define progression of ovarian cancer in patients with persistently elevated levels. J Clin Oncol (2001). , 19(20), 4054-7.

[9] Rustin, G. J. Follow-up with CA 125 after primary therapy of advanced ovarian cancer has major implications for treatment outcome and trial performances and should not be routinely performed. Ann Oncol (2011). Suppl 8:viiiviii48., 45.

[10] Yin, B. W, & Lloyd, K. O. Molecular cloning of the CA 125 ovarian cancer antigen: identification as a new mucin, MUC16. J Biol Chem (2001). , 276(29), 27371-5.

[11] Markman, M, Rothman, R, Hakes, T, et al. Second-line platinum therapy in patients with ovarian cancer previously treated with cisplatin. J Clin Oncol (1991). , 9(3), 389-93.

[12] Markman, M, & Hoskins, W. Responses to salvage chemotherapy in ovarian cancer: a critical need for precise definitions of the treated population. J Clin Oncol (1992). , 10(4), 513-4.

[13] Thigpen, J. T, & Vance, R. B. T. Khansur Second-line chemotherapy for recurrent carcinoma of the ovary. Cancer (1993). Suppl):, 1559-64.

[14] Berek, J. S, & Bertelsen, K. du Bois A, et al. Advanced epithelial ovarian cancer: 1998 consensus statements. Ann Oncol (1999). SS92., 87.

[15] Paclitaxelpegylated liposomal doxorubicin hydrochloride and topotecan for second-line or subsequent treatment of advanced ovarian cancer. Technology appraisal 91. London: National Institute for Health and Clinical Excellence; (2005). available at: http://www.nice.org.uk/nicemedia/pdf/TA091guidance.pdfAccessed Aug 17, 2012).

[16] Stuart, G, Kitchener, H, Bacon, M, et al. Gynecologic Cancer InterGroup (GCIG) Consensus Statement on Clinical Trials in Ovarian Cancer. Report From the Fourth Ovarian Cancer Consensus Conference. Int J Gynecol Cancer (2011). , 21(4), 750-55.

[17] Parmar, M. K, Ledermann, J. A, Colombo, N, et al. Paclitaxel plus platinum-based chemotherapy versus conventional platinum-based chemotherapy in women with relapsed ovarian cancer: the ICON4/AGO-OVAR-2.2 trial. Lancet (2003). , 361(9375), 2099-106.

[18] González-martín, A, Calvo, E, Bover, I, et al. Randomized phase II trial of carboplatin versus paclitaxel and carboplatin in platinum-sensitive recurrent advanced ovarian carcinoma: a GEICO (Grupo Español de Investigación en Cáncer de Ovario) study. Ann Oncol (2005). , 16, 749-55.

[19] Lee, J. J, & Swain, S. M. Peripheral neuropathy induced by microtubule-stabilizing agents. J Clin Oncol (2006). , 24(10), 1633-42.

[20] Jones, S. E, Erban, J, Overmoyer, B, et al. Randomized phase III study of docetaxel compared with paclitaxel in metastatic breast cancer. J Clin Oncol (2005). , 23(24), 5542-51.

[21] Pfisterer, J, Plante, M, Vergote, I, et al. Gemcitabine plus carboplatin compared with carboplatin in patients with platinum-sensitive recurrent ovarian cancer: an intergroup trial of the AGO-OVAR, the NCIC CTG, and the EORTC GCG. J Clin Oncol (2006). , 24(29), 4699-707.

[22] Pujade-lauraine, E, Wagner, U, Aavall-lundqvist, E, et al. Pegylated Liposomal Doxorubicin and Carboplatin compared with Paclitaxel and Carboplatin for patients

with platinum-sensitive ovarian cancer in late relapse. J Clin Oncol (2010). , 28(20), 3323-9.

[23] Wagner, U, Marth, C, Largillier, R, et al. Final overall survival results of phase III GCIG CALYPSO trial of pegylated liposomal doxorubicin and carboplatin vs paclitaxel and carboplatin in platinum-sensitive ovarian cancer patients. Br J Cancer (2012). , 107(4), 588-91.

[24] Brundage, M, Gropp, M, Mefti, F, et al. Health-related quality of life in recurrent platinum-sensitive ovarian cancer-- results from the CALYPSO trial. Ann Oncol (2012). , 23(8), 2020-7.

[25] Aghajanian, C, Blank, S. V, Goff, B. A, et al. OCEANS: A randomized, double-blind, placebo-controlled phase III trial of chemotherapy with or without bevacizumab in patients with platinum-sensitive recurrent epithelial ovarian, primary peritoneal, or fallopian tube cancer. J Clin Oncol (2012). , 30(17), 2039-45.

[26] Fong, P. C, Boss, D. S, Yap, T. A, et al. Inhibition of poly(ADP-ribose) polymerase in tumors from BRCA mutation carriers. N Engl J Med (2009). , 361(2), 123-34.

[27] Kaye, S. B, Lubinski, J, Matulonis, U, et al. Phase II, Open-Label, Randomized, Multicenter Study Comparing the Efficacy and Safety of Olaparib, a Poly (ADP-Ribose) Polymerase Inhibitor, and Pegylated Liposomal Doxorubicin in Patients With BRCA1 or BRCA2 Mutations and Recurrent Ovarian Cancer. J Clin Oncol (2012). , 30(4), 372-9.

[28] Ledermann, J, Harter, P, Gourley, C, et al. Olaparib maintenance therapy in platinum-sensitive relapsed ovarian cancer. N Engl J Med (2012). , 366(15), 1382-92.

[29] Tan, D. S, Rothermundt, C, Thomas, K, et al. BRCAness syndrome in ovarian cancer: a case-control study describing the clinical features and outcome of patients with epithelial ovarian cancer associated with BRCA1 and BRCA2 mutations. J Clin Oncol (2008). , 26(34), 5530-36.

[30] Garcia, A. A, Meara, O, & Bahador, A. A, et al. Phase II study of gemcitabine and weekly paclitaxel in recurrent platinum-resistant ovarian cancer. Gynecol Oncol (2004). , 93(2), 493-8.

[31] Sehouli, J, Stengel, D, Oskay-oezcelik, G, et al. Nonplatinum topotecan combinations versus topotecan alone for recurrent ovarian cancer: results of a phase III study of the North-Eastern German Society of Gynecological Oncology Ovarian Cancer Study Group. J Clin Oncol (2008). , 26(19), 3176-82.

[32] Joly, F, Petit, T, Pautier, P, et al. Weekly combination of topotecan and gemcitabine in early recurrent ovarian cancer patients: a French multicenter phase II study. Gynecol Oncol (2009). , 115(3), 382-8.

[33] Mirza, M. R, Lund, B, Lindegaard, J. C, et al. A phase II study of combination chemotherapy in early relapsed epithelial ovarian cancer using gemcitabine and pegylated liposomal doxorubicin. Gynecol Oncol (2010). , 26-31.

[34] Vergote, I, Finkler, N. J, Hall, J. B, et al. Randomized phase III study of canfosfamide in combination with pegylated liposomal doxorubicin compared with pegylated liposomal doxorubicin alone in platinum-resistant ovarian cancer. Int J Gynecol Cancer (2010). , 20(5), 772-80.

[35] Monk, B. J, Herzog, T. J, Kaye, S. B, et al. Trabectedin plus Pegylated Liposomal Doxorubicin in recurrent ovarian cancer. J Clin Oncol (2010). , 28(19), 3107-14.

[36] Monk, B. J, Herzog, T. J, Kaye, S. B, et al. Trabectedin plus pegylated liposomal doxorubicin (PLD) versus PLD in recurrent ovarian cancer: Overall survival analysis. Eur J Cancer (2012). , 2361-68.

[37] Garcia, A. A, Yessaian, A, Pham, H, et al. Phase II study of Gemcitabine and Docetaxel in recurrent platinum resistant ovarian cancer. Cancer Invest (2012). , 30(4), 295-9.

[38] Williams, C, Simera, I, & Bryant, A. Tamoxifen for relapse of ovarian cancer. Cochrane Database Syst Rev (2010). CD001034.

[39] Smyth, J. F, Gourley, C, Walker, G, et al. Antiestrogen therapy is active in selected ovarian cancer cases: the use of letrozole in estrogen receptor-positive patients. Clin Cancer Res (2007). , 13(12), 3617-22.

[40] Kristensen, G, Kaern, J, Baekelandt, M, et al. Chemotherapy versus hormonal treatment in patients with platinum and taxane resistant ovarian cancer: a NSGO study. J Clin Oncol (2008). suppl)[abstract 5508].

[41] ten Bokkel Huinink WGore M, Carmichael J, et al. Topotecan versus Paclitaxel for he treatment of recurrent epithelial ovarian cancer. J Clin Oncol (1997). , 15(6), 2183-93.

[42] ten Bokkel Huinink WLane SR, Ross GA, et al. Long-term survival in a phase III, randomised study of topotecan versus paclitaxel in advanced epithelial ovarian carcinoma. Ann Oncol (2004). , 15(1), 100-3.

[43] Gore, M. ten Bokkel Huinnink W, Carmichael J, et al. Clinical evidence for topotecan-paclitaxel non--cross-resistance in ovarian cancer. J Clin Oncol (2001). , 19(7), 1893-900.

[44] Byrne, O, Bliss, K. J, & Graham, P. JD, et al. A phase III study of Doxil/Caelyx versus paclitaxel in platinum-treated, taxane-naive relapsed ovarian cancer. Proc Am Soc Clin Oncol 21:(2002). abstr 808).

[45] Gordon, A. N, Fleagle, J. T, Guthrie, D, et al. Recurrent epithelial ovarian carcinoma: a randomized phase III study of pegylated liposomal doxorrubicin versus topotecan. J Clin Oncol (2001). , 19(14), 3312-22.

[46] Gordon, A. N, Tonda, M, Sun, S, et al. Long-term survival advantage for women treated with pegylated liposomal doxorrubicin compared with topotecan in a phase 3

randomized study of recurrent and refractory epithelial ovarian cancer. Gynecol Oncol (2004). , 95(1), 1-8.

[47] Mutch, D. G, Orlando, M, Goss, T, et al. Randomized phase III trial of gemcitabine compared with pegylated liposomal doxorrubicin in patients with platinum-resistant ovarian cancer. J Clin Oncol (2007). , 25(19), 2811-8.

[48] Ferrandina, G, Ludovisi, M, Lorusso, D, et al. Phase III Trial of Gemcitabine compared with Pegylated Liposomal Doxorubicin in progressive or recurrent ovarian cancer. J Clin Oncol (2008). , 26(6), 890-6.

[49] Vergote, I, & Finkler, N. del Campo J, et al. Phase 3 randomised study of canfosfamide (Telcyta®, TLK286) versus pegylated liposomal doxorubicin or topotecan as third-line therapy in patients with platinum-refractory or-resistant ovarian cancer. Eur J Cancer (2009). , 45(13), 2324-32.

[50] Colombo, N, & Gore, M. Treatment of recurrent ovarian cancer relapsing 6-12 months post platinum-based chemotherapy. Crit Rev Oncol Hematol (2007). , 64(2), 129-38.

[51] Bookman, M. A. Extending the platinum-free interval in recurrent ovarian cancer: the role of Topotecan in second-line chemotherapy. Oncologist (1999).

[52] Poveda, A, Vergote, I, Tjulandin, S, et al. Trabectedin plus pegylated liposomal doxorubicin in relapsed ovarian cancer: outcomes in the partially platinum-sensitive (platinum-free interval 6-12 months) subpopulation of OVA-301 phase III randomized trial. Ann Oncol (2011). , 22(1), 39-48.

[53] Kaye, S. B, Colombo, N, Monk, B. J, et al. Trabectedin plus pegylated liposomal doxorubicin in relapsed ovarian cancer delays third-line chemotherapy and prolongs the platinum-free interval. Ann Oncol (2011). , 22(1), 49-58.

Chapter 10

Molecular Mechanisms of Platinum Resistance in Ovarian Cancer

Gonzalo Tapia and Ivan Diaz-Padilla

Additional information is available at the end of the chapter

http://dx.doi.org/10.5772/55562

1. Introduction

In 2012, approximately 22,280 women will be diagnosed with ovarian carcinoma in the United States and roughly 15,500 will die from this disease, ranked the most common cause of death among gynecologic malignancies in developed countries [1]. Most women with epithelial ovarian cancer (EOC) present with advanced disease (stage III or IV) at the time of diagnosis. This phenomenon is mainly due to the lack of specific symptoms until disease has spread beyond the ovaries, at which time the chance of cure is dramatically reduced [2]. Current standard treatment of ovarian cancer, in both early and advanced stages, consists of complete cytoreductive surgery followed by chemotherapy, usually based on a platinum and a taxane doublet [3,4,5]. Initial response rate (RR) is high (70%-80%); but the majority of patients with advanced disease relapse within two years. Recurrent ovarian cancer is not curable, due to the development of chemoresistance [6,7]. The Gynecologic Oncology Group (GOG) adopted the definition of sensitivity to chemotherapy (or sensitivity to platinum) in EOC based on clinical criteria from retrospective case series [8]. When patients were re-challenged with a platinum compound the longer the interval from the last dose of platinum patients had received the better the response (and outcome) was. This clinical observation set the base for the current classification of platinum resistance in relapsed EOC (Figure 1), and allowed the commonly used stratification criteria in clinical trials of recurrent EOC. Platinum-resistant disease is also characterized by resistance to other cytotoxic agents, and not necessarily only resistant to platinum. However, current treatment for platinum-resistant EOC consists of chemotherapy agents whose mechanism of action is somewhat different from that of platinum compounds [9].

Since platinum compounds are the backbone in the systemic treatment of EOC, there is great interest in elucidate the molecular mechanisms contributing to platinum resistance in this disease. The present chapter will provide a comprehensive basic and translational update with

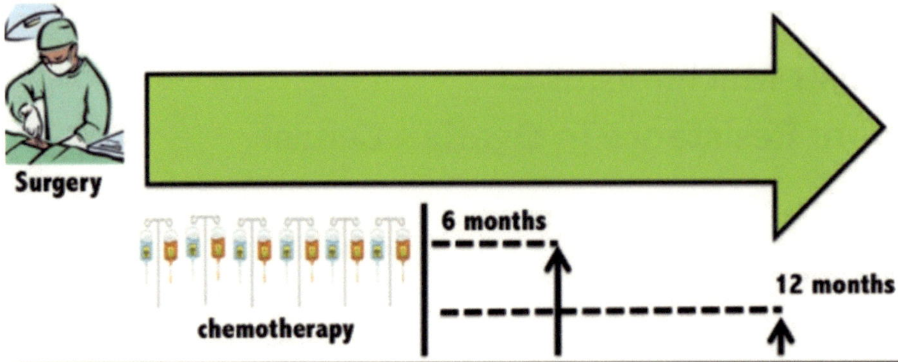

Platinum sensitivity classification	Refractory	Resistant	Partially sensitive	Sensitive
Probability of second platinum response	0%	< 10%	30%	> 50%

Figure 1. Platinum-resistance definition by the Gynecologic Oncology Group (GOG). Platinum sensitivity is classified as resistant, partially sensitive, or sensitive, according to the time relapsed since finishing first-line treatment. Probability of re-treatment response is shown for each group of patients.

regards to biological pathways implicated in the development of platinum resistance, focusing on ovarian cancer therapeutics.

2. Cisplatin: Mechanism of action

Once introduced actively into the cell mediated by a copper transporter (CTR1), the molecule is activated through a series of aquation reactions, in which one of the chloride ligands is slowly displaced by water. Aquated cisplatin avidly binds DNA, with a predilection for nucleophilic N7-sites on purine bases [10]. The first step of the reaction involves the formation of monoadducts. These monoadducts may then react further to form intra-strand and inter-strand crosslinks. The cytotoxic activity of platinum compounds has been related to binding with DNA and the production of intra-strand and inter-strand crosslinks, as well as the formation of adducts that cause conformational DNA changes, impeding the separation of both DNA strands, which subsequently impairs replication and inhibits DNA synthesis [11]. Intra-strand cross-links are the most abundant products of the interaction with DNA (around 70% of all platinum-DNA linking products). These lesions cause significant distortions in the DNA that can be recognized by one or more DNA binding proteins. These proteins can either initiate DNA damage repair or signal for apoptosis. Platinum-mediated programmed cell death is caused by cell cycle arrest in the G2-phase, although the pathways from platinum–DNA binding to apoptosis are not completely understood [12].

Other proposed mechanisms of cisplatin cytotoxicity include mitochondrial damage, decreased ATPase activity, and altered cellular transport mechanisms. Mitochondria seem to play a role in the cell death. This is believed to be mediated by their interaction with nuclear DNA [13]. Additionally, mitochondria are thought to be a major target of cisplatin and mitochondrial DNA is heavily damaged by cisplatin leading to mitochondrial loss of energy production and decreasing the ATPase activity [14,15]. Another proposed mechanism of action is the transporter-mediated uptake. Entering the cells is the first step for cisplatin to exert its toxic effects. In recent years there has been increasing evidence that the cellular uptake of cisplatin is mediated, at least in part, by transport proteins. Several transporters, which are expressed on the cell membranes, have been associated with cisplatin transport across the plasma membrane and across the cell: the copper transporter 1 (Ctr1), the copper transporter 2 (Ctr2), the P-type copper-transporting ATPases ATP7A and ATP7B [16,17].

3. Platinum analogues and ovarian cancer therapeutics

Despite the clear advantage in OS and PFS obtained with cisplatin–paclitaxel, it was immediately noted that this regimen carries a significant toxicity, namely peripheral neurotoxicity and nephrotoxicity [18]. Another important limitation of cisplatin–paclitaxel chemotherapy is the difficulty in administering it as an outpatient regimen. Prior to the introduction of paclitaxel, several studies had established that cisplatin and carboplatin are therapeutically equivalent in women with advanced epithelial ovarian cancer. Furthermore, carboplatin is associated with significantly lower neurotoxicity and renal toxicity and that the combination of carboplatin and 3-h infusion paclitaxel can be given as an outpatient schedule. This was also demonstrated in a Cochrane meta-analysis [19].

Three trials have investigated the equivalence of carboplatin and cisplatin in combination with paclitaxel in the first-line setting [20,21,22]. Given the evidence of a more favorable toxicity profile and ease of delivery, the carboplatin–paclitaxel combination has become an almost universal choice in the management of ovarian cancer, and is the standard comparator in all the recent trials performed in this disease.

4. Mechanisms of cellular resistance to platinum agents

Even though initial responsiveness to platinum-based therapy is high in ovarian cancer, the majority of patients relapse. Several mechanisms of cellular resistance to platinum compounds have been described. These mechanisms can be classified in two groups: 1) those that the limit the formation of cytotoxic platinum-DNA adducts, and 2) those that prevent cell death occurring after platinum-DNA adduct formation [11,23]. A better understanding of the molecular basis of cisplatin resistance may lead to new antitumor strategies that will sensitize unresponsive ovarian cancers to cisplatin-based chemotherapy.

4.1. Reduced intracellular drug accumulation

Decreased cellular uptake of cisplatin by resistant cells is one of the major mechanisms of resistance described in vitro. The mechanism responsible for reduced cisplatin accumulation in resistant cells may be ascribed to either an inhibition in drug uptake, an increase in drug efflux, or both. Cisplatin and its analogues may accumulate within cells by passive diffusion or facilitated transport. The copper transporter-1 (CTR1) regulates the influx of cisplatin and its analogues into the cell. This is supported by the evidence in cell lines of deletion of the yeast *CTR1* gene, which encodes a high-affinity copper transporter, results in increased cisplatin resistance and reduced intracellular accumulation of cisplatin in various cell lines including ovarian cancer [24,25]. In human ovarian cancer cell lines it has been demonstrated that copper and cisplatin are competitive inhibitors for the transport of each other into the cell and cause a rapid down-regulation of *CTR1* expression mediated by internalization of this transporter from the plasma membrane and subsequent [26]. Two copper exporters, ATP7A and ATP7B, have also been proposed to be involved in cellular resistance to cisplatin [27]. ATP7A is thought to sequester platinum agents in intracellular compartments, preventing their reaction with nuclear DNA. ATP7A is over-expressed in some cisplatin-resistant ovarian carcinoma cell lines. Additionally, ovarian cancer patients with ATP7A expression have a lower survival rate than patients with undetectable levels of expression, as determined by ATP7A immunostaining [28]. Over-expression of ATP7B in primary ovarian carcinomas and ovarian carcinoma cell lines resulted in resistance to cisplatin, with only 60% of the cisplatin accumulation present in ATP7B-expressing cells compared to vector control [29].

MRP-related transport proteins are involved in the active efflux of platinum drugs. MRP is a member of the ABC (adenosine triphosphate-binding cassette) family of transport proteins that participates in the efflux of anticancer drugs from cells. Thus, it has been speculated that deregulation of some of the MRP components may influence platinum resistance [30]. The MRP gene family is composed of at least seven members (MRP1–7) but recent reports reinforced the notion that MRP2 expression levels can be important in predicting the sensitivity of tumors to platinum-based therapies [31,32]. MDR1 encodes an integral membrane protein named P-glycoprotein (Pgp) or an ATP-binding cassette subfamily B, member 1, which acts as a drug efflux pump [33]. This protein is a transmembrane transporter that resides in the plasma membrane of many cells, including cancer cells that are multidrug resistant. Pgp recognizes a wide range of anticancer drugs and was shown to reduce intracellular concentrations of a variety of cytotoxic drugs, including platinum agents. Pgp activity results in blunted chemotherapy-induced cytotoxicity in vitro and in vivo. Moreover, anticancer drugs were found to induce MDR1 gene. Since Pgp alone can mediate resistance to a whole array of drugs through drug efflux, it is an attractive target for the improvement of anticancer therapy. In theory, co-administration of transporter inhibitors with Pgp-substrate anticancer drugs could reverse MDR and improve treatment outcome. Clinical trials aimed at specifically inhibiting the function of Pgp have given mixed results, but in at least some cases this inhibition has resulted in improved tumor shrinkage and increased patient survival. Unfortunately, Pgp inhibitors such as PSC-833 (Valspodar) induced pharmacokinetic interactions that limited drug clearance and metabolism of the concomitantly administered chemotherapy, thereby elevating plasma concentrations beyond acceptable toxicity [34]. It is thus clear that the Pgp overexpression can be a cause of failure of anticancer chemotherapy and be associated with worse prognosis in patients with ovarian and breast cancers, sarcomas and other malignancies [29,35,36].

4.2. Intracellular cisplatin inactivation

Glutathione (gamma-glutamylcysteinylglycine: GSH), the most abundant intracellular thiol, contributes (along with methionine, metallothionein and other cysteine-rich proteins) to detoxify many cellular toxins, including cisplatin and its analogues. Part of the cytoplasmic cisplatin reacts with DNA, which ultimately lead to the activation of the apoptosis cascade in response to DNA damage. However, a major fraction of intracellular cisplatin can be converted into cisplatin-thiol conjugates by GSH-S-transferase π, and these conjugates are ultimately inactivated. Both GSTπ and γ-glutamylcysteine synthetase (γ- GCS), the latter being the enzyme involved in GSH synthesis, have been associated with cisplatin resistance in ovarian, cervical and lung cancer cell lines [37,38,39].

Thus, reducing intracellular glutathione levels would seem a rational strategy to overcome platinum resistance. To that end, a novel glutathione analog prodrug, canfosfamide, initiated clinical development in ovarian cancer. Canfosfamide (TLK286) works by targeting tumors that over-express glutathione S-transferase (GST) P1-1, increasing the sensitivity of those tumors to the cytotoxic effects of canfosfamide. Following activation, the apoptotic activity of canfosfamide is mediated through the stress response pathway, resulting in the induction of cellular apoptosis. Human cancer cells exposed to canfosfamide demonstrate activation of mitogen- activated protein (MAP) kinase MKK4, p38 kinase, jun-N-terminal kinase (JNK) and caspase 3. The cytotoxic activity of canfosfamide has been demonstrated *in vitro* and *in vivo* against a variety of human cancer cell lines, including ovarian cancer cells (OVCAR3).

A phase II trial involving 34 patients with platinum-refractory or platinum-resistant ovarian cancer reported that 15% of patients had an objective response and 50% of patients had disease stabilization [40]. Three phase III trials in platinum-resistant ovarian cancer were undertaken in an attempt to define the potential role of canfosfamide in ovarian cancer therapeutics: TLK286 versus liposomal doxorubicin or topotecan (ASSIST-1,41); TLK286 plus carboplatin versus liposomal doxorubicin (ASSIST-3,42) and TLK286 plus liposomal doxorubicin versus liposomal doxorubicin alone (ASSIST-5,43). Unfortunately, none of these studies showed superior efficacy of canfosfamide compared to standard treatment.

4.3. Increased DNA repair

The cytotoxicity of cisplatin is attributed to the formation of cisplatin-DNA adducts, and to the induction of DNA damage. The balance between DNA damage to DNA repair dictates tumor cell death or survival after cisplatin therapy. Depending on the type of damage inflicted on the DNA structure, different DNA repair mechanisms have the ability to restore these lesions and remove the platinum-DNA adducts from the tumor DNA [44]. The major pathway in the repair of DNA damage is the nucleotide excision repair (NER) system. NER is one of five separate DNA repair mechanisms that also include mismatch repair (MMR), homologous recombination repair (HR), base excision repair (BER) and translesion synthesis. The preponderance of one repair mechanism over another may also change in different tumor types.

4.3.1. Nucleotide Excision Repair (NER)

The nucleotide excision repair (NER) pathway is predominantly responsible for repairing platinum-DNA adducts in cellular DNA. Several proteins interact in a coordinated fashion to recognize damage and further repair of the DNA (Figure 2). One of these proteins is excision repair cross-complementation group 1 (ERCC1). This 33-kD protein, mainly coupled with XPF (Xeroderma Pigmentosum-F protein) acts in the rate-limiting incision step that cleaves the DNA strand before DNA polymerases and ligases act to reconstitute double-strand integrity. Different studies with ovarian cancer cell lines have demonstrated that high ERCC1 mRNA expression is correlated with increased capacity of cells to repair cisplatin-induced DNA damage, thus conferring resistance to the drug. Further, transfection experiments using ERCC1 antisense vectors in both cell lines and mice have shown increased sensitivity to platinum [45,46,47].

There is growing interest in evaluating the potential role of ERCC1 as a biomarker of platinum resistance in ovarian cancer. However, despite multiple studies evaluating the association between ERCC1 protein expression or even single nucleotide polymorphisms and clinical outcome, no definitive conclusion has yet been reached regarding the predictive and/or prognostic role of ERRCC1 in the management of EOC [48,49].

4.3.2. DNA mismatch repair

The mismatch repair (MMR) system is a strand-specific DNA repair mechanism involved in the post-replicative repair of the errors made by DNA polymerases and in charge of eliminating single-base mismatches and insertion-deletion loops that have escaped the proofreading back-up mechanisms.

Loss of function of the cellular mismatch repair system (MMR) can partially contribute to develop DNA damage tolerance. Unaltered, MMR scans newly synthesized DNA and removes mismatches that result from nucleotide incorporation errors made by the DNA polymerases. The repair process consists of 3 steps—initiation, excision, and re-synthesis—that involve several proteins: MLH1, MSH2, MSH3, MSH6, and PMS2. Inactivation of MMR leads to the occurrence of unrepaired deletions in mononucleotide and dinucleotide repeats, resulting in variable length repeats. This phenomenon is called microsatellite instability (MSI), which can be caused by genetic or epigenetic inactivation and has been postulated as a potential marker for MMR deficiency. DNA methylation changes in plasma have been suggested as another rationale of chemotherapy resistance in OEC after treatment (acquired MLH1 methylation) [50].

MMR deficient human cancer cell lines tolerate cytotoxic drugs, suggesting that loss of MMR could cause platinum resistance [51]. Most MMR-deficient cancers have mutations in MLH1 or MSH2. Samimi et al [52] investigated MLH1 and MSH2 expression in paired ovarian tumor

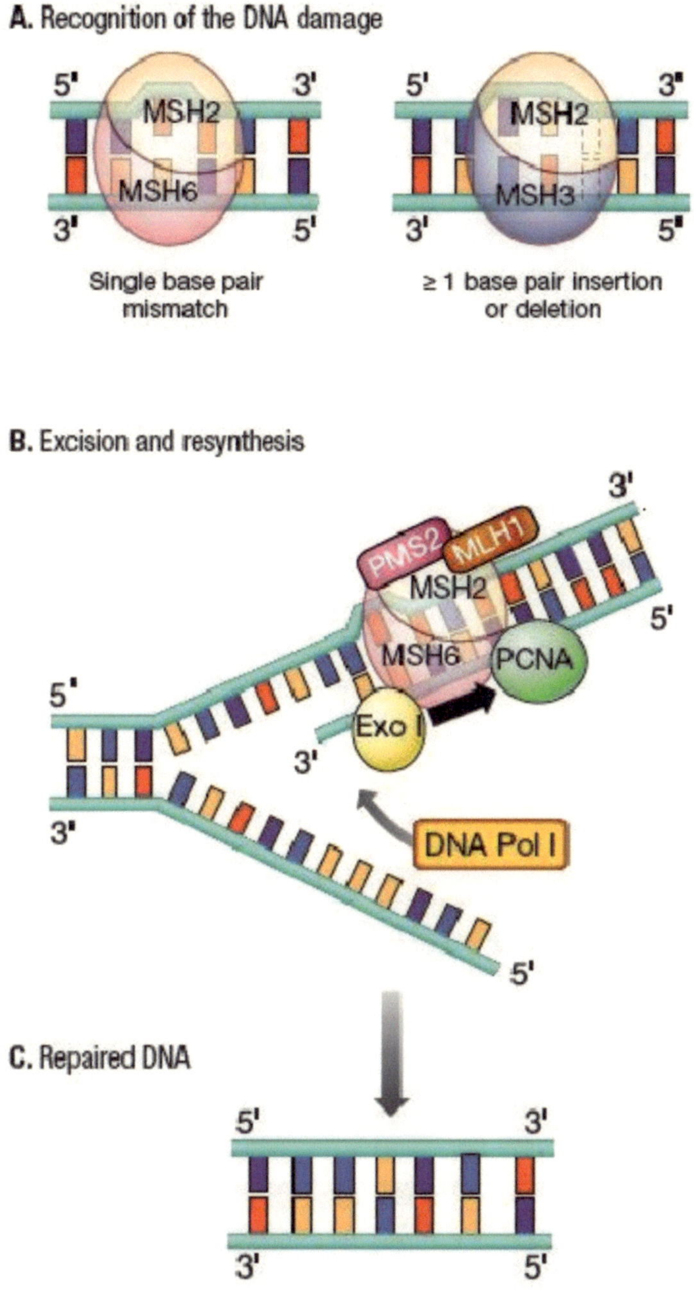

Figure 2. Schematic Representation of the Mismatch Repair Pathway (*Adapted with permission from Diaz-Padilla I, Poveda A. Clin Ovarian Cancer Other Gynecol Malig 2010, 3(1):29-35.*) Base-base mismatches are the most frequent errors associated with microsatellites (repetitive sequences of mononucleotide, dinucleotide, or higher-order nucleotide repeats distributed throughout the human genome). The mismatch repair system is responsible for the surveillance and correction of errors introduced in microsatellites. Mismatch repair proteins: MLH1, MSH2, MSH3, MSH6, PMS2. Exo 1, exonuclease; DNA Pol, DNA polymerase δ; PCNA, proliferating cell nuclear antigen.

sections from 54 ovarian cancer patients before and after platinum-based therapy by using immunohistochemical staining techniques. These authors demonstrated associations between MLH1 and MSH2 protein expression and clinical parameters known to be of prognostic significance as well as response to treatment and overall survival. MLH1 and MSH2 staining decreased significantly after platinum-based therapy. Hypermethylation of the MLH1 promoter has also been identified as a casual event in sporadic MMR-deficient malignant tumors. In ovarian cancer, it is estimated that about 10% of cases are related to this molecular pathway [53], although the methodology and definitions when assessing MSI in ovarian cancer are heterogeneous and not prospectively validated. The frequency of MMR dysfunction seems to vary depending on the histological subtype, being higher in endometrioid (19%) and mucinous (17%) subtypes. It is an assumption that MMR deficiency might be a tumor-initiating phenomenon in ovarian cancer, similar to colorectal and endometrial tumors. However, MMR deficient ovarian cancers have been only poorly characterized to date with respect to their epidemiological, molecular and clinical features.

Only a few studies have found a consistent relationship between MMR inactivation and platinum-based chemotherapy resistance (primarily down-regulation or mutations in MMR genes MLH1, MSH2 or MSH1) [50, 54,55,56].

This resistance to cisplatin can be circumvented using a DNA demethylating agent such as 2′-deoxy-5-azacytidine (decitabine; Dacoge, MGI Pharma) in combination with cisplatin or carboplatin to reverse this resistance mechanism [57]. Two phase II clinical trials have tested the combination of carboplatin and decitabine in recurrent Platinum-resistant OC patients with different conclusions [58,59].

4.3.3. Homologous recombination repair pathway

Platinum-based chemotherapy causes inter-strand DNA cross-linking which cause DNA double-strand breaks (DSBs) during DNA replication. DSBs are one of the most toxic lesions to DNA. This is because it affects both strands of the duplex, thus no intact complimentary strand is available as a template for repair. When such lesions are not repaired the cell undergoes apoptosis. If the reparation is not done appropriately, secondary lesions can occur, such as mutations and/or deletions. Cells have evolved two major pathways for the repair of DSBs: non-homologous end-joining (NHEJ) and homologous recombination (HR). The HR system is the preferred system by cells when it comes to repair DSBs. It is a highly conserved system, generally regarded as error-free, that requires an intact sister chromatid to act as template for correct repair of the break without loss of sequence information. As such, HR takes place in G2 and S phases of the cell cycle.

The *BRCA1* gene is located on chromosome 17q21. The BRCA1 protein is a component of a number of supercomplexes, each of which plays a role in DNA damage response activation, cell cycle checkpoint activation and/or DSB repair. Some of the key components of this repair process are proteins such as BRCA2, RAD51 and PALB2. Actually, the interaction between specific domains of BRCA1 and PALB2 is key in the reparation of DBSs. Thus, mutations in domains of BRCA1 can potentially abolish its PALB2-binding activity, resulting in compromised HR function. These mutations have been found in BRCA1-mutated tumors, implying that loss of this specific BRCA1 function in DSB repair is source of the genomic instability and tumorigenesis observed in this subset of BRCA1 mutation carriers.

The BRCA2 gene is located on chromosome 13q. The BRCA2 protein has its primary function in HR and its based upon its ability to bind to the strand invasion recombinase, RAD51. In fact, recruitment of RAD51 to sites of DNA damage requires BRCA2, and BRCA2-deficient cells exhibit genomic instability.

Despite only 5-10% of epithelial ovarian cancer has an inherited background, more than 90% of hereditary ovarian tumors bear BRCA1/2 mutations. It has been described that these tumors are generally of serous histology, and high-grade. They usually present at younger ages, and more recently, it has been described that BRCA-mutated tumors have better prognosis. [60,61,62]. It is relevant to note that up to 55% of sporadic epithelial ovarian tumors have some sort of BRCA dysfunction. This has been named as BRCAness, and it may have important clinical consequences. One of the reasons behind this better outcome relies on a higher sensitivity to platinum compounds [63,64]. However, BRCA1/2-mutated also develop platinum resistance. One possible explanation is in relation with the production of secondary intragenic mutations in BRCA1/2 that restore these genetic expressions and HR function correcting the open reading frames of mutated BRCA1/2 [65,66,67]. However BRCA1/2 restoration does not explain all cases of cisplatin resistance so investigations in other mechanisms of chemo-resistance in BRCA-deficient ovarian cancer cells are needed.

Recently, PARP inhibitors have been developed as an important novel strategy for the treatment of BRCA mutation-associated ovarian and breast cancer. The rationale for this approach is that by inhibiting BER, these agents can prevent repair that occurs after cytotoxic chemotherapy that causes single-strand DNA breaks, and also they can work by creating "synthetic lethality" in cells which have lost one mechanism of DNA repair. In the absence of HR, inhibition of PARP results in poor repair of these lesions and apoptosis, increasing around 1000-fold the sensitivity in cells that are BRCA1 or BRCA2 deficient [68,69,70]. Although olaparib and veliparib are the most widely studied in ovarian cancer [71,72,73,74,75], other PARP inhibitors are in development such as BSI-201, AG014699, CEP9722, MK4827, E7016, LT673, to name just a few.

5. Conclusion and future directions

Chemotherapy resistance is the ultimate reason for tumor recurrence. Relapsed ovarian cancer is an incurable disease where chemotherapy plays a major therapeutic role. Platinum agents, likely in conjunction with taxanes, are the most active cytotoxic drugs in ovarian cancer. Traditionally, ovarian cancer recurrence has been classified according to the time elapsed from the last dose of platinum. Thus, relapses occurring more than six months from the last dose of platinum are generally re-treated with a platinum combination. Responses to a platinum rechallenge tend to be similar to the initial response, and the longer the platinum-free interval is the better the responses are. The so-called "platinum-sensitive" patients have better prognosis than women whose relapse is shorter than six months. For this group of patients therapeutic options are limited and usually consist in non-platinum agents.

The development of platinum resistance is a multifactorial and complex molecular process. Understanding the molecular basis of this mechanism would help potentially in selecting patients who are likely to have platinum-resistance tumors for alternate non-platinum containing regimens. This would spare women from unnecessary toxic effects and ineffective treatments. One potential scenario where the application of a molecular selection of patients by platinum sensitivity would be at initial presentation. A substantial number of advanced ovarian cancer patients undergo neoadjuvant chemotherapy prior to debulking surgery. Such chemotherapy consists of platinum and a taxane doublet. Despite most patients do have a major response to primary chemotherapy, about 20-30% fail to respond or progress.

The development of platinum resistance seems a dynamic process. Patients who initially respond to platinum-based chemotherapy end up becoming resistant. This suggests that we may need to investigate the mechanisms at several time points of the disease course. It is likely that primary platinum resistance is a molecular phenomenon different from secondary (and subsequent) platinum resistance. At this point, it is key that reliable biomarkers can be identified to better define platinum resistance. The quest for a bona-fide biomarker of platinum resistance in ovarian cancer has been so far disappointing. It may well be the case that several markers need to be jointly studied, since platinum resistance is not a one-step molecular event. Further validation in large (ideally prospective) cohorts and in randomized phase III trials will be still needed. It will be difficult though to extrapolate results of platinum sensitivity when other agents are given concomitantly. It is not possible to rule out the potential influence of cytotoxics with similar mechanisms of action or biologics with the potential of modifying the tumor microenvironment. Unraveling the mechanisms of resistance to platinum (and other chemotherapy agents) in ovarian cancer is a very difficult task. However, its potential clinical benefits are worth such tremendous joint basic and clinical research effort.

Author details

Gonzalo Tapia[1] and Ivan Diaz-Padilla[2*]

*Address all correspondence to: ivandpadilla@hospitaldemadrid.com

1 Division of Medical Oncology, Gregorio Marañón University Hospital, Madrid, Spain

2 Division of Medical Oncology, Centro Integral Oncológico Clara Campal, Madrid, Spain

Disclosures: The authors have no conflict of interest

References

[1] Siegel R, Naishadham D, Jemal A. Cancer Statistics , 2012. Cancer Journal The (Internet). Wiley Online Library; 2012;62(1):10–29. Available from: http://www.ncbi.nlm.nih.gov/pubmed/22237781

[2] McGuire WP, Hoskins WJ, Brady MF, Kucera PR, Partridge EE, Look KY, et al. Cyclophosphamide and cisplatin compared with paclitaxel and cisplatin in patients with stage III and stage IV ovarian cancer. (Internet). The New England Journal of Medicine. 1996 p. 1–6. Available from: http://www.ncbi.nlm.nih.gov/pubmed/7494563

[3] Bristow RE, Tomacruz RS, Armstrong DK, Trimble EL, Montz FJ. Survival effect of maximal cytoreductive surgery for advanced ovarian carcinoma during the platinum era: a meta-analysis. Journal of Clinical Oncology (Internet). 2002;20(5):1248–59. Available from: http://www.ncbi.nlm.nih.gov/pubmed/11870167

[4] Muggia FM, Braly PS, Brady MF, Sutton G, Niemann TH, Lentz SL, et al. Phase III randomized study of cisplatin versus paclitaxel versus cisplatin and paclitaxel in patients with suboptimal stage III or IV ovarian cancer: a gynecologic oncology group study. (Internet). Journal of Clinical Oncology. 2000 p. 106–15. Available from: http://www.ncbi.nlm.nih.gov/pubmed/10623700

[5] Ozols RF, Bundy BN, Greer BE, Fowler JM, Clarke-Pearson D, Burger RA, et al. Phase III trial of carboplatin and paclitaxel compared with cisplatin and paclitaxel in patients with optimally resected stage III ovarian cancer: a Gynecologic Oncology Group study. (Internet). Journal of Clinical Oncology. Nature Publishing Group; 2003 p. 3194–200. Available from: http://www.ncbi.nlm.nih.gov/pubmed/12860964

[6] Thigpen JT, Vance RB, Khansur T. Second-line chemotherapy for recurrent carcinoma of the ovary. Cancer. 1993;71(4 Suppl):1559–64.

[7] Du Bois A, Quinn M, Thigpen T, Vermorken J, Avall-Lundqvist E, Bookman M, et al. 2004 consensus statements on the management of ovarian cancer: final document of the 3rd International Gynecologic Cancer Intergroup Ovarian Cancer Consensus Conference (GCIG OCCC 2004). Annals of oncology official journal of the European Society for Medical Oncology ESMO (Internet). 2005. p. viii7–viii12. Available from: http://www.ncbi.nlm.nih.gov/pubmed/16239238

[8] Ledermann JA, Kristeleit RS. Optimal treatment for relapsing ovarian cancer. Annals of oncology official journal of the European Society for Medical Oncology ESMO (Internet). OXFORD UNIV PRESS; 2010;21 Suppl 7(Supplement 7):vii218–i222. Available from: http://discovery.ucl.ac.uk/539589/

[9] Harter P, Du Bois A, Hahmann M, Hasenburg A, Burges A, Loibl S, et al. Surgery in recurrent ovarian cancer: the Arbeitsgemeinschaft Gynaekologische Onkologie

(AGO) DESKTOP OVAR trial. (Internet). Annals of Surgical Oncology. 2006 p. 1702–10. Available from: http://www.ncbi.nlm.nih.gov/pubmed/17009163

[10] Jamieson ER, Lippard SJ. Structure, Recognition, and Processing of Cisplatin–DNA Adducts. Chemical Reviews (Internet). 1999;99(9):2467–98. Available from: http://pubs.acs.org/doi/abs/10.1021/cr980421n

[11] Siddik ZH. Cisplatin: mode of cytotoxic action and molecular basis of resistance. Oncogene (Internet). Nature Publishing Group; 2003;22(47):7265–79. Available from: http://www.ncbi.nlm.nih.gov/pubmed/14576837

[12] Jordan P, Carmo-Fonseca M. Molecular mechanisms involved in cisplatin cytotoxicity. Cellular and Molecular Life Sciences (Internet). 2000;57(8):1229–35. Available from: http://dx.doi.org/10.1007/PL00000762

[13] Mitochondria F, Biochem EJ. The mitochondrion in apoptosis: how Pandora ' s box opens. Cell (Internet). 2001;2(January):67–71. Available from: http://www.ncbi.nlm.nih.gov/pubmed/11413468

[14] Olivero OA, Chang PK, Lopez-Larraza DM, Semino-Mora MC, Poirier MC. Preferential formation and decreased removal of cisplatin-DNA adducts in Chinese hamster ovary cell mitochondrial DNA as compared to nuclear DNA. Mutation Research. 1997;391(1-2):79–86.

[15] Murata T, Hibasami H, Maekawa S, Tagawa T, Nakashima K. Preferential binding of cisplatin to mitochondrial DNA and suppression of ATP generation in human malignant melanoma cells. Biochemistry International. 1990;20(5):949–55.

[16] Ishida S, Lee J, Thiele DJ, Herskowitz I. Uptake of the anticancer drug cisplatin mediated by the copper transporter Ctr1 in yeast and mammals. Proceedings of the National Academy of Sciences of the United States of America (Internet). National Academy of Sciences; 2002;99(22):14298–302. Available from: http://www.pubmedcentral.nih.gov/articlerender.fcgi?artid=137878&tool=pmcentrez&rendertype=abstract

[17] Safaei R, Otani S, Larson BJ, Rasmussen ML, Howell SB. Transport of cisplatin by the copper efflux transporter ATP7B. Molecular Pharmacology (Internet). 2008;73(2):461–8. Available from: http://www.ncbi.nlm.nih.gov/entrez/query.fcgi?cmd=Retrieve&db=PubMed&dopt=Citation&list_uids=17978167

[18] Tsang RY, Al-Fayea T, Au H-J. Cisplatin overdose: toxicities and management. Drug safety an international journal of medical toxicology and drug experience (Internet). Adis International Ltd (41 Centorian Drive, Private Bag 65901, Mairangi Bay, Auckland 10 1311, New Zealand); 2009;32(12):1109–22. Available from: http://www.ncbi.nlm.nih.gov/pubmed/19916578

[19] Stewart L, Advanced Ovarian Cancer Trialists Group. Chemotherapy for advanced ovarian cancer. Advanced Ovarian Cancer Trialists Group. Cochrane database of sys-

tematic reviews Online (Internet). 2000;(2):CD001418. Available from: http://www.ncbi.nlm.nih.gov/pubmed/10796788

[20] Neijt JP, Engelholm SA, Tuxen MK, Sorensen PG, Hansen M, Sessa C, et al. Exploratory phase III study of paclitaxel and cisplatin versus paclitaxel and carboplatin in advanced ovarian cancer. (Internet). Journal of Clinical Oncology. Nature Publishing Group; 2000 p. 3084–92. Available from: http://www.ncbi.nlm.nih.gov/pubmed/10963636

[21] Du Bois A, Lück H-J, Meier W, Adams H-P, Möbus V, Costa S, et al. A randomized clinical trial of cisplatin/paclitaxel versus carboplatin/paclitaxel as first-line treatment of ovarian cancer. (Internet). Journal Of The National Cancer Institute. 2003 p. 1320–9. Available from: http://www.ncbi.nlm.nih.gov/pubmed/20937992

[22] Aaronson NK, Ahmedzai S, Bergman B, Bullinger M, Cull A, Duez NJ, et al. The European Organization for Research and Treatment of Cancer QLQ-C30: a quality-of-life instrument for use in international clinical trials in oncology. Journal Of The National Cancer Institute (Internet). Oxford University Press; 1993;85(5):365–76. Available from: http://jnci.oxfordjournals.org/content/85/5/365.short

[23] Rabik CA, Dolan ME. Molecular mechanisms of resistance and toxicity associated with platinating agents. Cancer Treatment Reviews (Internet). 2007;33(1):9–23. Available from: http://www.pubmedcentral.nih.gov/articlerender.fcgi?artid=1855222&tool=pmcentrez&rendertype=abstract

[24] Holzer AK, Manorek GH, Howell SB. Contribution of the major copper influx transporter CTR1 to the cellular accumulation of cisplatin, carboplatin, and oxaliplatin. Molecular Pharmacology (Internet). ASPET; 2006;70(4):1390–4. Available from: http://molpharm.aspetjournals.org/cgi/content/abstract/70/4/1390

[25] Song I-S, Savaraj N, Siddik ZH, Liu P, Wei Y, Wu CJ, et al. Role of human copper transporter Ctr1 in the transport of platinum-based antitumor agents in cisplatin-sensitive and cisplatin-resistant cells. Molecular Cancer Therapeutics (Internet). AACR; 2004;3(12):1543–9. Available from: http://www.ncbi.nlm.nih.gov/entrez/query.fcgi?cmd=Retrieve&db=PubMed&dopt=Citation&list_uids=15634647

[26] Holzer AK, Katano K, Klomp LWJ, Howell SB. Cisplatin rapidly down-regulates its own influx transporter hCTR1 in cultured human ovarian carcinoma cells. Clinical Cancer Research (Internet). 2004;10(19):6744–9. Available from: http://www.ncbi.nlm.nih.gov/pubmed/15475465

[27] Samimi G, Katano K, Holzer AK, Safaei R, Howell SB. Modulation of the cellular pharmacology of cisplatin and its analogs by the copper exporters ATP7A and ATP7B. Molecular Pharmacology (Internet). 2004;66(1):25–32. Available from: http://molpharm.aspetjournals.org/cgi/content/abstract/66/1/25

[28] Samimi G, Varki NM, Wilczynski S, Safaei R, Alberts DS, Howell SB. Increase in expression of the copper transporter ATP7A during platinum drug-based treatment is

associated with poor survival in ovarian cancer patients. Clinical Cancer Research. 2003;9(16 Pt 1):5853–9.

[29] Nakayama K, Kanzaki A, Ogawa K, Miyazaki K, Neamati N, Takebayashi Y. Copper-transporting P-type adenosine triphosphatase (ATP7B) as a cisplatin based chemoresistance marker in ovarian carcinoma: comparative analysis with expression of MDR1, MRP1, MRP2, LRP and BCRP. International journal of cancer Journal international du cancer (Internet). 2002;101(5):488–95. Available from: http://www.ncbi.nlm.nih.gov/pubmed/12216079

[30] Borst P, Rottenberg S, Jonkers J. How do real tumors become resistant to cisplatin? Cell cycle Georgetown Tex (Internet). Landes Bioscience; 2008;7(10):1353–9. Available from: http://www.ncbi.nlm.nih.gov/pubmed/18418074

[31] Korita P V, Wakai T, Shirai Y, Matsuda Y, Sakata J, Takamura M, et al. Multidrug resistance-associated protein 2 determines the efficacy of cisplatin in patients with hepatocellular carcinoma. Oncology Reports. 2010 p. 965–72.

[32] Kool M, De Haas M, Scheffer GL, Scheper RJ, Van Eijk MJ, Juijn JA, et al. Analysis of expression of cMOAT (MRP2), MRP3, MRP4, and MRP5, homologues of the multidrug resistance-associated protein gene (MRP1), in human cancer cell lines. Cancer Research (Internet). 1997;57(16):3537–47. Available from: http://www.ncbi.nlm.nih.gov/pubmed/9270026

[33] Gottesman MM, Ling V. The molecular basis of multidrug resistance in cancer: the early years of P-glycoprotein research. FEBS Letters (Internet). 2006;580(4):998–1009. Available from: http://www.ncbi.nlm.nih.gov/pubmed/16405967

[34] Fracasso PM, Brady MF, Moore DH, Walker JL, Rose PG, Letvak L, et al. Phase II study of paclitaxel and valspodar (PSC 833) in refractory ovarian carcinoma: a gynecologic oncology group study. Journal of Clinical Oncology (Internet). 2001;19(12): 2975–82. Available from: www.ncbi.nlm.nih.gov/pubmed/11408492

[35] Hoffmann A-C, Wild P, Leicht C, Bertz S, Danenberg KD, Danenberg P V, et al. MDR1 and ERCC1 Expression Predict Outcome of Patients with Locally Advanced Bladder Cancer Receiving. Trial (Internet). 2010;12(8):628–36. Available from: http://www.pubmedcentral.nih.gov/articlerender.fcgi?artid=2915407&tool=pmcentrez&rendertype=abstract

[36] Rodrigues FFO, Santos RE, Melo MB, Silva MALG, Oliveira AL, Rozenowicz RL, et al. Correlation of polymorphism C3435T of the MDR-1 gene and the response of primary chemotherapy in women with locally advanced breast cancer. Genetics and molecular research GMR (Internet). 2008;7(1):1117–21. Available from: http://www.ncbi.nlm.nih.gov/entrez/query.fcgi?cmd=Retrieve&db=PubMed&dopt=Citation&list_uids=12684679

[37] Kelland L. The resurgence of platinum-based cancer chemotherapy. Nature Reviews Cancer (Internet). Nature Publishing Group; 2007;7(8):573–84. Available from: http://www.ncbi.nlm.nih.gov/pubmed/17625587

[38] Sakamoto M, Kondo A, Kawasaki K, Goto T, Sakamoto H, Miyake K, et al. Analysis of gene expression profiles associated with cisplatin resistance in human ovarian cancer cell lines and tissues using cDNA microarray. Human cell official journal of Human Cell Research Society (Internet). 2001;14(4):305–15. Available from: http://www.ncbi.nlm.nih.gov/entrez/query.fcgi?cmd=Retrieve&db=PubMed&dopt=Citation&list_uids=11925933

[39] Li M, Balch C, Montgomery JS, Jeong M, Chung JH, Yan P, et al. Integrated analysis of DNA methylation and gene expression reveals specific signaling pathways associated with platinum resistance in ovarian cancer. BMC medical genomics (Internet). BioMed Central; 2009;2(1):34. Available from: http://www.pubmedcentral.nih.gov/articlerender.fcgi?artid=2712480&tool=pmcentrez&rendertype=abstract

[40] Kavanagh JJ, Gershenson DM, Choi H, Lewis L, Patel K, Brown GL, et al. Multi-institutional phase 2 study of TLK286 (TELCYTA, a glutathione S-transferase P1-1 activated glutathione analog prodrug) in patients with platinum and paclitaxel refractory or resistant ovarian cancer. (Internet). International journal of gynecological cancer official journal of the International Gynecological Cancer Society. Nature Publishing Group; 2005 p. 593–600. Available from: http://dx.doi.org/10.1111/j.1525-1438.2005.00114.x

[41] Vergote I, Finkler N, Del Campo J, Lohr A, Hunter J, Matei D, et al. Phase 3 randomised study of canfosfamide (Telcyta, TLK286) versus pegylated liposomal doxorubicin or topotecan as third-line therapy in patients with platinum-refractory or -resistant ovarian cancer. (Internet). European Journal of Cancer. Elsevier Ltd; 2009 p. 2324–32. Available from: http://www.ncbi.nlm.nih.gov/pubmed/19515553

[42] Rose P. Canfosfamide (C, TLK286) plus carboplatin (P) vs. liposomal doxorubicin (D) as 2nd line therapy of platinum (P) resistant ovarian cancer (OC): phase 3 study results. Journal of Clinical Oncology. Nature Publishing Group; 2007;25(Suppl.):5529.

[43] Vergote I, Finkler NJ, Hall JB, Melnyk O, Edwards RP, Jones M, et al. Randomized phase III study of canfosfamide in combination with pegylated liposomal doxorubicin compared with pegylated liposomal doxorubicin alone in platinum-resistant ovarian cancer. (Internet). International journal of gynecological cancer official journal of the International Gynecological Cancer Society. 2010 p. 772–80. Available from: http://content.wkhealth.com/linkback/openurl?sid=WKPTLP:landingpage&an=00009577-201007000-00013

[44] Reed E. Platinum-DNA adduct, nucleotide excision repair and platinum based anticancer chemotherapy. Cancer Treatment Reviews (Internet). 1998;24(5):331–44. Available from: http://www.ncbi.nlm.nih.gov/pubmed/9861196

[45] Selvakumaran M, Pisarcik DA, Bao R, Yeung AT, Hamilton TC. Enhanced Cisplatin Cytotoxicity by Disturbing the Nucleotide Excision Repair Pathway in Ovarian Cancer Cell Lines. Cancer Research (Internet). 2003;63(6):1311–6. Available from: www.ncbi.nlm.nih.gov/pubmed/12649192

[46] Dabholkar M, Vionnet J, Bostick-Bruton F, Yu JJ, Reed E. Messenger RNA levels of XPAC and ERCC1 in ovarian cancer tissue correlate with response to platinum-based chemotherapy. Journal of Clinical Investigation (Internet). 1994;94(2):703–8. Available from: http://www.pubmedcentral.nih.gov/articlerender.fcgi?artid=296149&tool=pmcentrez&rendertype=abstract

[47] Kohn EC, Sarosy G, Bicher A, Link C, Christian M, Steinberg SM, et al. Dose-intense taxol: high response rate in patients with platinum-resistant recurrent ovarian cancer. (Internet). Journal Of The National Cancer Institute. 1994 p. 18–24. Available from: http://www.ncbi.nlm.nih.gov/pubmed/7505830

[48] Smith S, Su D, Rigault De La Longrais IA, Schwartz P, Puopolo M, Rutherford TJ, et al. ERCC1 genotype and phenotype in epithelial ovarian cancer identify patients likely to benefit from paclitaxel treatment in addition to platinum-based therapy. Journal of Clinical Oncology (Internet). 2007;25(33):5172–9. Available from: http://www.ncbi.nlm.nih.gov/pubmed/18024864

[49] Krivak TC, Tian C, Rose GS, Armstrong DK, Maxwell GL. A Gynecologic Oncology Group Study of serum CA-125 levels in patients with stage III optimally debulked ovarian cancer treated with intraperitoneal compared to intravenous chemotherapy: an analysis of patients enrolled in GOG 172. (Internet). Gynecologic Oncology. Elsevier Inc.; 2009 p. 81–5. Available from: http://www.ncbi.nlm.nih.gov/pubmed/19945740

[50] Gifford G, Paul J, Vasey PA, Kaye SB, Brown R. The acquisition of hMLH1 methylation in plasma DNA after chemotherapy predicts poor survival for ovarian cancer patients. Clinical Cancer Research (Internet). American Association for Cancer Research; 2004;10(13):4420–6. Available from: http://eprints.gla.ac.uk/18729/

[51] Anthoney DA, Kaye SB. Drug resistance: the clinical perspective. Methods in Molecular Medicine (Internet). 1999;28:1–15. Available from: http://www.ncbi.nlm.nih.gov/pubmed/21374022

[52] Samimi G, Fink D, Varki NM, Husain A, Hoskins WJ, Alberts DS, et al. Analysis of MLH1 and MSH2 expression in ovarian cancer before and after platinum drug-based chemotherapy. Clinical Cancer Research (Internet). 2000;6(4):1415–21. Available from: http://clincancerres.aacrjournals.org/cgi/content/full/6/4/1415

[53] Murphy MA, Wentzensen N. Frequency of mismatch repair deficiency in ovarian cancer: A systematic review. International journal of cancer Journal international du cancer (Internet). 2010;1–25. Available from: http://www.ncbi.nlm.nih.gov/entrez/query.fcgi?db=pubmed&cmd=Retrieve&dopt=AbstractPlus&list_uids=21140452

[54] Helleman J, Van Staveren IL, Dinjens WN, Van Kuijk PF, Ritstier K, Ewing PC, et al. Mismatch repair and treatment resistance in ovarian cancer. BMC Cancer (Internet). BioMed Central; 2006;6(1):201. Available from: http://www.pubmedcentral.nih.gov/articlerender.fcgi?artid=1557864&tool=pmcentrez&rendertype=abstract

[55] Watanabe Y, Koi M, Hemmi H, Hoshai H, Noda K. A change in microsatellite instability caused by cisplatin-based chemotherapy of ovarian cancer. British Journal of Cancer (Internet). Nature Publishing Group; 2001;85(7):1064–9. Available from: http://eutils.ncbi.nlm.nih.gov/entrez/eutils/elink.fcgi?dbfrom=pubmed&id=11592780&retmode=ref&cmd=prlinks

[56] Fink D, Nebel S, Norris PS, Baergen RN, Wilczynski SP, Costa MJ, et al. Enrichment for DNA mismatch repair-deficient cells during treatment with cisplatin. International journal of cancer Journal international du cancer. 1998;77(5):741–6.

[57] Brown R, Plumb JA. Demethylation of DNA by decitabine in cancer chemotherapy. Expert Review of Anticancer Therapy (Internet). 2010;4(4):501–10. Available from: http://eprints.gla.ac.uk/15879/

[58] Matei D, Fang F, Shen C, Schilder J, Arnold A, Zeng Y, et al. Epigenetic Resensitization to Platinum in Ovarian Cancer. Cancer Research (Internet). 2012;72(9):2197–205. Available from: http://cancerres.aacrjournals.org/cgi/doi/10.1158/0008-5472.CAN-11-3909

[59] Glasspool RM, Gore M, Rustin G, McNeish I, Wilson R, Pledge S, et al. Randomized phase II study of decitabine in combination with carboplatin compared with carboplatin alone in patients with recurrent advanced ovarian cancer. Journal of Clinical Oncology (Internet). 2009;27(15s):suppl; abstr 5562. Available from: http://eprints.gla.ac.uk/42722/

[60] Ben David Y, Chetrit A, Hirsh-Yechezkel G, Friedman E, Beck BD, Beller U, et al. Effect of BRCA mutations on the length of survival in epithelial ovarian tumors. Journal of Clinical Oncology (Internet). 2002;20(2):463–6. Available from: http://www.ncbi.nlm.nih.gov/pubmed/11786575

[61] Cass I, Baldwin RL, Varkey T, Moslehi R, Narod SA, Karlan BY. Improved survival in women with BRCA-associated ovarian carcinoma. Cancer (Internet). 2003;97(9):2187–95. Available from: http://www.ncbi.nlm.nih.gov/pubmed/12712470

[62] Tan DSP, Rothermundt C, Thomas K, Bancroft E, Eeles R, Shanley S, et al. "BRCAness" syndrome in ovarian cancer: a case-control study describing the clinical features and outcome of patients with epithelial ovarian cancer associated with BRCA1 and BRCA2 mutations. Journal of Clinical Oncology (Internet). 2008;26(34):5530–6. Available from: http://www.ncbi.nlm.nih.gov/pubmed/18955455

[63] Yang D, Khan S, Sun Y, Hess K, Shmulevich I, Sood AK, et al. Association of BRCA1 and BRCA2 mutations with survival, chemotherapy sensitivity, and gene mutator phenotype in patients with ovarian cancer. Jama The Journal Of The American Medi-

cal Association (Internet). 2011;306(14):1557–65. Available from: http://www.ncbi.nlm.nih.gov/pubmed/21990299

[64] Weberpals J, Garbuio K, O'Brien A, Clark-Knowles K, Doucette S, Antoniouk O, et al. The DNA repair proteins BRCA1 and ERCC1 as predictive markers in sporadic ovarian cancer. International journal of cancer Journal international du cancer (Internet). Wiley Subscription Services, Inc., A Wiley Company; 2009;124(4):806–15. Available from: http://www.ncbi.nlm.nih.gov/pubmed/19035454

[65] Edwards SL, Brough R, Lord CJ, Natrajan R, Vatcheva R, Levine DA, et al. Resistance to therapy caused by intragenic deletion in BRCA2. Nature (Internet). Nature Publishing Group; 2008;451(7182):1111–5. Available from: http://www.ncbi.nlm.nih.gov/pubmed/18264088

[66] Sakai W, Swisher EM, Karlan BY, Agarwal MK, Higgins J, Friedman C, et al. Secondary mutations as a mechanism of cisplatin resistance in BRCA2-mutated cancers. Nature (Internet). Nature Publishing Group; 2008;451(7182):1116–20. Available from: http://dx.doi.org/10.1038/nature06633

[67] Swisher EM, Sakai W, Karlan BY, Wurz K, Urban N, Taniguchi T. Secondary BRCA1 mutations in BRCA1-mutated ovarian carcinomas with platinum resistance. Cancer Research (Internet). 2008;68(8):2581–6. Available from: http://www.pubmedcentral.nih.gov/articlerender.fcgi?artid=2674369&tool=pmcentrez&rendertype=abstract

[68] Satoh MS, Poirier GG, Lindahl T. Dual function for poly(ADP-ribose) synthesis in response to DNA strand breakage. Biochemistry (Internet). 1994;33(23):7099–106. Available from: http://www.ncbi.nlm.nih.gov/pubmed/8003475

[69] Bryant HE, Schultz N, Thomas HD, Parker KM, Flower D, Lopez E, et al. Specific killing of BRCA2-deficient tumours with inhibitors of poly(ADP-ribose) polymerase. Nature (Internet). Nature Publishing Group; 2005;434(7035):913–7. Available from: http://www.ncbi.nlm.nih.gov/pubmed/15829966

[70] Farmer H, McCabe N, Lord CJ, Tutt ANJ, Johnson DA, Richardson TB, et al. Targeting the DNA repair defect in BRCA mutant cells as a therapeutic strategy. Nature (Internet). Nature Publishing Group; 2005;434(7035):917–21. Available from: http://www.ncbi.nlm.nih.gov/pubmed/15829967

[71] Yap TA, Boss DS, Fong PC, Roelvink M, Tutt A, Carmichael J, et al. First in human phase I pharmacokinetic (PK) and pharmacodynamic (PD) study of KU-0059436 (Ku), a small molecule inhibitor of poly ADP-ribose polymerase (PARP) in cancer patients (p), including BRCA1/2 mutation carriers. Journal of Clinical Oncology (Internet). Nature Publishing Group; 2007;25(Suppl.):3529. Available from: http://meeting.ascopubs.org/cgi/content/abstract/25/18_suppl/3529

[72] Fong PC, Spicer J, Reade S, Reid A, Vidal L, Schellens JH, et al. Phase I pharmacokinetic (PK) and pharmacodynamic (PD) evaluation of a small molecule inhibitor of Poly ADP-Ribose Polymerase (PARP), KU-0059436 (Ku) in patients (p) with ad-

vanced tumours. Journal of Clinical Oncology (Internet). Nature Publishing Group; 2006;24(Suppl.):3022. Available from: http://meeting.ascopubs.org/cgi/content/abstract/24/18_suppl/3022

[73] Audeh MW, Penson RT, Friedlander M, Powell B, Bell-McGuinn KM, Scott C, et al. Phase II trial of the oral PARP inhibitor olaparib (AZD2281) in BRCA-deficient advanced ovarian cancer. J Clin Oncol Meeting Abstracts (Internet). 2009;27(15S):5500. Available from: http://meeting.ascopubs.org/cgi/content/abstract/27/15S/5500

[74] Kaye S, Kaufman B, Lubinski J, Matulonis U, Gourley C, Karlan B, et al. Phase II study of the oral parp inhibitor olaparib (AZD2281) versus liposomal doxorubicin in ovarian cancer patients with brca1 and/or BRCA2 mutations. Annals of Oncology (Internet). 2010;21:viii304. Available from: http://www.embase.com/search/results?subaction=viewrecord&from=export&id=L70303663

[75] Kummar S, Jiuping J, Morgan RJ, Lenz H-JD, Puhalla SL, Belani CP, et al. A Phase I Study of Veliparib in Combination with Metronomic Cyclophosphamide in Adults with Refractory Solid Tumors and Lymphomas. Clinical Cancer Research (Internet). 2012; Available from: http://www.ncbi.nlm.nih.gov/pubmed/22307137

Section 4

Molecular Pathogenesis and Targeted Therapies

Chapter 11

Biological Significance of Apoptosis in Ovarian Cancer: TRAIL Therapeutic Targeting

Nadzeya Goncharenko-Khaider, Denis Lane,
Isabelle Matte, Claudine Rancourt and Alain Piché

Additional information is available at the end of the chapter

http://dx.doi.org/10.5772/53380

1. Introduction

An apoptotic program is present in almost all cell types. Functional characterization of the apoptotic cascade has revealed how the apoptotic program is activated in response to diverse stresses such as DNA damage, signaling imbalance provoked by oncogene activation, survival factors insufficiency or hypoxia. One of the hallmarks of tumor cells is their ability to resist apoptosis. The concept that apoptosis serves as a barrier to cancer development has been well established (Evan and Littlewood, 1998; Hengartner, 2000; Lowe et al., 2004; Adams and Cory, 2007). This is especially relevant for ovarian cancer (OC) where most patients presenting with advanced OC (most commonly high grade serous OC) will respond to the initial chemotherapy treatment suggesting that most tumor cells present are sensitive to chemotherapy. However, only 10-15% of these patients maintain a complete response to the initial therapy implying that a fraction of the tumor cells escaped apoptosis induced by chemotherapeutic drugs. Thus, one of the main obstacles to an effective treatment in OC is the failure of the initial chemotherapy to eradicate a sufficient number of tumor cells to prevent disease recurrence. Attenuation of apoptosis in those tumor cells contributes to the resistance to subsequent therapy and likely plays an important role in OC progression.

This chapter focuses on the molecular pathways that lead to apoptotic resistance and the need to move towards new targeted treatment in OC. Particular attention will be given to the tumor necrosis factor-related apoptosis-inducing ligand (TRAIL) signaling cascade. TRAIL is a cytokine that triggers apoptosis in a wide variety of tumor cells with apparent little effect on normal cells. We will discuss the various mechanisms that OC cells may develop to suppress TRAIL cytotoxicity. Furthermore, we will review the emerging TRAIL-targeting strategies for treating OC and provide information about the latest clinical studies of TRAIL agonists that are being conducted for the treatment of OC.

2. Treatment for ovarian cancer

Because of the limited efficacy of current treatments for advanced OC, novel and more effective therapies are being investigated. An emerging option for the treatment of OC is the targeting of the TRAIL signaling cascade. Because of its unique ability to trigger apoptosis in cancer cells and spare normal cells, in contrast to other cytokines such as FasL and TNFα, TRAIL is an attractive and promising treatment for cancer therapy. Preclinical studies in mice provided the first evidence that the soluble recombinant TRAIL suppresses the growth of human tumor xenografts with no apparent systemic toxicity (Walczak et al., 1999; Ashkenazi et al., 1999). More recently, recombinant TRAIL has entered clinical trials for the treatment of various malignancies (Ashkenazi, 2008; Ashkenazi et al., 2008; Abdulghani and El-Deiry, 2010; Hellwig and Rehm, 2012). In addition to soluble TRAIL, several agonistic antibodies targeting TRAIL R1 or TRAIL R2 death receptors have been developed and entered into clinical trials that included OC patients (Ashkenazi et al., 2008; Hellwig and Rehm, 2012). As for standard chemotherapy, tumor cells have developed various mechanisms to escape the apoptosis induced by TRAIL. This underscores the need to understand the mechanisms of TRAIL resistance, and based on this knowledge, identify and validate novel combinations that could be used with TRAIL to potentiate its therapeutic efficacy. For example, TRAIL resistance has been often associated with overexpression of anti-apoptotic proteins. Therefore, the identification of combination treatments that abrogate anti-apoptotic protein function is promising.

3. Apoptosis overview

Deregulation of the apoptotic cascade not only plays a key role in the pathogenesis and progression of cancer, but also leads to resistance to chemotherapy. There are two major cellular death pathways that transduce the effects of various death inducers: the extrinsic and the intrinsic pathway (Figure 1). The extrinsic pathway is triggered when TRAIL binds to TRAIL R1 or TRAIL R2. Receptor trimerization, along with the subsequent oligomerization and clustering of the receptors, leads to the recruitment of the adaptor protein Fas-associated protein with death domain (FADD). FADD allows the recruitment of the inactive pro-caspase-8 or –caspase-10 via a shared death effector domain (DED) leading to the formation of the death-inducing signaling complex (DISC). Depending on the cell type, apoptosis activation through the extrinsic pathways may or may not depend on the intrinsic pathway. For example, in type I cells, upon DISC activation, sufficient caspase-8 is activated and, in turn, directly activates the effector caspases (caspase-3, -6, -7) leading to the execution of apoptosis (Abdulghani and El-Deiry, 2010). FLICE-inhibitory protein (c-FLIP) shares structural homology with pro-caspase-8 and possesses a death effector domain that lacks protease activity. In specific conditions, its structure allows c-FLIP to be recruited to the DISC where it inhibits the processing and activation of pro-caspase-8. Although many isoforms of c-FLIP have been identified, only three are expressed in human cells (Djerbi et al., 2001). They consist of two short variants, c-FLIP$_S$ and c-FLIP$_R$, and a long splice variant, c-FLIP$_L$. Both c-FLIP$_L$ and c-FLIP$_S$ contain two DEDs and compete with pro-caspase-8 for association with FADD (Bagnoli et al., 2010). Depending on the level of c-FLIP$_L$ expression, its function at the DISC will vary. When present in high amounts, c-FLIP$_L$ will exert an anti-apoptotic effect at the DISC (Krueger et al., 2001). When present in low amounts, it may heterodimerize with caspase-8 at the DISC and promotes apoptosis (Chang et al., 2002). c-FLIP is thus seen as a major inhibitor of the extrinsic pathway of apoptosis. In so-called type II cells, less caspase-8 is activated at the DISC and efficient apoptosis requires further signal amplification via the intrinsic or mitochondrial pathway. This is achieved by caspase-8-mediated Bid cleavage to generate a truncated form of Bid (tBid) which subsequently engages Bax/Bak to activate the mitochondria.

The intrinsic pathway is usually triggered in response to DNA damage, hypoxia or oncogene overexpression. As a sensor of cellular stress, p53 is a critical initiator of the intrinsic pathway. In response to cellular damage, p53 translocates from the cytoplasm to the nucleus where it promotes the transcription of pro-apoptotic members of the Bcl-2 family. Pro-apoptotic Bcl-2 family members Bax and Bak form pores in the outer mitochondrial membrane causing the release of cytochrome c and other apoptogenic factors such as apoptosis inducing factor (AIF) and SMAC/DIABLO into the cytoplasm. The released of cytochrome c, along with apoptosis protease activating factor-1 (APAF-1) and pro-caspase-9 form the apoptosome. Within the apoptosome, clustered pro-caspase-9 gets activated and cleaves downstream effector caspases, leading to the hallmark of apoptosis (Youle and Strasser, 2008; Brunelle and Letai, 2009). The release of SMAC/DIABLO from the mitochondria promotes apoptosis by binding to and neutralizing members of the family of inhibitor of apoptosis proteins (IAPs), which can block caspase-3 activity through its baculovirus IAP repeat domains. Although the extrinsic and intrinsic pathways are activated by different mechanisms, these two pathways are interconnected (Figure 1). In type II cells, activated caspase-8 cleaves pro-apoptotic Bcl-2 family member Bid to form truncated Bid (tBid), which can then interact with Bax/Bak. This interaction increases the release of cytochrome c from the mitochondria. Thus, Bid provides a connection between extrinsic and intrinsic pathways (so called mitochondrial amplification loop). The reasons that determine whether tumor cells rely on type I or II signaling are not well understood but resistance has been attributed to dysfunction of different steps in the TRAIL-induced apoptosis pathway and/or elevation of survival signals (Zhang and Fang, 2005). In particular, it has been proposed that the levels of c-FLIP and XIAP relative to caspase-8 and SMAC/DIABLO might be important determinants (Kim et al., 2000).

Bcl-2 family proteins are involved in the regulation of apoptosis by controlling mitochondrial membrane permeability. Several studies have demonstrated that these proteins can interact with each other and these interactions can neutralize their pro- or anti-apoptotic functions. The balance between anti- and pro-apoptotic members dictates the fate of cell survival or death. Pro-apoptotic Bcl-2 members can be divided into 2 groups according to their function and the number of BH domains that they possess. Proteins containing BH domains 1-3 are known as multidomain pro-apoptotic proteins such as Bax, Bak and Bok (Youle and Strasser, 2008). BH-3-only pro-apoptotic proteins such as Bik, Bid, Bad, Bim, Bmf, Noxa, Puma and others can form heterodimers with the multidomain proteins Bax and Bak leading to the activation of the mitochondria. Anti-apoptotic proteins such as Bcl-2, Bcl-XL and Mcl-1 can also form hetero-dimeric interactions with Bax and Bak, thereby neutralizing their pro-apoptotic activity. Anti-apoptotic proteins can form hetero-dimers with BH-3-only proteins and this interaction neutralizes the pro-survival function of anti-apoptotic proteins.

4. TRAIL and its receptors

TRAIL is a member of the TNF ligand superfamily of cytokines and is a type II transmembrane protein, which is anchored to the plasma membrane and presented to the cell surface. The extracellular domain of TRAIL can be shed from the cell surface by cysteine proteases to produce soluble TRAIL. Both the soluble and the membrane-bounded TRAIL can trigger apoptosis by interacting with its cognate death receptors expressed by target cells. Of the five human TRAIL receptors that have been identified, both TRAIL R1 (DR4) and TRAIL R2 (DR5) contain a functional death domain in their intracellular portion, unlike decoy receptors TRAIL R3 (DcR1) and TRAIL R4 (DcR2), which lack a functional death domain and are thus incapable of transmitting an apoptotic signal (Pan et al., 1997a; Pan et al., 1997b; Sheridan et al., 1997; Marsters et al., 1997). Soluble TRAIL also binds with low affinity to soluble osteoprotegerin (OPG), which is a decoy receptor for RANKL that blocks the RANK-RANKL interaction (Hofbauer et al., 2000). OPG negatively regulates osteoclastogenesis and soluble OPG can act as a scavenger for soluble TRAIL and therefore inhibits TRAIL-induced apoptosis (Vitovski et al., 2007).

5. Expression of apoptosis-related proteins in ovarian cancer

Because the susceptibility of tumor cells to apoptosis appears to be determined, at least in part, by the ratio between pro- and anti-apoptotic proteins, the expression pattern of anti-apoptotic proteins, Bcl-2, Bcl-X_L and Mcl-1 has been assessed in OC tissues. For example, higher Bcl-2 expression has been generally associated with a favorable outcome in OC (Henriksen et al., 1995; Herod et al., 1996; Marx et al., 1997; Marone et al., 1998). This apparent paradox may be explained by the observation that high Bcl-2 expression delays cell cycle progression by promoting accumulation of cells in S phases without affecting the rate of apoptosis in OC cells (Bélanger et al., 2005). Bcl-X_L expression is generally higher in OC tissues when compared to normal tissues (Marone et al., 1998) but has not been consistently associated with worse outcome (Shigemasa et al., 2002; Williams et al., 2005). This could be related to the observation that the ability of Bcl-X_L to attenuate apoptosis appears to be cell context-dependent in OC (Dodier and Piché, 2006). In at least one study, increased Mcl-1 expression has been correlated with poor prognostic for patients with OC (Shigemasa et al., 2002). Elevated expression of c-FLIP$_L$ has been reported in a substantial percentage of OC tissues from patients with advanced diseases (Mezzanzanica et al., 2004; Horak et al., 2005a) and has been associated with adverse outcome in some studies (Ouellet et al, 2007; Bagnoli et al., 2009) whereas others have found no such association (Duiker et al., 2010).

In patients with OC, high TRAIL expression in either tumor or stromal cells is a predictor of overall survival (Lancaster et al., 2003; Horak et al., 2005a). Interestingly in Horak's study, almost 50% of the tumor analyzed expressed elevated level of c-FLIP$_L$ and about 80% of tumors displayed low expression of TRAIL R1 and/or TRAIL R2, which could contribute to protect OC cells from TRAIL-induced apoptosis. Loss of TRAIL expression has been associated with worse outcome (Duiker et al., 2010). Furthermore, this group reported that epigenetic silencing of TRAIL R1 occurred in 8% to 27% OC tumor samples (Horak et al., 2005b). Higher expression of TRAIL receptors in OC cells has been associated with a worse outcome (Ouellet et al., 2007; Dong et al., 2008) but other studies have found no correlation between TRAIL R1 or TRAIL R2 expression and survival (Duiker et al., 2010).

6. Resistance in OC cells

The mechanisms of resistance to TRAIL can be divided into three categories based on their mode of acquisition: intrinsic resistance, acquired resistance and environment-mediated resistance (Goncharenko-Khaider et al., 2012). Each of them will be discussed separately.

6.1. Intrinsic resistance

Intrinsic resistance is observed when tumor cells are resistant to a specific drug without previous exposure to this drug. The incidence of intrinsic resistance to TRAIL among patients presenting with OC is not known but intrinsic TRAIL resistance among OC cell lines and primary OC cells is roughly 50% (Cuello et al., 2001a; Vignati et al., 2002; Siervo-Sassi et al., 2003; Lane et al., 2004). Multiple mechanisms have been described for intrinsic TRAIL resistance in OC cells because the susceptibility to TRAIL-induced apoptosis can be regulated at multiple levels in the apoptotic signaling cascade. The loss of TRAIL R1 expression by epigenetic silencing correlated with resistance to TRAIL-induced apoptosis in OC cells (Horak et al., 2005b). Aberrant methylation of TRAIL receptors has been reported in up to 40% of OC tumors (Shivapurkar et al., 2004). Despite these observations in OC tissues, the levels of TRAIL receptors or decoy receptors do not usually correlate with sensitivity or resistance to TRAIL in OC cell lines (Cuello et al., 2001a; Vignati et al., 2002; Lane et al., 2004). However, the modulation of TRAIL receptors expression may sensitize tumor cells to TRAIL. For example, celestrol-induced upregulation of TRAIL R1 and TRAIL R2 enhances TRAIL-induced apoptosis (Zhu et al., 2010).

As mentioned earlier, c-FLIP is an important modulator of TRAIL sensitivity. Therefore, it is not surprising that c-FLIP overexpression has been associated with intrinsic TRAIL resistance in OC cells. A number of studies have demonstrated that the down-regulation of c-

$FLIP_L$ (through different means) enhances TRAIL-induced apoptosis in resistant OC cells (Lane et al., 2004; Clarke et al., 2007; Syed et al. 2007; Park et al., 2009). In addition, the knockdown of c-$FLIP_L$ inhibited human OC cell lines migratory phenotype in a TRAIL-dependent manner *in vitro* and inhibited the invasion of tumor cells into the peritoneal cavity (El-Gazzar et al., 2010a).

Activation of the PI3K/Akt promotes cell survival and resistance to chemotherapy in OC cells (Fraser et al., 2008; Abedini et al., 2010). The constitutive activation of Akt in OC cell lines and primary tumor cells also promotes resistance to TRAIL (Goncharenko-Khaider et al., 2010). There is a close correlation between the activation of Akt in OC cells and the degree of resistance to TRAIL (Goncharenko-Khaider et al., 2010; Lane et al., 2010). The inhibition of Akt phosphorylation reversed cellular resistance to TRAIL whereas the transfection of Akt in tumor cells with low Akt basal activity enhanced TRAIL resistance (Goncharenko-Khaider et al., 2010). Akt confers resistance, in part, by modulating TRAIL-induced Bid cleavage (Goncharenko-Khaider et al., 2010). The role of Akt in TRAIL resistance among OC cells is also supported by the observation that the inhibition of Akt activation by trastuzumab (Cuello et al., 2001b), an ErbB2 receptor inhibitor, or by a small molecule that inhibits hPEBP4 (Qiu et al., 2010), enhanced TRAIL-induced apoptosis.

TRAIL triggers changes in mitochondrial membrane permeability which results in the release of pro-apoptotic proteins such as cytochrome *c* and SMAC/DIABLO from the mitochondria. In a cohort of 75 patients, Mao et al. demonstrated decreased expression of SMAC/DIABLO and increased expression of XIAP in OC compared to normal ovarian tissues (Mao et al., 2007). However, they observed no difference in SMAC/DIABLO and XIAP expression between TRAIL sensitive and resistant cell lines. To assess the biological relevance of these observations, they stably transfected TRAIL resistant OC cell lines with a SMAC/DIABLO expression vector and showed enhanced TRAIL-induced apoptosis in transfected cells. Similarly, the treatment of TRAIL resistant OC cells with a small molecule SMAC/DIABLO mimic enhanced TRAIL- and TRAIL R1 or R2 agonist-induced apoptosis (Petrucci et al., 2007). Others have found a lack of correlation between XIAP protein expression and TRAIL sensitivity (Goncharenko-Khaider et al., 2010). Furthermore, down-regulation of XIAP in TRAIL resistant OC cells failed to enhance TRAIL-induced apoptosis (Goncharenko-Khaider et al., 2010) suggesting that XIAP is not a major factor contributing to TRAIL resistance in OC.

In summary, intrinsic TRAIL resistance appears to be multi-factorial and can be influenced by the activation of survival pathways such as Akt. In this context, the identification of informative and validated biomarkers of TRAIL resistance will be important for selecting patients and predicting the clinical outcome.

6.2. Acquired resistance

Acquired resistance is a mechanism by which tumor cells that were initially sensitive to a drug adapted to survive to prolonged exposure to this drug. Acquired drug resistance constitutes a major problem in the management of OC. This type of resistance is believed to be caused by sequential genetic alterations in tumor cells often associated with sub-lethal exposure to apoptosis-inducing drugs that eventually result in a therapy-resistant phenotype.

For example, in an OC cell line model, resistance to the anti-TRAIL-R2 antibody TRA-8 was induced by repeated exposure to non-apoptosis-inducing doses of the antibody (Li et al., 2006). Interestingly, the apoptotic responses induced by TRAIL, a TRAIL-R1 agonist antibody (2E12), and other apoptotic stimuli were not impaired. Lane et al. demonstrated that TRAIL acquired resistance was due to a rapid degradation of active caspase-3 subunits by the proteasome in the TRAIL resistant variant OC cells OVCAR3 (Lane et al., 2006). Interestingly, TRAIL resistant OVCAR3 cells remained sensitive to chemotherapeutic drugs.

One reassuring finding of these studies in OC and other in different tumor types is the fact that acquired TRAIL resistance does not confer cross-resistance to chemotherapeutic drugs such as cisplatin. In fact, combining standard chemotherapy with TRAIL treatment appears to be beneficial because treatment with platinum compounds upregulates the expression of TRAIL death receptors regardless of the p53 status which leads to increase apoptosis in OC cells (El-Gazzar et al., 2010b).

6.3. Environment-mediated resistance

Environment-mediated drug resistance (*de novo* resistance) is a form of resistance by which tumor cells are transiently protected from drug-induced apoptosis via the induction of survival signaling pathways (Meads et al., 2009). Soluble factors in the tumor environment may engage cell surface receptor to activate survival pathways. Evidence is accumulating that the tumor environment affects both tumor progression and response to chemotherapy in OC. The accumulation of peritoneal fluid that develops during OC progression, which contains a large mass of the tumor cells, represents a unique form of tumor environment. The floating malignant cells are capable of surviving and proliferating despite lacking immediate proximity to blood vessels presumably due to the permissive attributes of this environment. There are several indirect evidences to suggest that ascites alter drug resistance in tumor cells. Proteomic profiling of tumor cells from ascites before and after chemotherapy showed an increase in the activation of survival pathways such as Akt pathway (Davidson et al., 2006). Moreover, OC ascites attenuate TRAIL and drug-induced apoptosis *in vitro* (Lane et al., 2007; Lane et al., 2010a; Lane et al., 2010b). OC ascites contains significant levels of bioactive lipids such as lysophosphatidic acid (LPA), which exceed levels required to activate LPA receptors (Yamada et al., 2004; Lane et al., 2010a). LPA, one of the ligands of G-protein coupled receptors, has been shown to induce cell survival signaling pathways through different mechanisms including PI3K/Akt activation and regulation of DR4 and c-FLIP (Tanyi et al., 2003; Kang et al., 2004; Ishdorj et al., 2008). Furthermore, LPA inhibits cisplatin-induced apoptosis (Tanyi et al., 2003). The role of LPA, as a component of ascites, in modulating drug resistance in OC cells remains however uncertain. For example, the blockade of LPA cascade did not altered TRAIL-induced apoptosis in OC cells (Lane et al., 2010a) and incubation of OC cells with LPA did not protect them from TRAIL-induced apoptosis (Lane et al., 2010).

A wide variety of cytokines can be measured in OC ascites and interleukin-6 (IL-6) and interleukin-8 (IL-8) are among the most abundant (Giuntoli et al., 2009; Lane et al., 2011; Matte et al., 2012). A number of studies have reported an association between serum levels of IL-6 and prognosis, where elevated levels correlated with a poor relapse-free and overall survival (Plante et al., 1994; Scambia et al., 1995; Tempfer et al., 1997). Interestingly, it was recently shown that elevated ascites levels of IL-6, but not IL-8, were an independent predictor of shorter progression-free survival (Lane et al., 2011). Whether IL-6 is a critical soluble factor in ascites-mediated TRAIL resistance is unclear but a recent study suggests that IL-6 may indeed be an important component of the tumor environment that support tumor growth (Kulbe et al., 2012). Recently, high levels of IL-10, OPG and leptin in ascites were found to correlate with shorter PFS (Matte et al., 2012). Furthermore, in this study, Il-10 neutralizing antibodies attenuated the protective effect of ascites against TRAIL-induced apoptosis suggesting that IL-10 is one of the factors in ascites that promote ascites-induced TRAIL resistance.

The role of integrins in mediating cell proliferation, migration and survival in ovarian cancer is well established (Carreiras et al., 1999; Cruet-Hennequart et al., 2003; Lane et al., 2008). Integrins transmit signals directly through ligation-dependent recruitment of non-receptor tyrosine kinases from the focal adhesion kinase (FAK) leading to the activation of several cell signaling pathways including the PI3K/Akt pathway (Stupack and Cheresh, 2002). Recently, it has been shown that the PI3K/Akt cascade is activated by OC ascites (Lane et al., 2010a). The ability of different ascites to induce Akt phosphorylation in tumor cells strongly correlates with their ability to inhibit TRAIL-induced apoptosis. The PI3K/Akt pathway most likely couples signals from ascites-activated cell surface receptors which regulate the expression and/or phosphorylation of apoptosis-regulating targets. Ascites-induced activation of $\alpha v\beta 5$ integrins leads to focal adhesion kinase (FAK) phosphorylation and FAK induces the activation of Akt (Lane et al., 2010a). This leads to Akt-mediated up-regulation of c-FLIPs expression in ovarian cancer cells (Lane et al., 2007).

Collectively, these data support the role of ascites to promote resistance to TRAIL-induced apoptosis, at least *in vitro*. Whether this is relevant *in vivo* remains unclear for the moment. However, the prosurvival activity of ascites against TRAIL-induced apoptosis has been associated with shorter PFS in women with OC suggesting that ascites-mediated resistance might be clinically relevant (Lane et al., 2010b).

7. TRAIL targeting agents

Different strategies have been used to activate the TRAIL signaling pathway in cancer therapy. A variety of recombinant forms of soluble TRAIL have been developed and fused with different tags (Pitti et al., 1996; Schneider et al., 2000; Ganten et al., 2006). Major limitations however of recombinant soluble TRAIL (rsTRAIL) include the short half-life *in vivo* and relative lack of specificity as rsTRAIL can also bind decoy receptors TRAIL R3 and TRAIL R4. Despite these potential limitations, rsTRAIL (dulanermin) has entered phase I and phase II clinical trials. Alternatively, various humanized TRAIL receptor agonist antibodies have been developed which target TRAIL R1 (Mapatumumab) or TRAIL R2 (Apomab, Conatumumab, Lexatumumab, Tigatuzumab and LBY-135), and are currently being evaluated clinically (Table 1). These antibodies have a significantly increased half-life and consequently their bioavailability is increased at the tumor site.

Name	**Targets**	**Compagny**	**Clinical stage development**
Apomab/Drozitumab (PRO95780) (human monoclonal antibody agonist)	TRAIL R2	Genetech	Phase II
Conatumumab (AMG 655) (human monoclonal antibody agonist)	TRAIL R2	Amgen	Phase I/II
Dulanermin (rs TRAIL)	TRAIL R1 and TRAIL R2	Amgen/Genetech	Phase I/II
Lexatumumab (HGS-ETR2) (monoclonal antibody agonist)	TRAIL R2	Human Genome Sciences	Phase I
Mapatumumab (TRM 1, HGS-ETR1)	TRAIL R1	Human Genome Sciences	Phase II
Tigatuzumab (CS-1008) (humanized monoclonal antibody agonist)	TRAIL R2	Daiichi Sankyo	Phase I/II
LBY-135 (humanized monoclonal antibody agonist)	TRAIL R2	Novartis	Phase I

Table 1. TRAIL-targeting agents

8. Therapeutic potential of TRAIL agonistic agents in ovarian cancer: Preclinical studies

8.1. Monotherapy

The anti-tumor activity of dulanermin has been extensively evaluated in preclinical models (Ashkenazi et al., 1999; Hylander et al., 2005; Pollack et al., 2001). Furthermore, preclinical *in vitro* studies have demonstrated that OC cell lines displayed variable sensitivity to recombinant human TRAIL (Cuello et al., 2001; Vignati et al., 2002; Siervo-Sassi et al., 2003; Lane et al., 2004). TRAIL-resistant cell lines usually remain sensitive to chemotherapy and conversely, cisplatin-resistant cell lines may be sensitive to TRAIL. Collectively, these results suggest that both platinum-sensitive and platinum-resistant OC are candidates for TRAIL-targeting therapy (Tomek et al., 2004). To increase cancer cell-directed toxicity of TRAIL, fusion proteins of rsTRAIL with target moiety to epidermal growth factor receptor (EGFR) have been developed and were shown to have superior pro-apoptotic activity compared to soluble TRAIL in tumor cells that expressed high levels of EGFR such as the OC cell line OVCAR3 (Bremer et al., 2008).

8.2. Combination therapy

Several studies demonstrated that the combination of TRAIL with cisplatin was more efficient than either molecule alone in various OC cell lines *in vitro* (Cuello et al., 2001; Vignati et al., 2002; Siervo-Sassi et al., 2003; Tomek et al., 2004; Liu et al., 2006). In a mouse model of OC, treatment with rhTRAIL-DR5 or rhTRAIL in combination with cisplatin significantly reduced tumor growth compared to rhTRAIL-DR5 alone (97% and 85% reduction in the combination arms versus 63% reduction in the rhTRAIL-DR5 arm alone) (Duiker et al., 2009). In this study, the beneficial effect of combined treatment was related to the observation that cisplatin strongly enhanced TRAIL R2 surface expression. Similar to cisplatin, proteasome inhibitors and nelfinavir, an HIV protease inhibitor, up-regulate TRAIL R2 and enhance the sensitivity of ovarian cancer cells and tissue explants to an apoptosis-inducing TRAIL receptor antibody (Saulle et al., 2007; Brüning et al., 2008; Brüning et al., 2009; Pasquini et al., 2010). For example, mapatumumab (TRAIL R1 agonist) and lexatumumab (TRAIL R2 agonist) were more efficient than TRAIL to induce apoptosis in primary OC cells and enhanced apoptosis induced by the proteasome inhibitor bortezomid (Pasquini et al., 2010). Using a model of acquired cisplatin resistant cell lines, Duiker et al. showed that cisplatin enhances TRAIL-induced apoptosis in cisplatin-resistant ovarian cancer cells, and induction of caspase-8 protein expression is the key factor of TRAIL sensitization (Duiker et al., 2011). Estes et al. evaluated the cytotoxicity of TRAIL R2 agonist (TRA-8) in nineteen chemotherapy-naive primary ovarian tumor samples (stage III/IV) (Estes et al., 2007). Using a similar ex vivo model, increased cytotoxicity was observed when TRA-8 was used in combination with chemotherapeutic drugs (Frederick et al., 2009). The potential of TRA-8 was further evaluated in a xenograft mouse model of OC (Bevis et al., 2011). When used alone, TRA-8 produced only a modest benefit in terms of tumor growth inhibition. However, animals treated with the combination of carboplatin, docetaxel and TRA-8 demonstrated a better outcome when compared to carboplatin and docetaxel only.

Because TRAIL cytotoxicity in OC cells relies on the activation of both the extrinsic and the intrinsic apoptosis pathways, the combination of TRAIL with pro-apoptotic proteins is of interest. For example, SMAC/DIABLO or LBW242, a SMAC/DIABLO mimic, sensitizes OC cell lines to the antitumor effects of TRAIL and anticancer drugs commonly used in clinic (Mao et al., 2007; Petrucci et al., 2007; Petrucci et al., 2012). These observations suggest that the LBW242 could be of value for the development of experimental strategies for treatment of ovarian cancer. Radicicol, an Hsp90 inhibitor, potentiate the apoptotic effect of TRAIL on ovarian carcinoma cell lines by increasing the activation of the caspase-8- and Bid-dependent pathway and the mitochondria-mediated apoptotic pathway, leading to caspase activation (Kim et al., 2012).

The enhanced efficacy of TRAIL in combination with other agents in preclinical models is encouraging and suggests that combination therapies with TRAIL probably represent the best clinical option at this point. Because TRAIL resistance in OC can be induced by various pathways, a combination of molecules that targets critical steps in the TRAIL signaling cascade is likely to be the most efficient approach.

9. Clinical trials with TRAIL targeting agents in OC patients

A large number of phase I/II clinical trials have been undertaken with TRAIL targeting agents either as monotherapy or in combination with chemotherapeutic drugs in a wide range of solid and haematological malignancies (Table 2). For the purpose of this discussion, we have only considered clinical studies with TRAIL targeting agents that included patients with OC.

Name	Status	Clinical stage	Clinical Trials Identifier
Apomab/Drozitumab			
A study of PRO95780 in patients with previously untreated, advanced-stage NSCLC	Completed	Phase II	NCT00480831
A study of PRO95780 in combination with Rituximab in patients with NHL that has progressed following previous Rituximab therapy	Completed	Phase II	NCT00517049
A study of PRO95780 in combination with Cetuximab and Irinotecan chemotherapy or the FOLFIRI regimen with Bevacizumab in patients with previously treated metastatic colorectal cancer	Completed	Phase I	NCT00497497
A study of PRO95780 administered in combination with the FOLFOX regimen and Bevacizumab in patients with previously untreated, locally advanced, recurrent, and metastatic colorectal Cancer	Completed	Phase I	NCT00851136
Conatumumab			
Phase I/II study of Conatumumab and Gemcitabine Hydrochloride followed by Conatumumab, Capecitabine, and 3-dimensional conformal radiotherapy in patients with locally advanced pancreatic cancer	Approved – not yet active	Phase I	NCT01017822
A phase 1b/2 study of AMG 655 in combination with Paclitaxel and Carboplatin for the first-line treatment of advanced NSCLC	Completed	Phase I/II	NCT00534027
Phase 1b/2 study of AMG 655 with mFOLFOX6 and Bevacizumab for first-line metastatic colorectal cancer	Completed	Phase I/II	NCT00625651
Phase 1b/2 study of AMG 655 with Doxorubicin for the first-line treatment of unresectable soft tissue sarcoma	Completed	Phase I/II	NCT00626704

Name	Status	Clinical stage	Clinical Trials Identifier
A study of AMG 655 or AMG 479 in combination with Gemcitabine for treatment of metastatic pancreatic cancer	Completed	Phase I/II	NCT00630552
AMG655/Panitumumab combination in metastatic colorectal cancer study	Completed	Phase I/II	NCT00630786
AMG 655 in combination with AMG 479 in advanced, refractory solid tumors	Completed	Phase I/II	NCT00819169
Phase 2 safety & efficacy of FOLFIRI in combination with AMG 479 or AMG 655 vs FOLFIRI in KRAS-mutant metastatic colorectal carcinoma	Completed	Phase II	NCT00813605
Phase 1b Lymphoma Study of AMG 655 in Combination With Bortezomib or Vorinostat	Completed	Phase I	NCT00791011
Dulanermin			
A study of AMG 951 [rhApo2L/TRAIL] in subjects with previously untreated NSCLC treated with chemotherapy +/- Bevacizumab	Completed	Phase II	NCT00508625
A study of Dulanermin administered in combination with Camptosar®/Erbitux® chemotherapy or FOLFIRI (with or without Bevacizumab) in subjects with previously treated metastatic colorectal cancer	Completed	Phase I	NCT00671372
A study of Dulanermin administered in combination with the FOLFOX regimen and Bevacizumab in patients with previously untreated, locally advanced, recurrent, or metastatic colorectal cancer	Completed	Phase I	NCT00873756
Lexatumumab			
Phase I study of Lexatumumab with or without recombinant interferon gamma in pediatric patients with relapsed or refractory solid tumors or lymphoma	Completed	Phase I	NCT00428272
Mapatumumab Mapatumumab, Cisplatin and radiotherapy for advanced cervical cancer	Active	Phase I/II	NCT01088347
Study of TRM-1 (TRAIL-R1 monoclonal antibody) in subject with relapsed or refractory NSCLC	Completed	Phase II	NCT00092924
Study of TRM-1 (TRAIL-R1 monoclonal antibody) in subjects with relapsed or refractory NHL	Completed	Phase II	NCT00094848

Name	Status	Clinical stage	Clinical Trials Identifier
Study of Mapatumumab in combination with Bortezomib (Velcade) and Bortezomib alone in subjects with relapsed or refractory multiple myeloma	Completed	Phase II	NCT00315757
A Study of Mapatumumab in combination with Paclitaxel and Carboplatin in Subjects With NSCLC	Completed	Phase II	NCT00583830
Study of Mapatumumab in combination with Sorafenib in subjects with advanced hepatocellular carcinoma	Completed	Phase II	NCT01258608
Tigatuzumab			
An imaging and pharmacodynamic trial of CS-1008 in patients with metastatic colorectal cancer	Active	Phase I	NCT01220999
Open-label study of CS1008 for subjects with untreated and unresectable pancreatic cancer	Completed	Phase II	NCT00521404
Combination chemotherapy with CS-1008 to treat ovarian cancer	Completed	Phase II	NCT00945191
CS-1008 with Carboplatin/Paclitaxel in chemotherapy naive subjects with metastatic or unresectable NSCLC	Completed	Phase II	NCT00991796
CS1008- in combination with Sorafenib compared to Sorafenib alone in subjects with advanced liver cancer	Completed	Phase II	NCT01033240
Abraxane with or without Tigatuzumab in patients with metastatic, triple negative breast cancer	Completed	Phase II	NCT01307891
Study of CS-1008 in patients with advanced solid malignancies and lymphomas (without leukemic component)	Completed	Phase I	NCT00320827
Study of CS-1008 in combination with FOLFIRI in patients who have failed other treatments	Completed	Phase I	NCT01124630

Abbreviations: NHL, non Hodgkin lymphoma; NSCLC, non-small cell lung cancer

Table 2. Active or completed clinical trials with TRAIL targeting agents

TRAIL-based treatment strategies that entered clinical studies have included dulanermin. In a phase I study involving 71 patients with advanced or metastatic solid tumors or non-Hodgkin lymphoma (NHL), dulanermin appeared safe and well tolerated (Herbst et al., 2010). Partial response and stable disease were observed in 3% and 53% of patients respectively in this study. Additonal clinical studies with dulanermin in combination with other drugs have been performed most often in patients with lung cancer (Soria et al., 2010; Soria et al., 2011).

Although there have been several published early-phase trials with antibody targeting TRAIL-R1 or TRAIL-R2, only two have included patients with OC. The feasibility of intravenous mapatumumab administration, as a single-agent, has been examined in a phase I pharmacokinetic and biological correlative study in patients with advanced solid malignancies refractory to standard therapy (Tolcher et al., 2007). Of the 49 patients enrolled in the study, two had advanced OC. Mapatumumab dosing ranged from 0.01 to 10 mg/kg and was administered every 2-4 weeks. Overall, mapatumumab was well tolerated and toxicity was generally limited to grade 1-2 events. No objective response was observed for mapatumumab in this unselected phase I study. Hotte et al. evaluated the safety and tolerability of mapatumumab in a phase I clinical trial involving 41 patients with malignant solid tumors refractory to conventional therapy in which 22% of the patients had OC (Hotte et al., 2008). Mapatumumab was administered intravenously every 4 weeks and patients received a median of 2 cycles (range, 1-33) with mapatumumab doses ranging from 0.01 to 20 mg/kg. The patient that received 33 cycles of mapatumumab had a diagnosis of borderline OC. She experienced no cumulative toxicity. Indeed, mapatumumab was generally well tolerated and common adverse events included fatigue, hypotension, nausea and fever. No objective response was observed. Conatumumab (AMG 655), a TRAIL R2-specific antibody is currently being evaluated in patients with advanced refractory solid tumors that includes ovarian tumors in combination with ganitumab, a fully human monoclonal antibody against insulin-like growth factor receptor 1 (National Cancer Institute (NCI) Clinical Trials Identifier Number : NCT00819169).

Of the two studies published with mapatumumab in combination with chemotherapy, one included a patient with OC (primary peritoneal carcinoma) (Leong et al., 2009). A phase II using tigatuzumab (CS-1008), a humanized TRAIL-R2 antibody, in combination with paclitaxel and carboplatin is underway (NCI Clinical Trials Identifier Number: NCT00945191).

10. Conclusions and future directions

The inherent properties of TRAIL or its agonists offer a new targeted therapy for OC. Preclinical studies using TRAIL or its agonists have demonstrated the therapeutic potential of these molecules and formed the basis of ongoing phase I/II clinical trials. Although these treatments appear to be clinically well tolerated so far, intrinsic, acquired and environment-mediated resistance may limit the effectiveness of these approaches. However, the development of combination treatments appears to be capable of overcoming, at least in part, some of these limitations. As the search for more effective treatment for OC continues, the morbidity and mortality will hopefully improve. TRAIL treatment strategies have been used so far in the context of salvage treatment and the optimal patient population that will mostly benefit from these treatments remains to be defined. Although significant progress has been made in our understanding of the molecular basis of TRAIL resistance in OC, efforts should continue to further improve this knowledge as this will likely lead to the development of specific biomarkers of resistance and more efficient targeted therapies.

http://dx.doi.org/10.5772/53380

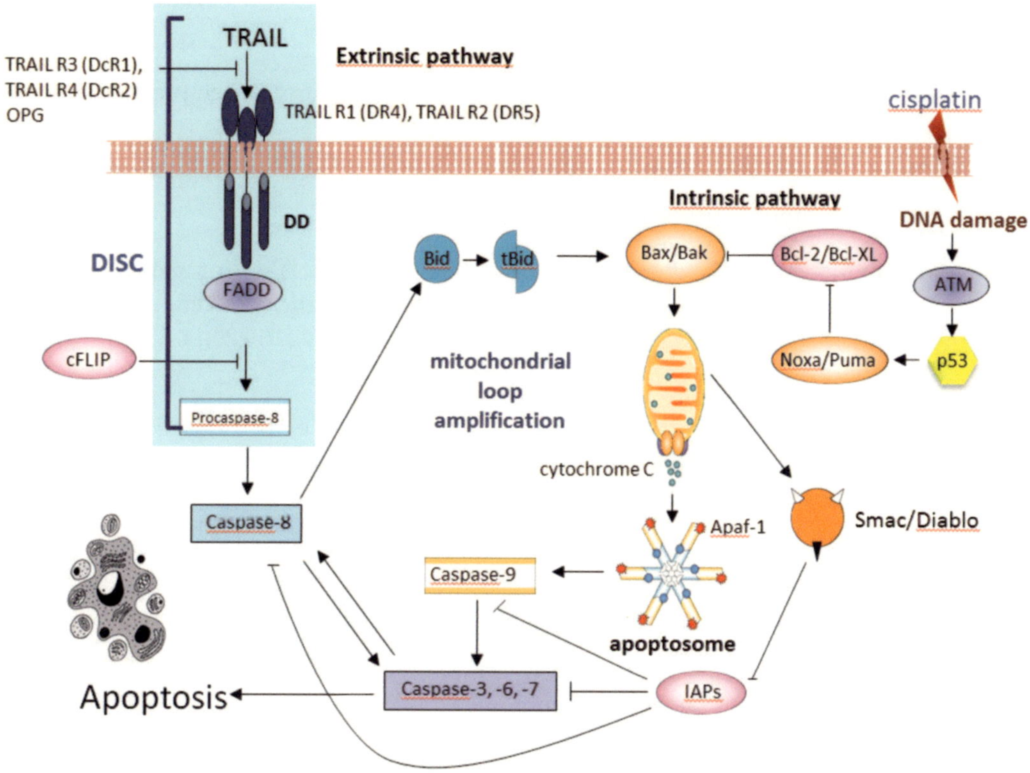

Figure 1. Apoptotic pathways. Binding of TRAIL to death receptors (TRAIL R1, TRAIL R2) leads to the recruitment of the adaptor molecule, FADD. Pro-caspase-8 binds to FADD leading to DISC formation and resulting in its activation. Activated caspase-8 directly activates executioner caspases (caspase-3, -6, and -7) (type I cells) or cleaves Bid (type II cells). Translocation of the truncated Bid (tBid) to the mitochondria promotes the assembly of Bax-Bak oligomers and mitochondria outer membrane permeability changes. Cytochrome c is released into cytosol resulting in apoptosome assembly. Active caspase-9 then propagates a proteolytic cascade of effector caspases activation that leads to morphological hallmarks of apoptosis. Further cleavage of pro-caspase-8 by effector caspases generates a mitochondrial amplification loop that further enhances apoptosis. When FLIP levels are elevated in cells, caspase-8 preferentially recruits FLIP to form a caspase-8-FLIP heterodimer which does not trigger apoptosis. Chemotherapeutic drugs such as cisplatin cause DNA damage which is sensed by the ataxia telangiectasia mutated homolog (ATM) leading to the activation of p53 dependent activation of genes such as PUMA and Noxa which can bind to anti-apoptotic proteins Bcl-2/Bcl-XL thereby opposing their effect. This leads to mitochondrial permeabilization and activation.

Author details

Nadzeya Goncharenko-Khaider, Denis Lane, Isabelle Matte, Claudine Rancourt and Alain Piché*

*Address all correspondence to: Alain.Piche@USherbrooke.ca

Département de Microbiologie et Infectiologie, Faculté de Médecine et des Sciences de la Santé, Université de Sherbrooke, Sherbrooke, Canada

References

[1] Adams JM and Cory S. The Bcl-2 apoptotic switch in cancer development and therapy. Oncogene 2007;26:1324–1337.

[2] Abdulghani J and El-Deiry WS. TRAIL receptor signaling and therapeutics. Expert Opin Ther Targets 2010;14:1091-1108.

[3] Abedini MR, Muller EJ, Bergeron R, Gray DA, Tsang BK. Akt promotes chemoresistance in human ovarian cancer cells by modulating cisplatin-induced, p53-dependent ubiquitination of FLICE-like inhibitory protein. Oncogene 2010;29:11-25.

[4] Ashkenazi A, Pai RC, Fong S, Leung S, Lawrence DA, Marsters SA, Blackie C, Chang L, McMurtrey AE, Hebert A, DeForge L, Koumenis IL, Lewis D, Harris L, Bussiere J, Koeppen H, Shahrokh Z, Schwall RH. Safety and antitumor activity of recombinant soluble Apo2 ligand. J Clin Invest 1999;104:155-162.

[5] Ashkenazi A, Holland P, Eckhardt SG. Ligand-based targeting of apoptosis in cancer: the potential of recombinant human apoptosis ligand 2/tumor necrosis factor-related apoptosis-inducing ligand (rhApo2L/TRAIL). J Clin Oncol 2008;26:3621–3630.

[6] Ashkenazi A. Directing cancer cells to self-destruct with pro-apoptotic receptor agonists. Nat Rev Drug Discov 2008;7:1001-1012.

[7] Bagnoli M, Ambrogi F, Pilotti S, Alberti P, Ditto A, Barbareschi M, Galligioni E, Biganzoli E, Canevari S, Mezzanzanica D. c-FLIPL expression defines two ovarian cancer patient subsets and is a prognostic factor of adverse outcome. Endocr Relat Cancer 2009; 16:443-453.

[8] Bagnoli M, Canevari S. Mezzanzanica D. Cellular FLICE-inhibitory protein (c-FLIP) signalling: a key regulator of receptor-mediated apoptosis in physiologic context and in cancer. Int J Biochem Cell Biol 2010;42:210-213.

[9] Bélanger S, Côté M, Lane D, L'Espérance S, Rancourt C, Piché A. Bcl-2 decreases cell proliferation and promotes accumulation of cells in S phase without affecting the rate of apoptosis in human ovarian carcinoma cells. Gynecol Oncol 2005;97:796-806.

[10] Bevis KS, McNally LR, Sellers JC, Della Manna D, Londoño Joshi A, Amm H, Straughn JM Jr, Buchsbaum DJ. Anti-tumor activity of an anti-DR5 monoclonal antibody, TRA-8, in combination with taxane/platinum-based chemotherapy in an ovarian cancer model. Gynecol Oncol 2011;121:193-199.

[11] Bremer E, de Bruyn M, Samplonius DF, Bijma T, ten Cate B, de Leij LF, Helfrich W. Targeted delivery of a designed sTRAIL mutant results in superior apoptotic activity towards EGFR-positive tumor cells. J Mol Med 2008;86:909-924.

[12] Brunelle JK, Letai A. Control of mitochondrial apoptosis by the Bcl-2 family. J Cell Sci 2009;122:437-441.

[13] Brüning A, Vogel M, Burger P, Rahmeh M, Gingelmaier A, Friese K, Lenhard M, Burges A. Nelfinavir induces TRAIL receptor upregulation in ovarian cancer cells. Biochem Biophys Res Commun 2008;377:1309-1314.

[14] Brüning A, Burger P, Vogel M, Rahmeh M, Friese K, Lenhard M, Burges A. Bortezomib treatment of ovarian cancer cells mediates endoplasmic reticulum stress, cell cycle arrest, and apoptosis. Invest New Drugs 2009;27:543-551.

[15] Carreiras F, Rigot V, Cruet S, Andre F, Gauduchon P, Marvaldi J. Migration properties of the human ovarian adenocarcinoma cell line IGROV1: importance of alpha(V)beta3 integrins and vitronectin. Int J Cancer 1999;80:285-294.

[16] Chang DW, Xing Z, Pan Y, Algeciras-Schimnich A, Barnhart BC, Yaish-Ohad S, Peter ME, Yang X. c-FLIP(L) is a dual function regulator for caspase-8 activation and CD95-mediated apoptosis. Embo J 2002;21:3704-3714.

[17] Clarke P, Tyler KL. Down-regulation of cFLIP following reovirus infection sensitizes human ovarian cancer cells to TRAIL-induced apoptosis. Apoptosis 2007;12:211-223.

[18] Colombo N, Van Gorp T, Parma G, Amant F, Gatta G, Sessa C, Vergote I. Ovarian cancer. Crit Rev Oncol Hematol 2006;60:159-179.

[19] Cruet-Hennequart S, Maubant S, Luis J, Gauduchon P, Staedel C, Dedhar S. Alpha(v) integrins regulate cell proliferation through integrin-linked kinase (ILK) in ovarian cancer cells. Oncogene 2003;22:1688-1702.

[20] Cuello M, Ettenberg SA, Nau MM, Lipkowitz S. Synergistic induction of apoptosis by the combination of TRAIL and chemotherapy in chemoresistant ovarian cancer cells. Gynecol Oncol 2001;81:380-390.

[21] Cuello M, Ettenberg SA, Clark AS, Keane MM, Posner RH, Nau MM, Dennis PA, Lipkowitz S. Down-regulation of the erbB-2 receptor by trastuzumab (herceptin) enhances tumor necrosis factor-related apoptosis-inducing ligand-mediated apoptosis in breast and ovarian cancer cell lines that overexpress erbB-2. Cancer Res 2001;61:4892-4900.

[22] Davidson B, Espina V, Steinberg SM, Flørenes VA, Liotta LA, Kristensen GB, Tropé CG, Berner A, Kohn EC. Proteomic analysis of malignant ovarian cancer effusions as a tool for biologic and prognostic profiling. Clin Cancer Res 2006;12:791-799.

[23] Djerbi M, Darreh-Shori T, Zhivotovsky B, Grandien A. Characterization of the human FLICE-inhibitory protein locus and comparison of the anti-apoptotic activity of four different flip isoforms. Scand J Immunol 2001;54:180-189.

[24] Dodier P and Piché A. Bcl-X(L) is functionally non-equivalent for the regulation of growth and survival in human ovarian cancer cells. Gynecol Oncol 2006;100:254-263.

[25] Dong HP, Kleinberg L, Silins I, Flørnes, Tropé CG, Risberg B, Nesland JM, Davidson B. Death receptor expression is associated with poor response to chemotherapy and shorter survival in metastatic ovarian carcinoma. Cancer 2008;112:84-93.

[26] Duiker EW, de Vries EG, Mahalingam D, Meersma GJ, Boersma-van Ek W, Hollema H, Lub-de Hooge MN, van Dam GM, Cool RH, Quax WJ, Samali A, van der Zee AG, de Jong S. Enhanced antitumor efficacy of a DR5-specific TRAIL variant over recombinant human TRAIL in a bioluminescent ovarian cancer xenograft model. Clin Cancer Res 2009;15:2048-2057.

[27] Duiker EW, van der Zee AG, de Graeff P, Boersma-van Ek W, Hollema H, de Bock GH, de Jong S, de Vries EG. The extrinsic apoptosis pathway and its prognostic impact in ovarian cancer. Gynecol Oncol 2010;116:549-555.

[28] Duiker EW, Meijer A, van der Bilt AR, Meersma GJ, Kooi N, van der Zee AG, de Vries EG, de Jong S. Drug-induced caspase 8 upregulation sensitises cisplatin-resistant ovarian carcinoma cells to rhTRAIL-induced apoptosis. Br J Cancer. 2011;104:1278-1287.

[29] El-Gazzar A, Wittinger M, Perco P, Anees M, Horvat R, Mikulits W, Grunt TW, Mayer B, Krainer M. The role of c-FLIP(L) in ovarian cancer: chaperoning tumor cells from immunosurveillance and increasing their invasive potential. Gynecol Oncol 2010;117:451-459.

[30] El-Gazzar A, Perco P, Eckelhart E, Anees M, Sexl V, Mayer B, Liu Y, Mikulits W, Horvat R, Pangerl T, Zheng D, Krainer M. Natural immunity enhances the activity of a DR5 agonistic antibody and carboplatin in the treatment of ovarian cancer. Mol Cancer Ther 2010;9:1007-1018.

[31] Estes JM, Oliver PG, Straughn JM Jr, Zhou T, Wang W, Grizzle WE, Alvarez RD, Stockard CR, LoBuglio AF, Buchsbaum DJ. Efficacy of anti-death receptor 5 (DR5) antibody (TRA-8) against primary human ovarian carcinoma using a novel ex vivo tissue slice model. Gynecol Oncol 2007;105:291-298.

[32] Evan G, Littlewood T. A matter of life and cell death. Science 1998;281:1317–1322.

[33] Fraser M, Bai T, Tsang BK. Akt promotes cisplatin resistance in human ovarian cancer cells through inhibition of p53 phosphorylation and nuclear function. Int J Cancer 2008;122:534-546.

[34] Frederick PJ, Kendrick JE, Straughn JM Jr, Della Manna DL, Oliver PG, Lin HY, Grizzle WE, Stockard CR, Alvarez RD, Zhou T, LoBuglio AF, Buchsbaum DJ. Effect of TRA-8 anti-death receptor 5 antibody in combination with chemotherapy in an ex vivo human ovarian cancer model. Int J Gynecol Cancer 2009;19:814-819.

[35] Ganten TM, Koschny R, Sykora J, Schulze-Bergkamen H, Büchler P, Haas TL, Schader MB, Untergasser A, Stremmel W, Walzack H. Preclinical differentiation between apparently safe and potentially hepatotoxic applications of TRAIL either alone or in combination with chemotherapeutic drugs. Clin Cancer Res 2006;12:2640-2646.

[36] Giuntoli RL 2nd, Webb TJ, Zoso A, Rogers O, Diaz-Montes TP, Bristow RE, Oelke M. Ovarian cancer-associated ascites demonstrates altered immune environment: implications for antitumor immunity. Anticancer Res 2009; 29:2875-2884.

[37] Goncharenko-Khaider N, Lane D, Matte I, Rancourt C, Piché A. The inhibition of Bid expression by Akt leads to resistance to TRAIL-induced apoptosis in ovarian cancer cells. Oncogene 2010;29:5523-5536.

[38] Goncharenko-Khaider N, Lane D, Matte I, Rancourt C, Piché A. Targeted ovarian cancer treatment: the TRAILs of resistance. Am J Cancer Res 2012;2:75-92.

[39] Hellwig CT, Rehm M. TRAIL signaling and synergy mechanisms used in TRAIL-based combination therapies. Mol Cancer Ther 2012;11:3-13.

[40] Hengartner MO. The biochemistry of apoptosis. Nature 2000;407:770–6.

[41] Henriksen R, Wilander E, Oberg K. Expression and prognostic significance of Bcl-2 in ovarian tumours. Br J Cancer 1995;72:1324-1329.

[42] Herbst RS, Eckhardt SG, Kurzrock R, Ebbinghaus S, O'Dwyer PJ, Gordon MS, Novotny W, Goldwasser MA, Tohnya TM, Lum BL, Ashkenazi A, Jubb AM, Mendelson DS. Phase I dose-escalation study of recombinant human Apo2L/TRAIL, a dual proapoptotic receptor agonist, in patients with advanced cancer. J Clin Oncol 2010;28:2839-46.

[43] Herod JJ, Eliopoulos AG, Warwick J, Niedobitek G, Young LS, Kerr DJ. The prognostic significance of Bcl-2 and p53 expression in ovarian carcinoma. Cancer Res 1996;56:2178-2184.

[44] Herzog TJ. Recurrent ovarian cancer: how important is it to treat to disease progression? Clin Cancer Res 2004;10:7439-7449.

[45] Hofbauer LC, Heufelder AE. Role of receptor activator of nuclear factor-kappaB ligand and osteoprotegerin in the pathogenesis and treatment of metabolic bone diseases. J Clin Endocrinol Metab 2000;85:2355-2363.

[46] Horak P, Pils D, Kaider A, Pinter A, Elandt K, Sax C, Zielinski CC, Horvat R, Zeillinger R, Reinthaller A, Krainer M. Pertubation of the tumor necrosis factor-related apoptosis-inducing ligand cascade in ovarian cancer: overexpression of FLIPL and deregulation of the functional receptors DR4 and DR5. Clin Cancer Res 2005;11:8585-8591.

[47] Horak P, Pils D, Haller G, Pribill I, Röessler M, Tomek S, Horvat R, Zeillinger R, Zielinski C, Krainer M. Contribution of epigenetic silencing of tumor necrosis factor-related apoptosis-inducing ligand receptor 1 (DR4) to TRAIL resistance and ovarian cancer. Mol Cancer Res 2005;3:335-343.

[48] Hotte SJ, Hirte HW, Chen EX, Siu LL, Le LH, Corey A, Iacobucci A, MacLean M, Lo L, Fox NL, Oza AM. A phase I study of mapatumumab (fully human monoclonal antibody to TRAIL-R1) in patients with advanced solid malignancies. Clin Cancer Res 2008;14:3450-3455.

[49] Hylander BL, Pitoniak R, Penetrante RB, Gibbs JF, Otkay D, Cheng J, Repasky EA. The anti-tumor effect of Apo2L/TRAIL on patient pancreatic adenocarcinomas grown as xenografts in SCID mice. J Transl Med 2005;3:22.

[50] Ishdorj G, Graham BA, Hu X, Chen J, Johnston JB, Fang X, Gibson SB. Lysophosphatidic acid protects cancer cells from histone deacetylase (HDAC) inhibitor-induced apoptosis through activation of HDAC. J Biol Chem 2008;283:16818-16829.

[51] Kang YC, Kim KM, Lee KS, Namkoong S, Lee SJ, Han JA, Jeoung D, Ha KS, Kwon YG, Kim YM. Serum bioactive lysophospholipids prevent TRAIL-induced apoptosis via PI3K/Akt-dependent cFLIP expression and Bad phosphorylation. Cell Death Differ 2004; 11:1287-1298.

[52] Kim K, Fisher MJ, Xu SQ, el-Deiry WS. Molecular determinants of response to TRAIL in killing of normal and cancer cells. Clin Cancer Res 2000;6:335-346.

[53] Kim YJ, Lee SA, Myung SC, Kim W, Lee CS. Radicicol, an inhibitor of Hsp90, enhances TRAIL-induced apoptosis in human epithelial ovarian carcinoma cells by promoting activation of apoptosis-related proteins. Mol Cell Biochem. 2012;359:33-43.

[54] Krueger A, Baumann S, Krammer PH, Kirchhoff S. FLICE-inhibitory proteins : regulators of death receptor-mediated apoptosis. Mol Cell Biol 2001;21:8247-8254.

[55] Kulbe H, Chakravarty P, Leinster DA, Charles KA, Kwong J, Thompson RG, Coward JI, Schioppa T, Robinson SC, Gallagher WM, Galletta L; Australian Ovarian Cancer Study Group, Salako MA, Smyth JF, Hagemann T, Brennan DJ, Bowtell DD, Balkwill FR. A dynamic inflammatory cytokine network in the human ovarian cancer microenvironment. Cancer Res 2012;72:66-75.

[56] Lancaster JM, Sayer R, Blanchette C, Calingaert B, Whitaker R, Schildkraut J, Marks J, Berchuck A. High expression of tumor necrosis factor-related apoptosis-inducing ligand is associated with favorable ovarian cancer survival. Clin Cancer Res 2003;9:762-766.

[57] Lane D, Cartier A, L'Espérance S, Côté M, Rancourt C, Piché A. Differential induction of apoptosis by tumor necrosis factor-related apoptosis-inducing ligand in human ovarian carcinoma cells. Gynecol Oncol 2004;93:594-604.

[58] Lane D, Côté M, Grondin R, Couture MC, Piché A. Acquired resistance to TRAIL-induced apoptosis in human ovarian cancer cells is conferred by increased turnover of mature caspase-3. Mol Cancer Ther 2006;5:509-521.

[59] Lane D, Robert V, Grondin R, Rancourt C, Piché A. Malignant ascites protect against TRAIL-induced apoptosis by activating the PI3K/Akt pathway in human ovarian carcinoma cells. Int J Cancer 2007;121:1227-1237.

[60] Lane D, Cartier AC, Rancourt C, Piché A. Cell detachment modulates TRAIL resistance in ovarian cancer cells by downregulating the phosphatidylinositol 3-kinase/Akt pathway. Int J Gynecol Cancer 2008;18:670-676.

[61] Lane D, Goncharenko-Khaider N, Rancourt C, Piché A. Ovarian cancer ascites protects from TRAIL-induced cell death through αVβ5 integrin-mediated focal adhesion kinase and Akt activation. Oncogene 2010;29:3519-3531.

[62] Lane D, Matte I, Rancourt C, Piché A. The prosurvival activity of ascites against TRAIL is associated with a shorter disease-free interval in patients with ovarian cancer. J Ovarian Res 2010;3:1.

[63] Lane D, Matte I, Rancourt C, Piché A. Prognostic significance of IL-6 and IL-8 ascites levels in ovarian cancer patients. BMC Cancer 2011;11:210.

[64] Leong S, Cohen RB, Gustafson DL, Langer CJ, Camidge DR, Padavic K, Gore L, Smith M, Chow LQ, von Mehren M, O'Bryant C, Hariharan S, Diab S, Fox NL, Miceli R, Eckhardt SG. Mapatumumab, an antibody targeting TRAIL-R1, in combination with paclitaxel and carboplatin in patients with advanced solid malignancies: results of a phase I and pharmacokinetic study. J Clin Oncol 2009;27:4413-4421.

[65] Li Y, Wang H, Wang Z, Makhija S, Buchsbaum D, LoBuglio A, Kimberly R, Zhou T. Inducible resistance of tumor cells to tumor necrosis factor-related apoptosis-inducing ligand receptor 2-mediated apoptosis by generation of a blockade at the death domain function. Cancer Res 2006;66:8520-8528.

[66] Liu P, Mao H, Hou P. Synergistic antitumor effect of tumor necrosis factor-related apoptosis-inducing ligand combined with cisplatin in ovarian carcinoma cell lines *in vitro* and *in vivo*. Int J Gynecol Cancer 2006;16:538-548.

[67] Lowe SW, Cepero E, Evan G. Intrinsic tumour suppression. Nature 2004;432:307–315.

[68] Mao HL, Liu PS, Zheng JF, Zhang PH, Zhou LG, Xin G, Liu C. Transfection of Smac/DIABLO sensitizes drug-resistant tumor cells to TRAIL or paclitaxel-induced apoptosis in vitro. Pharmacol Res 2007;56:483-492.

[69] Marone M, Scambia G, Mozzetti S, Ferrandina G, Iacovella S, De Pasqua A, Benedetti-Panici P, Mancuso S. Bcl-2, Bax, Bcl-XL, and Bcl-XS expression in normal and neoplastic ovarian tissues. Clin Cancer Res 1998;4:517-524.

[70] Marsters SA, Sheridan JP, Pitti RM, Huang A, Skubatch M, Baldwin D, Yuan J, Gurney A, Goddard AD, Godowski P, Ashkenazi A. A novel receptor for Apo2L/TRAIL contains a truncated death domain. Curr Biol 1997;7:1003–1006.

[71] Marx D, Binder C, Meden H, Lenthe T, Ziemek T, Hiddemann T, Kuhn W, Schauer A. Differential expression of apoptosis associated genes bax and bcl-2 in ovarian cancer. Anticancer Res 1997;17:2233-2240.

[72] McGuire WP, Hoskins WJ, Brady MF, Kucera PR, Partridge EE, Look KY, Clarke-Pearson DL, Davidson M. Cyclophosphamide and cisplatin compared with paclitaxel and cisplatin in patients with stage III and stage IV ovarian cancer. N Engl J Med 1996;334:1-6.

[73] Matte I, Lane D, Laplante C, Rancourt C, Piché A. Profiling of cytokines in human epithelial ovarian cancer ascites. Am J Cancer Res 2012;2:566-580.

[74] Meads MB, Gatenby RA, Dalton WS. Environment-mediated drug resistance: a major contributor to minimal residual disease. Nat Rev Cancer 2009;9:665-674.

[75] Mezzanzanica D, Balladore E, Turatti F, Luison E, Alberti P, Bagnoli M, Figini M, Mazzoni A, Raspagliesi F, Oggionni M, Pilotti S, Canevari S. CD95-mediated apoptosis is impaired at receptor level by cellular FLICE-inhibitory protein (long form) in wild-type p53 human ovarian carcinoma. Clin Cancer Res 2004;10:5202-5214.

[76] Ouellet V, Le Page C, Madore J, Guyot MC, Barrès V, Lussier C, Tonin PN, Provencher DM, Mes-Masson AM. An apoptotic molecular network identified by microarray: on the TRAIL to new insights in epithelial ovarian cancer. Cancer. 2007;110:297-308.

[77] Pan G, O'Rourke K, Chinnaiyan AM, Gentz R, Ebner R, Ni J, Dixit VM. The receptor for the cytotoxic ligand TRAIL. Science 1997;276:111–113.

[78] Pan G, Ni J, Wei YF, Yu G, Gentz R, Dixit VM. An antagonist decoy receptor and a death domain-containing receptor for TRAIL. Science 1997;277:815–818.

[79] Park SJ, Kim MJ, Kim HB, Sohn HY, Bae JH, Kang CD, Kim SH. Trichostatin A sensitizes human ovarian cancer cells to TRAIL-induced apoptosis by down-regulation of c-FLIPL via inhibition of EGFR pathway. Biochem Pharmacol 2009;77:1328-1336.

[80] Pasquini L, Petronelli A, Petrucci E, Saulle E, Mariani G, Scambia G, Benedetti-Panici P, Greggi S, Cognetti F, Testa U. Primary ovarian cancer cells are sensitive to the proaptotic effects of proteasome inhibitors. Int J Oncol 2010;36:707-713.

[81] Petrucci E, Pasquini L, Petronelli A, Saulle E, Mariani G, Riccioni R, Biffoni M, Ferretti G, Benedetti-Panici P, Cognetti F, Scambia G, Humphreys R, Peschle C, Testa U. A small molecule Smac mimic potentiates TRAIL-mediated cell death of ovarian cancer cells. Gynecol Oncol 2007;105:481-492.

[82] Petrucci E, Pasquini L, Bernabei M, Saulle E, Biffoni M, Accarpio F, Sibio S, Di Giorgio A, Di Donato V, Casorelli A, Benedetti-Panici P, Testa U. A small molecule SMAC mimic LBW242 potentiates TRAIL- and anticancer drug-mediated cell death of ovarian cancer cells. PLoS One. 2012;7:e35073.

[83] Pitti RM, Marsters SA, Ruppert S, Donahue CJ, Moore A, Ashkenazi A. Induction of apoptosis by Apo-2 ligand, a new member of the tumor necrosis factor cytokine family. J Biol Chem 1996;271:12687-12690.

[84] Plante M, Rubin SC, Wong GY, Federici MG, Finstad CL, Gastl GA. Interleukin-6 level in serum and ascites as a prognostic factor in patients with epithelial ovarian cancer. Cancer 1994;73:1882-1888.

[85] Pollack IF, Erff M, Ashkenazi A. Direct stimulation of apoptotic signaling by soluble Apo2l/tumor necrosis factor-related apoptosis-inducing ligand leads to selective killing of glioma cells. Clin Cancer Res 2001;7:1362-1369.

[86] Qiu J, Xiao J, Han C, Li N, Shen X, Jiang H, Cao X. Potentiation of tumor necrosis factor-alpha-induced tumor cell apoptosis by a small molecule inhibitor for anti-apoptotic protein hPEBP4. J Biol Chem 2010;285:12241-12247.

[87] Saulle E, Petronelli A, Pasquini L, Petrucci E, Mariani G, Biffoni M, Ferretti G, Scambia G, Benedetti-Panici P, Cognetti F, Humphreys R, Peschle C, Testa U. Proteasome inhibitors sensitize ovarian cancer cells to TRAIL induced apoptosis. Apoptosis 2007;12:635-655.

[88] Scambia G, Testa U, Benedetti Panici P, Foti E, Martucci R, Gadducci A, Perillo A, Facchini V, Peschle C, Mancuso S. Prognostic significance of interleukin 6 serum levels in patients with ovarian cancer. Br J Cancer 1995;71:354-356.

[89] Schneider P. Production of recombinant TRAIL and TRAIL receptor: Fc chimeric proteins. Methods Enzymol 2000;322:325-345.

[90] Sheridan JP, Marsters SA, Pitti RM, Gurney A, Skubatch M, Baldwin D, Ramakrishnan L, Gray CL, Baker K, Wood WI, Goddard AD, Godowski P, Ashkenazi A. Control of TRAIL-induced apoptosis by a family of signaling and decoy receptors. Science 1997;277:818–821.

[91] Shigemasa K, Katoh O, Shiroyama Y, Mihara S, Mukai K, Nagai N, Ohama K. Increased MCL-1 expression is associated with poor prognosis in ovarian carcinomas. Jpn J Cancer Res. 2002;93:542-550.

[92] Shivapurkar N, Toyooka S, Toyooka KO, Reddy J, Miyajima K, Suzuki M, Shigematsu H, Takahashi T, Parikh G, Pass HI, Chaudhary PM, Gazdar AF. Aberrant methylation of TRAIL decoy receptor genes is frequent in multiple tumor types. Int J Cancer 2004; 109:786-792.

[93] Siervo-Sassi RR, Marrangoni AM, Feng X, Naoumova N, Winans M, Edwards RP, Lokshin A. Physiological and molecular effects of Apo2L/TRAIL and cisplatin in ovarian carcinoma cell lines. Cancer Lett 2003;190:61-72

[94] Soria JC, Smit E, Khayat D, Besse B, Yang X, Hsu CP, Reese D, Wiezorek J, Blackhall F. Phase 1b study of dulanermin (recombinant human Apo2L/TRAIL) in combination with paclitaxel, carboplatin, and bevacizumab in patients with advanced non-squamous non-small-cell lung cancer. J Clin Oncol 2010;28:1527-1533.

[95] Soria JC, Márk Z, Zatloukal P, Szima B, Albert I, Juhász E, Pujol JL, Kozielski J, Baker N, Smethurst D, Hei YJ, Ashkenazi A, Stern H, Amler L, Pan Y, Blackhall F. Randomized phase II study of dulanermin in combination with paclitaxel, carboplatin, and bevacizumab in advanced non-small-cell lung cancer. J Clin Oncol 2011;29:4442-4451.

[96] Stupack DG, Cheresh DA. Get a ligand, get a life: integrins, signaling and cell survival. J Cell Sci 2002;115:3729-3738.

[97] Syed V, Mukherjee K, Godoy-Tundidor S, Ho SM. Progesterone induces apoptosis in TRAIL-resistant ovarian cancer cells by circumventing c-FLIPL overexpression. J Cell Biochem 2007;102:442-452.

[98] Tanyi JL, Hasegawa Y, Lapushin R, Morris AJ, Wolf JK, Berchuck A, Lu K, Smith DI, Kalli K, Hartmann LC, McCune K, Fishman D, Broaddus R, Cheng KW, Atkinson EN, Yamal JM, Bast RC, Felix EA, Newman RA, Mills GB. Role of decreased levels of lipid phosphate phosphatase-1 in accumulation of lysophosphatidic acid in ovarian cancer. Clin Cancer Res 2003;9:3534-3545.

[99] Tempfer C, Zeisler H, Sliutz G, Haeusler G, Hanzal E, Kainz C. Serum evaluation of interleukin 6 in ovarian cancer patients. Gynecol Oncol 1997;66:27-30.

[100] Tolcher AW, Mita M, Meropol NJ, von Mehren M, Patnaik A, Padavic K, Hill M, Mays T, McCoy T, Fox NL, Halpern W, Corey A, Cohen RB. Phase I pharmacokinetic and biologic correlative study of mapatumumab, a fully human monoclonal antibody with agonist activity to tumor necrosis factor-related apoptosis-inducing ligand receptor-1. J Clin Oncol 2007;25:1390-1395.

[101] Vignati S, Codegoni A, Polato F, Broggini M. TRAIL activity in human ovarian cancer cells: potentiation of the action of cytotoxic drugs. Eur J Cancer 2002:38:177-183.

[102] Vitovski S, Phillips JS, Sayers J, Croucher PI. Investigating the interaction between osteoprotegerin and receptor activator of NF-KappaB or tumor-necrosis factor-related apoptosis-inducing ligand: evidence for a pivotal role for osteoprotegerin in regulating two distinct pathways. J Biol Chem 2007;282:31601-31609.

[103] Walczak H, Miller RE, Ariail K, Gliniak B, Griffith TS, Kubin M, Chin W, Jones J, Woodward A, Le T, Smith C, Smolak P, Goodwin RG, Rauch CT, Schuh JC, Lynch DH. Tumoricidal activity of tumor necrosis factor-related apoptosis-inducing ligand in vivo. Nat Med 1999;5:157-163.

[104] Williams J, Lucas PC, Griffith KA, Choi M, Fogoros S, Hu YY, Liu JR. Expression of Bcl-xL in ovarian carcinoma is associated with chemoresistance and recurrent disease. Gynecol Oncol 2005;96:287-295.

[105] Yamada T, Sato K, Komachi M, Malchinkhuu E, Tobo M, Kimura T, Kuwabara A, Yanagita Y, Ikeya T, Tanahashi Y, Ogawa T, Ohwada S, Morishita Y, Ohta H, Im DS, Tamoto K, Tomura H, Okajima F. Lysophosphatidic acid (LPA) in malignant ascites stimulates motility of human pancreatic cancer cells through LPA1. J Biol Chem 2004; 279:6595-6605.

[106] Youle RJ and Strasser A. The BCL-2 protein family: opposing activities that mediate cell death. Nat Rev Mol Cell Biol 2008;9:47-59.

[107] Zhang L, Fang B. Mechanisms of resistance to TRAIL-induced apoptosis in cancer. Cancer Gene Ther 2005;12:228–37.

[108] Zhu H, Liu XW, Ding WJ, Xu DQ, Zhao YC, Lu W, He QJ, Yang B. Up-regulation of death receptor 4 and 5 by celastrol enhances the anti-cancer activity of TRAIL/ Apo-2L. Cancer Lett 2010;297:155-164.

Chapter 12

Protein Kinase G-Iα Hyperactivation and VASP Phosphorylation in Promoting Ovarian Cancer Cell Migration and Platinum Resistance

Janica C. Wong and Ronald R. Fiscus

Additional information is available at the end of the chapter

http://dx.doi.org/10.5772/53468

1. Introduction

Platinum-based drugs such as cisplatin (*cis*-diammine-dichloro-platinum, also commonly known as CDDP) have dominated the drug therapy of ovarian cancer during the past three decades [1]. Cisplatin interacts with DNA to form intrastrand crosslink adducts, and its molecular mechanism involves regulation of p53 and the mitogen-activated protein kinase (MAPK) signaling pathway [2]. The phosphatidylinositol-3-kinase (PI3K)/Akt signaling pathway is crucial for regulation of survival and for progression and chemoresistance in ovarian cancer, leading to the development of new chemotherapeutic inhibitors targeting the PI3K/Akt pathway and the downstream serine/threonine protein kinase mTOR. [3]. Inhibition of PI3K pathway signaling using PI3K or mTOR inhibitors has been shown to sensitize ovarian cancer cell lines to the apoptosis-inducing effect of platinum compounds [4, 5]. In addition, activation of the PI3K/Akt/mTOR pathway in ovarian cancer cell lines contributes to cisplatin resistance [6]. The anti-apoptotic, pro-angiogenic effects of PI3K/Akt/mTOR may be mediated, at least in part, through a downstream signaling pathway involving endogenous endothelial-form nitric oxide synthase (eNOS, also called NOS3), and subsequently soluble guanylyl cyclase (sGC) and protein kinase G (PKG). Studies have shown that Akt activates eNOS by phosphorylating human eNOS at Ser1177 (equivalent to bovine eNOS at Ser1179), leading to an increase in nitric oxide (NO) production in endothelial cells [7, 8]. In the cases of vascular endothelial growth factor (VEGF) [9, 10], sphingosine 1-phosphate [11, 12], and estrogen [13, 14], there are vast evidences suggesting PI3K-activation of Akt is responsible for regulating the phosphorylation and activation of eNOS. In bovine aortic endothelial cells, eNOS co-immunoprecipitates with Akt, indicating that the two enzymes associate *in vivo*, and Akt directly activates eNOS, increasing eNOS activity by 15-20 fold

[15]. This signaling pathway has been shown to play an essential role in promoting angiogenesis or tumor vascularization [16]. In a very recent study, microgravity stimulated tube formation and migration in human umbilical vein endothelial cells (HUVEC), and the process was mediated through the PI3K-Akt-eNOS signal pathway [17].

Our early studies of the NO/cyclic GMP (cGMP)/PKG signaling pathway have identified PKG as a key mediator of vasodilation and anti-hypertensive effects induced by NO as well as atrial natriuretic peptide (ANP) [18-21]. Recent studies from our laboratory have shown that the PKG-Iα splice variant of PKG, at basal or moderately elevated activity, plays an important cytoprotective role in preventing spontaneous apoptosis and promoting cell proliferation in many types of mammalian cells, including neural cells [22-27], human ovarian cancer cells [28-30], primary murine vascular smooth muscle cells [31] and murine bone marrow mesenchymal (stromal) stem cells [32]. Evidence from our laboratory suggested that basal activation of PKG-Iα leads to increased attachment of cells to the extracellular matrix and increased cell migration, shown in bone marrow-derived mesenchymal (stromal) stem cells [32]. We have identified certain intracellular proteins that are directly phosphorylated and functionally regulated by PKG-Iα, including 1) the apoptosis-regulating protein BAD [26], 2) vasodilator-stimulated phosphoprotein (VASP) [28, 31, 32], 3) the oncogenic tyrosine kinase c-Src [28, 33] and 4) the transcription factor cAMP responsive element binding protein (CREB) [24, 34], which may contribute to the exaggerated proliferation, enhanced chemoresistance and increased cell migration and invasion in ovarian cancer cells (Figure 1). Our recent studies have shown that cisplatin regulates the endogenous expression of nitric oxide synthases (NOSs) in human ovarian cancer cells, upregulating inducible nitric oxide synthase (iNOS, also called NOS2) expression but dramatically downregulating the expression of eNOS and neural-form nitric oxide synthase (nNOS, also called NOS1), which is involved in determining cisplatin resistance in ovarian cancer cells [30]. Our studies show that the chemoresistance/cytoprotective effects of endogenous eNOS involve hyperactivation of PKG-Iα in the ovarian cancer cells [28].

Studies from our laboratory suggest that PKG-Iα promotes proliferation in ovarian cancer cells, which involves the enhancement of the tyrosine kinase activity of c-Src [28], an oncogenic protein often overexpressed and/or hyperactivated in many types of cancer cells. We showed that PKG-Iα plays a key role in activating c-Src and promoting cell proliferation, using the short interfering RNA (siRNA) or RNA interference (RNAi) technique, to knockdown the expression of PKG-Iα in ovarian cancer cells [28]. We found that epidermal growth factor (EGF)-induced activation of c-Src tyrosine kinase activity causes tyrosine phosphorylation of PKG-Iα, increasing the serine/threonine kinase activity of PKG-Iα and its growth-promoting effects in ovarian cancer cells [28]. Later, we have found that PKG-Iα directly phosphorylates c-Src at Ser17, which enhances the tyrosine kinase activity of c-Src in both *in vitro* and intact-cell experiments [33]. This novel interaction between PKG-Iα and c-Src causes reciprocal phosphorylation, which means PKG-Iα and c-Src phosphorylate each other, potentially setting up an "oncogenic reinforcement" resulting in exaggerated DNA synthesis and cell proliferation (Figure 1).

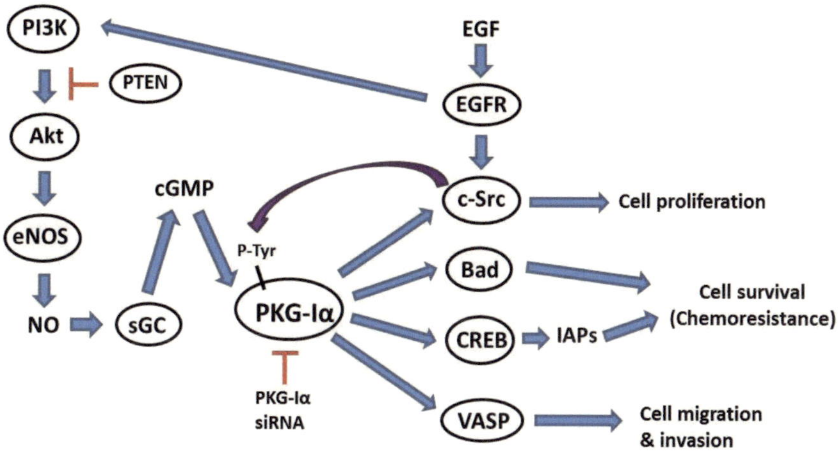

Figure 1. Model of the biological role of PKG-Iα in ovarian cancer cells illustrating the effects of growth factors (e.g. EGF), which stimulates both the PI3K/Akt pathway, enhancing eNOS activity and low-level NO generation and the activation of c-Src. The low, physiological levels of NO activate sGC, elevating cGMP levels that enhance the activation of PKG-Iα. PKG-Iα is further activated (hyperactivated) by the combined effects of cGMP allosteric stimulation and the tyrosine phosphorylation by c-Src. PKG-Iα phosphorylates several downstream proteins, including c-Src, Bad, CREB and VASP, leading to enhanced cell proliferation and cytoprotection, contributing to chemoresistance in ovarian cancer cells and increased cell migration and invasion.

2. Phosphorylation of the vasodilator-stimulated phosphoprotein (VASP) at Ser239 as a useful indicator of endogeneous PKG kinase activity

Vasodilator-stimulated phosphoprotein (VASP) was first described in 1987 as a protein phosphorylated in platelets in response to vasodilators such as sodium nitroprusside, nitroglycerin and various prostaglandins that elevate cAMP and cGMP [35]. VASP belongs to the Ena/VASP family which includes VASP, Mena (mammalian enabled) and EVL (Ena VASP-like). The Ena/VASP family proteins function as anti-capping proteins [36, 37], regulating the actin cytoskeleton dynamics [38-42] and are therefore important for actin-based adhesion [43, 44], migration [45-47] and cell–cell interaction [48-50]. Many studies from others have suggested the involvement of VASP in invasion, angiogenesis and tumorigenesis. In an *in vitro* model of capillary morphogenesis using human umbilical vein endothelial cells (HUVECs) in three-dimensional collagen gels, the differentiated endothelial cells showed 2 to 3-fold increase in migration with increased VASP mRNA and protein expression [51]. A study on human placenta development showed that VASP may participate in vasculogenesis and endothelial sprouting during placental vasculogenesis, and VASP expression was stimulated by vascular endothelial growth factor (VEGF) and interleukin-8 (IL-8) [52]. NIH-3T3 fibroblast deficient in VASP showed loss of contact inhibition, and continued cell division past confluence, while overproduction of VASP by transfection in NIH-3T3 fibroblasts resulted in neoplastic transformation, suggesting a role of VASP in tumorigenesis and/or cancer progression [53]. In human osteocarcinoma specimans, higher VASP expression was associated with metastasis and increased migration, and VASP expression was regulated by Rac1 [54]. In lung adenocarcinomas tissues, VASP expression was increased compared to normal lung tissues, and was significantly increased with more advanced tumor stage [55]. Elevated VASP expression was also reported in human breast cancer tissues [56] and was implicated on invasion and migration in breast cancer cells involving the Rac1 pathway [57]. Moreover, it was shown that in mice lacking VASP, melanoma growth was greatly impaired [58]. In gastric cancer cells, VASP was upregulated by epidermal growth factor (EGF) and promoted migration and invasion. Using microRNA (miRNA) expression profiling of the paired normal/tumor gastric tissues, the same group identified miR-610 as a novel miRNA regulated by EGF that targets VASP in gastric cancer cells [59].

VASP has been reported to be phosphorylated by cAMP-dependent protein kinase (PKA) and cGMP-dependent protein kinase (PKG) [35, 60]. VASP was found to be primarily present as a 46 kDa membrane-associated protein in its dephosphorylated form in platelets, and VASP is converted to an apparent 50 kDa phosphoprotein upon phosphorylation, as observed on Western blot [61, 62]. VASP contains three phosphorylation sites, Ser157, Ser239 and Thr274, all of which can be phosphorylated by either PKA or PKG [63]. Ser157 is the preferred site of phosphorylation for PKA, Ser239 is the preferred site for PKG, and Ser157 was the site responsible for the phosphorylation-induced mobility shift of VASP on Western blots [63]. Because it was well-characterized that VASP at Ser239 is the preferred phosphorylation site for PKG *in vitro* and in mammalian cells, VASP phosphorylation at Ser239 has been proposed to be a useful indicator of endogenous PKG kinase activity [61, 63, 64]. In fact, VASP at Ser239 was shown to be a functional biomarker of endothelial nitric oxide/cyclic GMP signaling [65], and could be used to indicate defective nitric oxide/cGMP signaling and endothelial dysfunction [66]. In colon cancer cells, VASP Ser239 phosphorylation was used as a biomarker for the action of the anticancer drug Exisulind, an inhibitor of type-5 phosphodiesterase (PDE-5) that elevates cGMP and stimulates PKG activation, and that constitutively activated mutants of PKG resulted in direct *in vivo* phosphorylation of VASP Ser239 [67].

We had shown that the endogenous NO/cGMP signaling pathway in ovarian cancer cells causes a constitutive downregulation of p53 protein expression, which likely contributes to the chemoresistance and exaggerated cell proliferation in these cells [29]. Furthermore, we have previously identified that PKG-Iα is the predominant isoform of PKG in both OV2008 (cisplatin-sensitive, wild-type p53) and A2780cp (cisplatin-resistant, mutated p53) ovarian cancer cells as determined by Western blot analysis as well as using the new, ultrasensitive NanoPro100 capillary electrophoresis-based nano-fluidic protein analysis system [28, 68, 69]. Our more recent data now show that the chemoresistance and exaggerated cell proliferation are likely mediated by the constitutive hyperactivation of PKG-Iα (reflected in the high levels of VASP phosphorylation at Ser239) in ovarian cancer cells, and that the PKG-Iα is already activated to approximately 90% of maximal activity, described in our previous book chapter [68]. In our recent study, epidermal growth factor (EGF)-induced activation of Src family kinase (SFK) was found to tyrosine-phosphorylate PKG-Iα increasing its serine/threonine kinase activity in ovarian cancer cells. The EGF-stimulated increase in PKG-Iα kinase activity (indicated by VASP Ser239 phosphorylation) was blocked by both SKI-1 and SU6656 (SFK inhibitors). Using the specific PKG-Iα kinase inhibitor DT-2 and small interfering RNA (siRNA) PKG-Iα gene knockdown, we showed that the inhibition of endogenous PKG-Iα kinase activity reduced VASP Ser239 phosphorylation and DNA synthesis rate in ovarian cancer cells [28]. New data from our laboratory show that the knockdown of PKG-Iα expression inhibits the EGF-stimulated increases in VASP Ser239 phosphorylation and Src/SFK autophosphorylation at the equivalent of Tyr416 (the phosphorylation site for activating the tyrosine kinase activity) in A2780cp (cisplatin-resistant, mutated p53) ovarian cancer cells (see Figure 2 below).

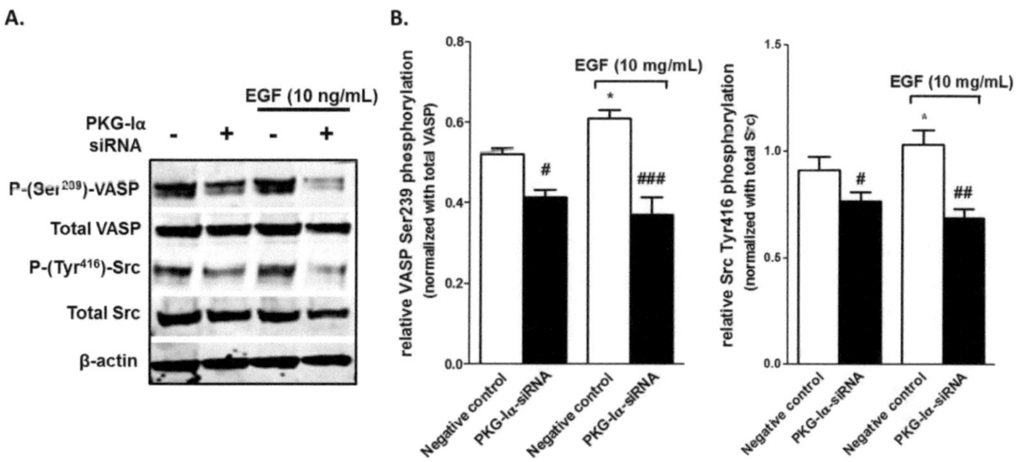

Figure 2. A, EGF (10 ng/mL) elevated VASP Ser239 phosphorylation and Src Tyr416 phosphorylation in A2780cp cells, assessed by Western blot analysis. Gene knockdown of PKG-Iα by PKG-Iα-siRNA partially inhibited the basal VASP phosphorylation and Src/SFK autophosphorylation and completely inhibited the EGF-stimulated increases in VASP phosphorylation and Src/SFK autophosphorylation. The Western blot shown is representative of four experiments. B, Quantification of the relative levels of VASP and Src phosphorylation from Western blot. Bar graphs show mean ± SEM from four independent experiments. *, P< 0.05, compared with no EGF control; #, P<0.05; ##, P<0.01; ###, P < 0.001, compared with negative control.

3. Role of PKG in invasion/migration in A2780cp ovarian cancer cells

The role of NO/cGMP/PKG pathway in invasion/migration in cancer cells is largely unknown. However, a significant number of reports have shown that the NO/cGMP/PKG pathway plays a key role in endothelial cell migration and angiogenesis, involving the downstream activation of the mitogen-activated protein kinase (MAPK) family. It has been shown that NO promotes endothelial cell migration and neovascularization by activating the PI3K/Akt signaling pathway in a PKG-dependent manner [70]. Activation of the NO/cGMP/PKG pathway also promoted endothelial cell angiogenesis and increased extracellular signal regulated kinase 1/2 (ERK1/2) and p38 phosphorylation [71, 72], which were blocked by soluble guanylyl cyclase (sGC) inhibitor, 1H-

[1,2,4]oxadiazolo[4,3-a]quinoxalin-1-one (ODQ), or PKG inhibitor DT-3 [73-75]. Moreover, the mitogenic effect of vascular endothelial growth factor (VEGF) on endothelial cells appears to be mediated by endogenous NO (from eNOS) and cGMP, which results in PKG activation and PKG-mediated downstream stimulation of MEK and ERK [76, 77]. Although it has not yet been reported which isoform of PKG is involved in the multiple pro-angiogenesis responses of endothelial cells, our recent studies suggest that endothelial cells express predominantly the PKG-Iα isoform (unpublished observations by J.C. Wong and R.R. Fiscus), which likely mediates the stimulation of downstream growth-promoting and pro-angiogenesis pathways in endothelial cells.

Interestingly, in colon cancer cells, recent studies showed that activation of PKG inhibited cell migration [78], and cGMP-dependent VASP phosphorylation suppressed the number and length of locomotory (filopodia) and invasive (invadopodia) actin-based organelles [79], suggesting a role of VASP Ser239 in invasion and migration. Our studies suggest that the opposite roles of PKG in regulating apoptosis, proliferation and migration reported by others are likely dependent on cell type, growth conditions (presence of different growth factors), as well as the differential expression of PKG-Iα and PKG-Iβ isoforms. The two splice variants of PKG-I, PKG-Iα and PKG-Iβ, are activated by different concentration ranges of NO and are localized to different subcellular locations within cells. Therefore, the two PKG-I isoforms can phosphorylate different sets of downstream target proteins and can mediate completely different biological responses. The very different biological roles of the two PKG-I isoforms are reviewed in further detail elsewhere in another recent book chapter from our laboratory [68]. For example, PKG-Iα (K_{act} = 0.1 μM by cGMP allosteric activation) is activated at low, physiological levels of NO, whereas PKG-Iβ is activated at higher, pathological levels of NO and requires at least 10-times higher levels of cGMP for activation (K_{act} = 1 μM) [68, 72, 80, 81].

In our hypothesis, the PKG-Iα and PKG-Iβ isoforms mediate opposite biological effects on cell proliferation and apoptosis, based on observations in two types of cells that express one isoform of PKG-I or the other. Our studies have shown that human ovarian cancer cells express predominantly the PKG-Iα isoform, and that the activation of this kinase by endogenous low-level NO (0.01 – 1 nM), generated by endogenous eNOS and nNOS, would selectively activate the PKG-Iα isoform within ovarian cancer cells from our laboratory, promoting DNA synthesis/cell proliferation and suppressing apoptosis, thus contributing to chemoresistance [28, 30, 68]. Studies in our laboratory, using both normal and malignant cells, including vascular smooth muscle cells, bone marrow-derived mesenchymal (stromal) stem cells and neuroblastoma cells, have suggested that a major role of the low-level-NO/cGMP/PKG-Iα signaling pathway is to protect these cells against the toxic/pro-apoptotic effects of high-level NO, as might occur during inflammation and exposure of cells to pro-inflammatory cytokines [22, 24, 25, 31, 32]. In contrast, based in part on published data from the laboratories of Weinstein and Thompson, it appears that when PKG-Iβ is activated by the higher levels of NO, the growth-inhibitory and pro-apoptotic effects of PKG-Iβ predominate over the growth-stimulatory and anti-apoptotic effects mediated by PKG-Iα. Their laboratories have shown that in colon cancer cells, PKG-Iβ is the predominant PKG-I isoform expressed. Upon activation, PKG-Iβ phosphorylates two downstream target proteins, β-catenin and MEKK1, resulting in inhibition of cell proliferation and induction of apoptosis [78, 82, 83].

As stated above, we have previously determined that PKG-Iα is the predominant isoform in A2780cp ovarian cancer cells [30, 68, 69]. To study whether PKG-Iα plays a role in cell migration/invasion in ovarian cancer cells, we performed experiments using small interfering RNA (siRNA) gene knockdown against PKG-Iα in transwell migration studies. Figure 3 shows that siRNA gene knockdown of PKG-Iα dramatically decreases no EGF as well as EGF-stimulated cell migration (as reflected by the quantity of migrated cells at the bottom of the transwell, stained with crystal violet) in A2780cp cisplatin-resistant ovarian cancer cells. These data confirm the role of endogenous PKG-Iα activity, potentially via VASP Ser239 phosphorylation, in promoting cell migration/invasion in ovarian cancer.

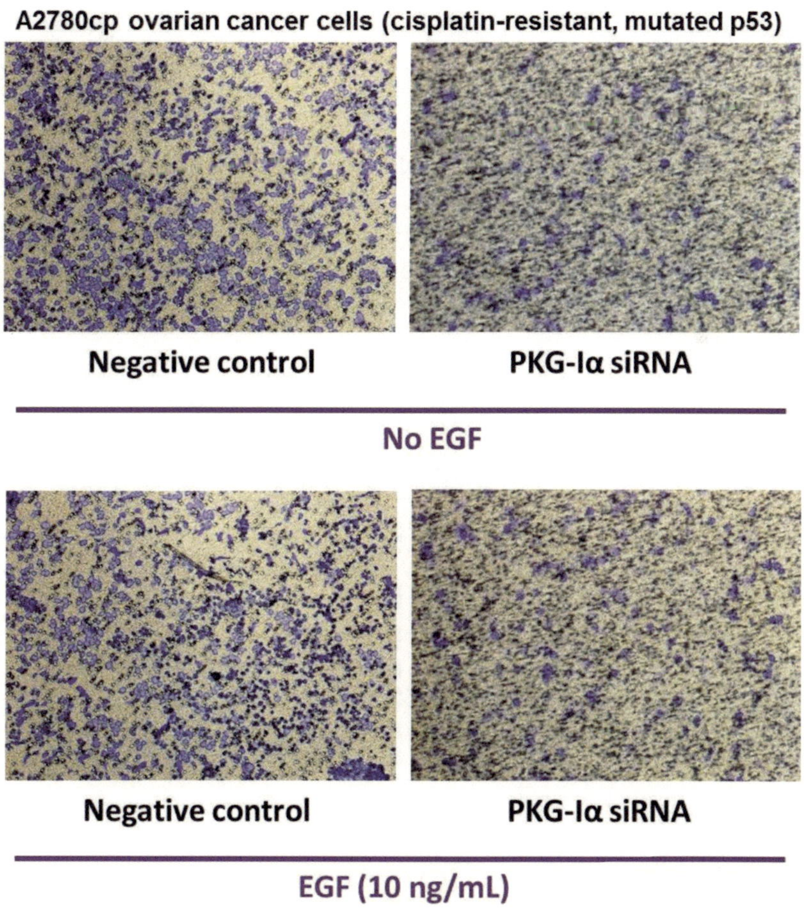

Figure 3. PKG-Iα siRNA gene knockdown in A2780cp cells decreased both basal and EGF-stimulated cell migration assessed by *in vitro* cell migration (invasion) assay. Migration of cells was assessed using transwells (Corning) with 8 μM pore polycarbonated inserts, coated with growth factor-reduced matrigel (BD Bioscience). The upper chamber contained 4 x 10^4 cells and the lower chamber contained 0.6 ml of complete medium with or without EGF. Migration through the membrane was determined after 24 h of incubation at 37°C. Cells remaining on the topside of the transwell membrane were removed using a cotton swab, and cells migrated to bottom were stained with 0.5% crystal violet.

4. Inhibition of the PKG-Iα signaling pathway enhances sensitivity of ovarian cancer cells to cisplatin-induced apoptosis – Potential involvement of cAMP-response-element-binding protein (CREB) and inhibitor of apoptosis proteins (IAPs)

Platinum-based drugs such as cisplatin have dominated the drug therapy of ovarian cancer during the past three decades [1]. Cisplatin interacts with DNA to form intrastrand crosslink adducts, and its molecular mechanism involves regulation of p53 and the mitogen-activated protein kinase (MAPK) signaling pathway [2]. It has been shown that inhibition of ERK1/2 activation with the mitogen-activated protein kinase/ERK kinase 1 (MEK1) inhibitor PD98059 resulted in decreased p53 protein half-life and diminished accumulation of p53 protein during exposure to cisplatin [84]. Our data have shown that human ovarian cancer cells express all of the key components of the NO/cGMP/PKG signaling pathway, including all three isoforms of NOSs, thus providing an endogenous source of NO [30]. Furthermore, ovarian cancer cells continuously produce NO at low physiological levels, activating the heme-dependent soluble guanylyl cyclase (sGC) [29], elevating cGMP levels sufficiently enough to cause continuous high-level activation of PKG [28]. Our data suggested that such basal sGC/cGMP activity regulates p53 expression, and promotes cell survival in part through regulation of caspase-3 [29] (now thought to be mediated by downstream hyperactivation of PKG-Iα).

Cisplatin is also widely employed in chemotherapy on treating solid tumors such as lung cancer. Recently, we showed that, in NCI-H460 and A549 non-small cell lung cancer (NSCLC) cells, PKG-Iα phosphorylates cAMP-response-element-binding protein (CREB) at Ser133 [34]. CREB was first shown to be phosphorylated by PKG *in vitro* by Colbran et al., which showed that PKG effectively phosphorylates CREB at Ser133, although at a slower rate compared to PKA [85]. Interestingly, NO was shown to regulate the c-fos promoter involving soluble guanylyl cyclase (sGC) and PKG [86] in a CREB-dependent manner [87]. They also showed that transfection of PKG in baby hamster kidney (BHK) cells activated the c-fos promoter [88], which required nuclear translocation of PKG and phosphorylation of CREB at Ser133 by PKG [87, 89, 90]. In our recent study, inhibition of the sGC/PKG-Iα signaling pathway by ODQ (sGC inhibitor), DT-2 (PKG-Iα kinase inhibitor) and PKG-Iα-siRNA gene knockdown showed that PKG-Iα kinase activity is necessary for maintaining higher levels of CREB phosphorylation at Ser133 and the protein expression of certain inhibitor of apoptosis proteins (IAPs), specifically c-IAP1, livin and survivin, as well as the anti-apoptotic Bcl-2 family member Mcl-1, preventing spontaneous apoptosis and promoting colony formation [34]. In the same study, we discovered that DT-2 and cisplatin have a synergistic effect on the induction of apoptosis, with DT-2 dramatically enhancing the pro-apoptotic effects of cisplatin in A549 cells (a NSCLC cell line that requires higher levels of cisplatin to induce apoptosis). We also showed that prior activation of PKG-Iα by 8-bromo-cGMP (8-Br-GMP), a cell-permeable cGMP analog that directly activates PKG [22, 24], has cytoprotective effects against cisplatin. PKG-Iα activity stimulated by 8-Br-cGMP was reflected by increased VASP phosphorylation at Ser239. Pretreatment of A549 cells with 8-Br-cGMP caused significant protection against cisplatin-induced apoptosis, even at higher concentrations of cisplatin. Interestingly, when the same treatments were used on PKG-Iα knockdown cells, the cytoprotective effects of 8-Br-cGMP against cisplatin-induced apoptosis was completely abolished, confirming that the cytoprotection (chemoresistance) was mediated by PKG-Iα [34].

To investigate whether such synergism occurs in ovarian cancer cells, we tested the combined treatment of the specific PKG-Iα kinase inhibitor, DT-2, and cisplatin in the A2780cp cisplatin-resistant ovarian cancer cell line. Our new preliminary data presented in this book chapter (illustrated in Figure 4) verified the synergistic effects of DT-2 and cisplatin. Figure 4 shows the level of apoptosis in A2780cp cells after a 24-hr co-treatment of DT-2 (5 or 10 μM) and cisplatin (2 μM). The Cell Death Detection ELISA[PLUS] assay (Roche Applied Science), based on quantitative sandwich-enzyme-immunoassay-principle with monoclonal antibodies directed against DNA and histones, were used to quantify apoptotic fragments. DT-2 (5 μM) or cisplatin (2 μM) alone did not cause significant increase in apoptosis. However, combined treatment of DT-2 (5 or 10 μM) and cisplatin (2 μM) significantly (###P<0.001) increased apoptosis, showing a synergistic effect.

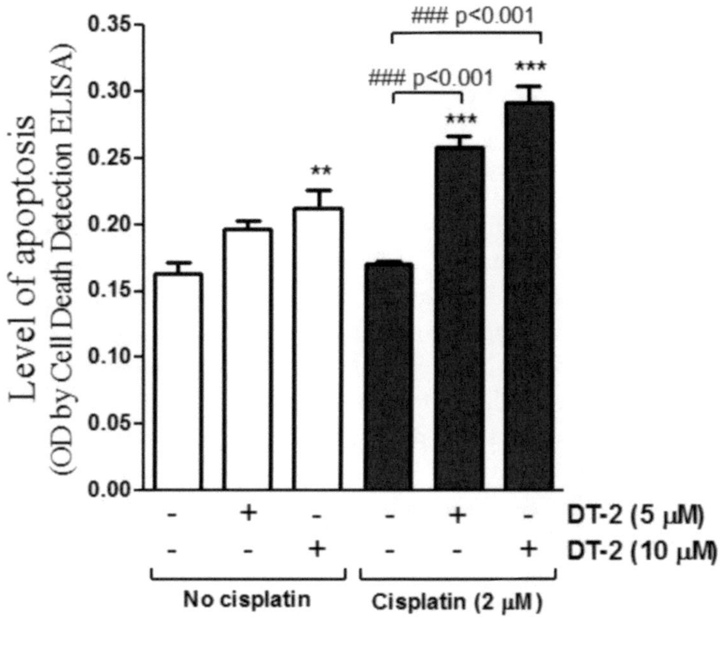

Figure 4. Synergistic effect of DT-2 with cisplatin in A2780cp human ovarian cancer cells. Combined treatment of DT-2 (5 or 10 μM) and cisplatin (2 μM) significantly (###P<0.001) increased apoptosis, compared to cisplatin (2 μM) alone. **P<0.01, ***P<0.001, compared to no DT-2 control. Statistical analysis was performed by one-way ANOVA, followed by Newman-Keuls Multiple Comparison Test using GraphPad (PRISM software). Results were expressed as the mean ± SEM of at least six different samples.

Based on our study of the roles of sGC/PKG-Iα/CREB/IAPs in cisplatin resistant non-small lung cancer cells, we have proposed the anti-apoptotic role of PKG-Iα observed in A2780cp cells is likely mediated through PKG-Iα downstream phosphorylation of CREB at Ser133 and activation of certain IAPs. IAPs have been shown to regulate apoptosis and tumorigenesis [91]. Although how CREB regulates apoptosis through IAPs is largely unknown, it was shown that CREB phosphorylation is a key event in the induction of certain IAPs, c-IAP2 and livin, via multiple protein kinases, PKA, ERK1/2 and p38 MAPK, in colon cancer cells [92, 93]. In ovarian cancer cells, X-linked inhibitor of apoptosis protein (XIAP) has been shown to control ovarian tumor growth and regulate Akt activity and caspase-3 in cisplatin-induced apoptosis [94-96], and the ability of cisplatin to down-regulate XIAP may be an important determinant of chemosensitivity [97]. Down-regulation of XIAP sensitized cells to cisplatin in the presence of wild-type p53, and both XIAP and Akt modulated cisplatin sensitivity individually but that XIAP required Akt for its full function [98]. Inhibition of PI3K/Akt/mTOR signaling has been shown to activate apoptosis and inhibit migration and invasion in ovarian cancer cells [3, 4, 99-104]. Furthermore, inhibition of PI3K pathway signaling using PI3K or mTOR inhibitors has been shown to sensitize ovarian cancer cell lines to induction of apoptosis by platinum compounds [4, 5]. Several recent evidences have suggested that such effects involve the matrix-metalloproteinases (MMPs) [105-107], which are zinc-dependent endopeptidases capable of degradation of extracellular matrix proteins.

5. Overall model of NO/cGMP/PKG-Iα signaling pathway in ovarian cancer

Figure 5 illustrates our overall model showing the involvement of the NO/cGMP/PKG-Iα pathway in promoting cell proliferation and suppressing apoptosis in human ovarian cancer cells, which would contribute to enhanced tumor growth and chemoresistance. Our early studies of the NO/cGMP/PKG pathway have identified PKG as a key mediator of vasodilation and anti-hypertensive effects induced by NO as well as atrial natriuretic peptide (ANP) [18-21]. Recent studies from our laboratory have shown that basal or moderately elevated PKG-Iα activity plays a cytoprotective role in preventing spontaneous apoptosis and promoting cell proliferation in many types of mammalian cells, including neural cells [22-27], human ovarian cancer cells [28-30], primary murine vascular smooth muscle cells [31] and murine bone marrow stromal cells [32]. We found that murine bone marrow-derived mesenchymal (stromal) stem cells endogenously produced ANP and that basal NO/cGMP/PKG-Iα activity and autocrine ANP/cGMP/PKG-Iα activity are necessary for preserving cell survival and promoting cell proliferation and migration in the OP9 bone marrow stromal cell line [32]. Recently, we have identified certain intracellular proteins phosphorylated by PKG-Iα, including BAD [26], vasodilator-stimulated phosphoprotein (VASP) [28, 31, 32], c-Src [28] and cAMP responsive element binding protein (CREB) [34]. We have recently shown that PKG-Iα directly phosphorylates BAD at Ser155, using *in vitro* experiments, and have further shown that a large part of the Ser155 phosphorylation of BAD within neuroblastoma cells is dependent on endogenous PKG-Iα kinase activity, contributing to decreased caspase-3 activity and inhibition of apoptosis [26].

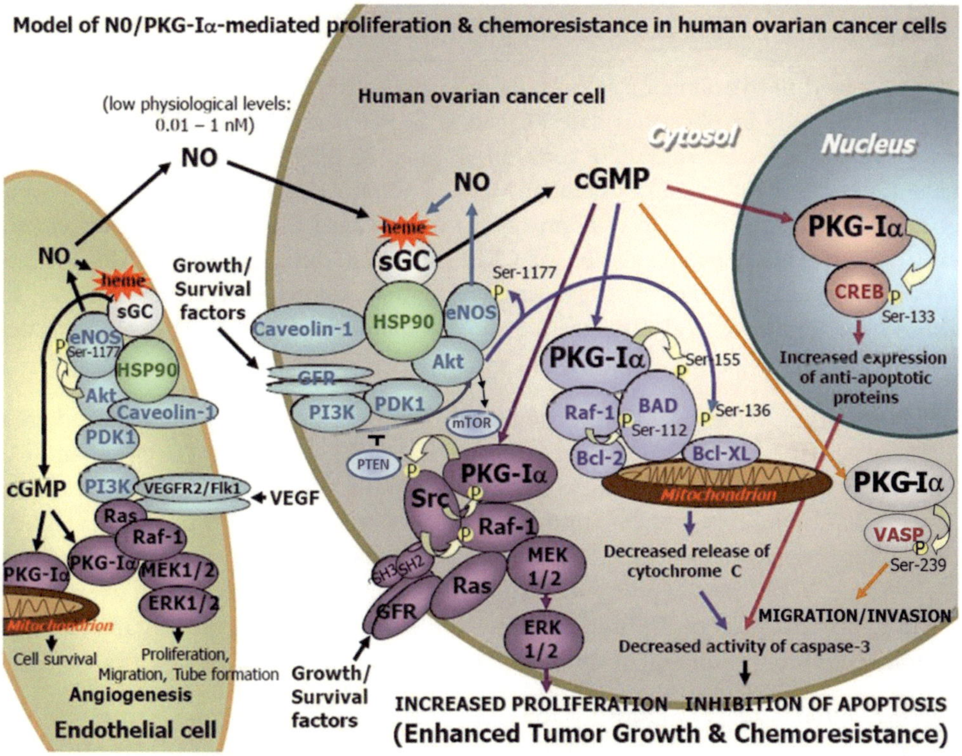

Figure 5. Cellular model of the involvement of the NO/cGMP/PKG-Iα signaling pathway in promoting chemoresistance, tumor growth and angiogenesis in ovarian cancer. A special role of VASP phosphorylation at Ser239 may contribute to enhanced ovarian cancer cell migration and invasion.

As illustrated in the model of Figure 5, we have also identified an important role of c-Src/PKG-Iα interaction in promoting DNA synthesis and cell proliferation in human ovarian cancer cells. Previous studies have shown that PKG-I binds Raf-1 and promotes downstream activation of MEK and ERK1/2 in endothelial cells [76]. In ovarian cancer cells, we proposed that PKG-Iα binds to Raf-1 at the internal surface of the plasma membrane, bringing PKG-Iα in close proximity to one of its downstream target proteins c-Src. This leads to downstream activation of the Raf-1/MEK/ERK signaling pathway, promoting cell proliferation. We found that PKG-Iα directly phosphorylates c-Src at Ser17, which enhances the tyrosine kinase activity of c-Src in both *in vitro* and intact-cell experiments [33]. Our recent studies have shown a clear role of the PKG-Iα-mediated phosphorylation of c-Src at Ser17 in preventing apoptosis and promoting proliferation, attachment and migration in the mesothelioma and NSCLC cells. It is very likely that a similar PKG-Iα catalyzed phosphorylation of c-Src at Ser17 occurs in human ovarian cancer cells, which can explain the dependence of the c-Src activation by EGF on the presence of PKG-Iα [28]. Epidermal growth factor (EGF)-induced activation of c-Src tyrosine kinase activity was found to cause tyrosine phosphorylation of PKG-Iα, increasing the serine/threonine kinase activity of PKG-Iα (indicated by phosphorylation of the PKG substrate VASP at Ser239) and its growth-promoting effects in ovarian cancer cells [28]. In human ovarian cancer cells, the c-Src-mediated tyrosine-phosphorylation of the EGF receptor was found to be highly dependent on PKG-Iα kinase activity [28].

We hypothesized in ovarian cancer cells, as reported in the lung cancer cells in our recent study [34], that PKG-Iα phosphorylated CREB at Ser133, and the cGMP/PKG-Iα signaling pathway maintains the expression of certain IAPs such as c-IAP1, livin and survivin as well as the anti-apoptotic Bcl-2 family member Mcl-1, leading to decreased activity of caspase-3 and promoting cell survival. In ovarian cancer cells where PKG-Iα is hyperactivated, increased downstream phosphorylation of CREB at Ser133 and increased IAPs expression may explain the development of resistance to cisplatin-induced apoptosis. Moreover, PKG-Iα siRNA gene knockdown also decreased both basal and EGF-stimulated cell migration in A2780cp ovarian cancer cells, as shown in Figure 3.

VASP phosphorylation at Ser239 has been shown to be a useful indicator of endogenous PKG kinase activity, both in our recent studies [28, 31, 32] and reports from others [61, 63, 64]. In the current study in this book chapter, we show that siRNA gene knockdown of PKG-Iα expression inhibited EGF-stimulated increases in VASP Ser239 phosphorylation and Src/SFK autophosphorylation in A2780cp (cisplatin-resistant, mutated p53) ovarian cancer cells. Therefore, VASP Ser239 phosphorylation may be a useful biomarker in ovarian cancer cells, and hyperactivation of the unique NO/sGC/PKG-Iα signaling pathway may be a novel therapeutic target for regulation of cancer cell migration/invasion.

Also shown in the model of Figure 5 is the role of endothelial cells, which would provide an additional source of endogenous NO within the growing tumor, potentially contributing to the "angiogenic switch", i.e. the increased tumor growth that occurs after the invasion of endothelial cells into the tumor. Endothelial cells also play another important role in tumor growth by providing new blood vessels needed for the vascularization and blood perfusion of the growing tumor. In endothelial cells, heat shock protein 90 (HSP90) and Akt activate eNOS involving the formation of a HSP90-Akt-Calmodulin (CaM)-eNOS complex, leading to an increase in NO production [108-111]. Interestingly, HSP90 activation of eNOS can be Ca^{2+}-dependent [112] or Ca^{2+}-independent [109, 113].

6. Future experiments

Our future studies will need to determine: 1) whether PKG-Iα is the only isoform of PKG expressed in other human ovarian cancer cell lines as well as in tumor samples of ovarian cancer patients, 2) the subcellular localization of PKG-Iα (and possibly PKG-Iβ), for example, membrane, nuclear, and/or cytosolic localization, 3) the roles of PKG-Iα, its downstream phosphorylation of CREB at Ser133 (and other transcription factors), expression of the IAPs and anti-apoptotic Bcl-2 family proteins in ovarian cancer cells.

7. Conclusions

The NO/cGMP/PKG-Iα pathway and the downstream phosphorylation of the actin-filament/focal-adhesion-regulating protein VASP at Ser239 appear to promote migration/invasion and the downstream phosphorylation of BAD at ser155, CREB at ser133 and c-Src at ser17 appear to promote DNA synthesis, cell proliferation and platinum resistance in ovarian cancer cells. The unique features of this signaling pathway in ovarian cancer cells may provide a novel therapeutic target for disrupting tumor growth and the metastasis and secondary tumor formation during ovarian cancer progression.

Acknowledgements

Financial. support for the research and the preparation of this book chapter was provided by Internal Funding from Roseman University of Health Sciences (formerly named University of Southern Nevada), Henderson, Nevada, USA, U.S. Department of Defense (DOD) grant W81XWH-07-1-0543 and Start-up Funding from the Nevada Cancer Institute, Las Vegas, Nevada, USA, awarded to Dr. Fiscus.

Author details

Janica C. Wong[1,2,3] and Ronald R. Fiscus[1,3]

1 Center for Diabetes & Obesity Prevention, Treatment, Research & Education, Cancer Research Program, and College of Pharmacy (Pharmaceutical Sciences), Roseman University of Health Sciences, Henderson, Nevada, and South Jordan, USA

2 Department of Chemistry, University of Nevada, Las Vegas, Nevada, USA

3 Cancer Molecular Biology Section, Nevada Cancer Institute, Las Vegas, Nevada, USA

References

[1] Gershenson. DM. Management of ovarian germ cell tumors. J Clin Oncol. 2007 Jul 10;25(20):2938-43.

[2] Siddik ZH. Cisplatin: mode of cytotoxic action and molecular basis of resistance. Oncogene. 2003 Oct 20;22(47):7265-79.

[3] Diaz-Padilla I, Duran I, Clarke BA, Oza AM. Biologic rationale and clinical activity of mTOR inhibitors in gynecological cancer. Cancer Treat Rev. 2012 Oct;38(6):767-75.

[4] Altomare DA, Wang HQ, Skele KL, De Rienzo A, Klein-Szanto AJ, Godwin AK, et al. AKT and mTOR phosphorylation is frequently detected in ovarian cancer and can be targeted to disrupt ovarian tumor cell growth. Oncogene. 2004 Jul 29;23(34):5853-7.

[5] Winograd-Katz SE, Levitzki A. Cisplatin induces PKB/Akt activation and p38(MAPK) phosphorylation of the EGF receptor. Oncogene. 2006 Nov 30;25(56): 7381-90.

[6] Lee S, Choi EJ, Jin C, Kim DH. Activation of PI3K/Akt pathway by PTEN reduction and PIK3CA mRNA amplification contributes to cisplatin resistance in an ovarian cancer cell line. Gynecol Oncol. 2005 Apr;97(1):26-34.

[7] Dimmeler S, Fleming I, Fisslthaler B, Hermann C, Busse R, Zeiher AM. Activation of nitric oxide synthase in endothelial cells by Akt-dependent phosphorylation. Nature. 1999 Jun 10;399(6736):601-5.

[8] Fulton D, Gratton JP, McCabe TJ, Fontana J, Fujio Y, Walsh K, et al. Regulation of endothelium-derived nitric oxide production by the protein kinase Akt. Nature. 1999 Jun 10;399(6736):597-601.

[9] Jesmin S, Mowa CN, Sultana SN, Mia S, Islam R, Zaedi S, et al. Estrogen receptor alpha and beta are both involved in the cerebral VEGF/Akt/NO pathway and cerebral angiogenesis in female mice. Biomed Res. 2010 Dec;31(6):337-46.

[10] Feliers D, Chen X, Akis N, Choudhury GG, Madaio M, Kasinath BS. VEGF regulation of endothelial nitric oxide synthase in glomerular endothelial cells. Kidney Int. 2005 Oct;68(4):1648-59.

[11] Igarashi J, Michel T. Sphingosine 1-phosphate and isoform-specific activation of phosphoinositide 3-kinase beta. Evidence for divergence and convergence of receptor-regulated endothelial nitric-oxide synthase signaling pathways. J Biol Chem. 2001 Sep 28;276(39):36281-8.

[12] Igarashi J, Bernier SG, Michel T. Sphingosine 1-phosphate and activation of endothelial nitric-oxide synthase. differential regulation of Akt and MAP kinase pathways by EDG and bradykinin receptors in vascular endothelial cells. J Biol Chem. 2001 Apr 13;276(15):12420-6.

[13] Hisamoto K, Ohmichi M, Kurachi H, Hayakawa J, Kanda Y, Nishio Y, et al. Estrogen induces the Akt-dependent activation of endothelial nitric-oxide synthase in vascular endothelial cells. J Biol Chem. 2001 Feb 2;276(5):3459-67.

[14] Haynes MP, Sinha D, Russell KS, Collinge M, Fulton D, Morales-Ruiz M, et al. Membrane estrogen receptor engagement activates endothelial nitric oxide synthase via the PI3-kinase-Akt pathway in human endothelial cells. Circ Res. 2000 Oct 13;87(8): 677-82.

[15] Gallis B, Corthals GL, Goodlett DR, Ueba H, Kim F, Presnell SR, et al. Identification of flow-dependent endothelial nitric-oxide synthase phosphorylation sites by mass

spectrometry and regulation of phosphorylation and nitric oxide production by the phosphatidylinositol 3-kinase inhibitor LY294002. J Biol Chem. 1999 Oct 15;274(42): 30101-8.

[16] Michell BJ, Griffiths JE, Mitchelhill KI, Rodriguez-Crespo I, Tiganis T, Bozinovski S, et al. The Akt kinase signals directly to endothelial nitric oxide synthase. Curr Biol. 1999 Jul 29-Aug 12;9(15):845-8.

[17] Shi F, Wang YC, Zhao TZ, Zhang S, Du TY, Yang CB, et al. Effects of Simulated Microgravity on Human Umbilical Vein Endothelial Cell Angiogenesis and Role of the PI3K-Akt-eNOS Signal Pathway. PLoS One. 2012;7(7):e40365.

[18] Fiscus RR, Murad F. cGMP-dependent protein kinase activation in intact tissues. Methods Enzymol. 1988;159:150-9.

[19] Fiscus RR, Rapoport RM, Murad F. Endothelium-dependent and nitrovasodilator-induced activation of cyclic GMP-dependent protein kinase in rat aorta. J Cyclic Nucleotide Protein Phosphor Res. 1983;9(6):415-25.

[20] Fiscus RR, Rapoport RM, Waldman SA, Murad F. Atriopeptin II elevates cyclic GMP, activates cyclic GMP-dependent protein kinase and causes relaxation in rat thoracic aorta. Biochim Biophys Acta. 1985 Jul 30;846(1):179-84.

[21] Fung E, Fiscus RR, Yim AP, Angelini GD, Arifi AA. The potential use of type-5 phosphodiesterase inhibitors in coronary artery bypass graft surgery. Chest. 2005 Oct; 128(4):3065-73.

[22] Fiscus RR. Involvement of cyclic GMP and protein kinase G in the regulation of apoptosis and survival in neural cells. Neurosignals. 2002 Jul-Aug;11(4):175-90.

[23] Fiscus RR, Tu AW, Chew SB. Natriuretic peptides inhibit apoptosis and prolong the survival of serum-deprived PC12 cells. Neuroreport. 2001 Feb 12;12(2):185-9.

[24] Fiscus RR, Yuen JP, Chan SL, Kwong JH, Chew SB. Nitric oxide and cyclic GMP as pro- and anti-apoptotic agents. J Card Surg. 2002 Jul-Aug;17(4):336-9.

[25] Cheng Chew SB, Leung PY, Fiscus RR. Preincubation with atrial natriuretic peptide protects NG108-15 cells against the toxic/proapoptotic effects of the nitric oxide donor S-nitroso- N-acetylpenicillamine. Histochem Cell Biol. 2003 Sep;120(3):163-71.

[26] Johlfs MG, Fiscus RR. Protein kinase G type-Ialpha phosphorylates the apoptosis-regulating protein Bad at serine 155 and protects against apoptosis in N1E-115 cells. Neurochem Int. 2010 Mar;56(4):546-53.

[27] Barger SW, Fiscus RR, Ruth P, Hofmann F, Mattson MP. Role of cyclic GMP in the regulation of neuronal calcium and survival by secreted forms of beta-amyloid precursor. J Neurochem. 1995 May;64(5):2087-96.

[28] Leung EL, Wong JC, Johlfs MG, Tsang BK, Fiscus RR. Protein kinase G type Ialpha activity in human ovarian cancer cells significantly contributes to enhanced Src activation and DNA synthesis/cell proliferation. Mol Cancer Res. 2010 Apr;8(4):578-91.

[29] Fraser M, Chan SL, Chan SS, Fiscus RR, Tsang BK. Regulation of p53 and suppression of apoptosis by the soluble guanylyl cyclase/cGMP pathway in human ovarian cancer cells. Oncogene. 2006 Apr 6;25(15):2203-12.

[30] Leung EL, Fraser M, Fiscus RR, Tsang BK. Cisplatin alters nitric oxide synthase levels in human ovarian cancer cells: involvement in p53 regulation and cisplatin resistance. Br J Cancer. 2008 Jun 3;98(11):1803-9.

[31] Wong JC, Fiscus RR. Protein kinase G activity prevents pathological-level nitric oxide-induced apoptosis and promotes DNA synthesis/cell proliferation in vascular smooth muscle cells. Cardiovasc Pathol. 2010 Nov-Dec;19(6):e221-31.

[32] Wong JC, Fiscus RR. Essential roles of the nitric oxide (NO)/cGMP/protein kinase G type-Ialpha (PKG-Ialpha) signaling pathway and the atrial natriuretic peptide (ANP)/cGMP/PKG-Ialpha autocrine loop in promoting proliferation and cell survival of OP9 bone marrow stromal cells. J Cell Biochem. 2011 Mar;112(3):829-39.

[33] Fiscus RR, Johlfs MG. Protein kinase G type-I phosphorylates c-Src at serine-17 and promotes cell survival, proliferation and attachment in human mesothelioma and non-small cell lung cancer cells.. BMC Pharmacology 2011;11(Suppl. 1): 031.

[34] Wong JC, Bathina M, Fiscus RR. Cyclic GMP/protein kinase G type-Ialpha (PKG-Ialpha) signaling pathway promotes CREB phosphorylation and maintains higher c-IAP1, livin, survivin and Mcl-1 expression and the inhibition of PKG-Ialpha kinase activity synergizes with cisplatin in non-small cell lung cancer cells. J Cell Biochem. 2012 (In Press).

[35] Waldmann R, Nieberding M, Walter U. Vasodilator-stimulated protein phosphorylation in platelets is mediated by cAMP- and cGMP-dependent protein kinases. Eur J Biochem. 1987 Sep 15;167(3):441-8.

[36] Bear JE, Svitkina TM, Krause M, Schafer DA, Loureiro JJ, Strasser GA, et al. Antagonism between Ena/VASP proteins and actin filament capping regulates fibroblast motility. Cell. 2002 May 17;109(4):509-21.

[37] Applewhite DA, Barzik M, Kojima S, Svitkina TM, Gertler FB, Borisy GG. Ena/VASP proteins have an anti-capping independent function in filopodia formation. Mol Biol Cell. 2007 Jul;18(7):2579-91.

[38] Walders-Harbeck B, Khaitlina SY, Hinssen H, Jockusch BM, Illenberger S. The vasodilator-stimulated phosphoprotein promotes actin polymerisation through direct binding to monomeric actin. FEBS Lett. 2002 Oct 9;529(2-3):275-80.

[39] Reinhard M, Rudiger M, Jockusch BM, Walter U. VASP interaction with vinculin: a recurring theme of interactions with proline-rich motifs. FEBS Lett. 1996 Dec 9;399(1-2):103-7.

[40] Jenzora A, Behrendt B, Small JV, Wehland J, Stradal TE. PREL1 provides a link from Ras signalling to the actin cytoskeleton via Ena/VASP proteins. FEBS Lett. 2005 Jan 17;579(2):455-63.

[41] Pasic L, Kotova T, Schafer DA. Ena/VASP proteins capture actin filament barbed ends. J Biol Chem. 2008 Apr 11;283(15):9814-9.

[42] Sechi AS, Wehland J. ENA/VASP proteins: multifunctional regulators of actin cytoskeleton dynamics. Front Biosci. 2004 May 1;9:1294-310.

[43] Brindle NP, Holt MR, Davies JE, Price CJ, Critchley DR. The focal-adhesion vasodilator-stimulated phosphoprotein (VASP) binds to the proline-rich domain in vinculin. Biochem J. 1996 Sep 15;318 (Pt 3):753-7.

[44] Galler AB, Garcia Arguinzonis MI, Baumgartner W, Kuhn M, Smolenski A, Simm A, et al. VASP-dependent regulation of actin cytoskeleton rigidity, cell adhesion, and detachment. Histochem Cell Biol. 2006 May;125(5):457-74.

[45] Zhang Y, Tu Y, Gkretsi V, Wu C. Migfilin interacts with vasodilator-stimulated phosphoprotein (VASP) and regulates VASP localization to cell-matrix adhesions and migration. J Biol Chem. 2006 May 5;281(18):12397-407.

[46] Loureiro JJ, Rubinson DA, Bear JE, Baltus GA, Kwiatkowski AV, Gertler FB. Critical roles of phosphorylation and actin binding motifs, but not the central proline-rich region, for Ena/vasodilator-stimulated phosphoprotein (VASP) function during cell migration. Mol Biol Cell. 2002 Jul;13(7):2533-46.

[47] Samarin S, Romero S, Kocks C, Didry D, Pantaloni D, Carlier MF. How VASP enhances actin-based motility. J Cell Biol. 2003 Oct 13;163(1):131-42.

[48] Krause M, Dent EW, Bear JE, Loureiro JJ, Gertler FB. Ena/VASP proteins: regulators of the actin cytoskeleton and cell migration. Annu Rev Cell Dev Biol. 2003;19:541-64.

[49] Kwiatkowski AV, Gertler FB, Loureiro JJ. Function and regulation of Ena/VASP proteins. Trends Cell Biol. 2003 Jul;13(7):386-92.

[50] Scott JA, Shewan AM, den Elzen NR, Loureiro JJ, Gertler FB, Yap AS. Ena/VASP proteins can regulate distinct modes of actin organization at cadherin-adhesive contacts. Mol Biol Cell. 2006 Mar;17(3):1085-95.

[51] Salazar R, Bell SE, Davis GE. Coordinate induction of the actin cytoskeletal regulatory proteins gelsolin, vasodilator-stimulated phosphoprotein, and profilin during capillary morphogenesis in vitro. Exp Cell Res. 1999 May 25;249(1):22-32.

[52] Kayisli UA, Demir R, Erguler G, Arici A. Vasodilator-stimulated phosphoprotein expression and its cytokine-mediated regulation in vasculogenesis during human placental development. Mol Hum Reprod. 2002 Nov;8(11):1023-30.

[53] Liu K, Li L, Nisson PE, Gruber C, Jessee J, Cohen SN. Reversible tumorigenesis induced by deficiency of vasodilator-stimulated phosphoprotein. Mol Cell Biol. 1999 May;19(5):3696-703.

[54] Wu G, Wei L, Yu A, Zhang M, Qi B, Su K, et al. Vasodilator-stimulated phosphoprotein regulates osteosarcoma cell migration. Oncol Rep. 2011 Dec;26(6):1609-15.

[55] Dertsiz L, Ozbilim G, Kayisli Y, Gokhan GA, Demircan A, Kayisli UA. Differential expression of VASP in normal lung tissue and lung adenocarcinomas. Thorax. 2005 Jul;60(7):576-81.

[56] Hu LD, Zou HF, Zhan SX, Cao KM. EVL (Ena/VASP-like) expression is up-regulated in human breast cancer and its relative expression level is correlated with clinical stages. Oncol Rep. 2008 Apr;19(4):1015-20.

[57] Han G, Fan B, Zhang Y, Zhou X, Wang Y, Dong H, et al. Positive regulation of migration and invasion by vasodilator-stimulated phosphoprotein via Rac1 pathway in human breast cancer cells. Oncol Rep. 2008 Oct;20(4):929-39.

[58] Kim YM, Renne C, Seifert S, Schuh K, Renne T. Impaired melanoma growth in VASP deficient mice. FEBS Lett. 2011 Aug 4;585(15):2533-6.

[59] Wang J, Zhang J, Wu J, Luo D, Su K, Shi W, et al. MicroRNA-610 inhibits the migration and invasion of gastric cancer cells by suppressing the expression of vasodilator-stimulated phosphoprotein. Eur J Cancer. 2012 Aug;48(12):1904-13.

[60] Halbrugge M, Walter U. Purification of a vasodilator-regulated phosphoprotein from human platelets. Eur J Biochem. 1989 Oct 20;185(1):41-50.

[61] Eigenthaler M, Nolte C, Halbrugge M, Walter U. Concentration and regulation of cyclic nucleotides, cyclic-nucleotide-dependent protein kinases and one of their major substrates in human platelets. Estimating the rate of cAMP-regulated and cGMP-regulated protein phosphorylation in intact cells. Eur J Biochem. 1992 Apr 15;205(2): 471-81.

[62] Halbrugge M, Friedrich C, Eigenthaler M, Schanzenbacher P, Walter U. Stoichiometric and reversible phosphorylation of a 46-kDa protein in human platelets in response to cGMP- and cAMP-elevating vasodilators. J Biol Chem. 1990 Feb 25;265(6): 3088-93.

[63] Butt E, Abel K, Krieger M, Palm D, Hoppe V, Hoppe J, et al. cAMP- and cGMP-dependent protein kinase phosphorylation sites of the focal adhesion vasodilator-stimulated phosphoprotein (VASP) in vitro and in intact human platelets. J Biol Chem. 1994 May 20;269(20):14509-17.

[64] Smolenski A, Bachmann C, Reinhard K, Honig-Liedl P, Jarchau T, Hoschuetzky H, et al. Analysis and regulation of vasodilator-stimulated phosphoprotein serine 239 phosphorylation in vitro and in intact cells using a phosphospecific monoclonal antibody. J Biol Chem. 1998 Aug 7;273(32):20029-35.

[65] Ibarra-Alvarado C, Galle J, Melichar VO, Mameghani A, Schmidt HH. Phosphorylation of blood vessel vasodilator-stimulated phosphoprotein at serine 239 as a functional biochemical marker of endothelial nitric oxide/cyclic GMP signaling. Mol Pharmacol. 2002 Feb;61(2):312-9.

[66] Oelze M, Mollnau H, Hoffmann N, Warnholtz A, Bodenschatz M, Smolenski A, et al. Vasodilator-stimulated phosphoprotein serine 239 phosphorylation as a sensitive

monitor of defective nitric oxide/cGMP signaling and endothelial dysfunction. Circ Res. 2000 Nov 24;87(11):999-1005.

[67] Deguchi A, Soh JW, Li H, Pamukcu R, Thompson WJ, Weinstein IB. Vasodilator-stimulated phosphoprotein (VASP) phosphorylation provides a biomarker for the action of exisulind and related agents that activate protein kinase G. Mol Cancer Ther. 2002 Aug;1(10):803-9.

[68] Fiscus RR, Leung EL, Wong JC, Johlfs MG. Nitric oxide/protein kinase G-Iα promotes c-Src activation, proliferation and chemoresistance in ovarian cancer. In: Farghaly S, editor. Ovarian Cancer - Basic Science Perspective: Intech Open Access Publisher; 2012. p. 315-34.

[69] Fiscus RR, Johlfs. MG. Protein kinase G (PKG): Involvement in promoting neural cell survival, proliferation, synaptogenesis and synaptic plasticity and the use of new ultrasensitive capillary-electrophoresis-based methodologies for measuring PKG expression and molecular actions.. In: Mukai H, editor. Protein Kinase Technologies (in the series NEUROMETHODS), Springer; 2012. p. 319-48.

[70] Kawasaki K, Smith RS, Jr., Hsieh CM, Sun J, Chao J, Liao JK. Activation of the phosphatidylinositol 3-kinase/protein kinase Akt pathway mediates nitric oxide-induced endothelial cell migration and angiogenesis. Mol Cell Biol. 2003 Aug;23(16):5726-37.

[71] Zaragoza C, Soria E, Lopez E, Browning D, Balbin M, Lopez-Otin C, et al. Activation of the mitogen activated protein kinase extracellular signal-regulated kinase 1 and 2 by the nitric oxide-cGMP-cGMP-dependent protein kinase axis regulates the expression of matrix metalloproteinase 13 in vascular endothelial cells. Mol Pharmacol. 2002 Oct;62(4):927-35.

[72] Pilz RB, Casteel DE. Regulation of gene expression by cyclic GMP. Circ Res. 2003 Nov 28;93(11):1034-46.

[73] Pyriochou A, Zhou Z, Koika V, Petrou C, Cordopatis P, Sessa WC, et al. The phosphodiesterase 5 inhibitor sildenafil stimulates angiogenesis through a protein kinase G/MAPK pathway. J Cell Physiol. 2007 Apr;211(1):197-204.

[74] Pyriochou A, Vassilakopoulos T, Zhou Z, Papapetropoulos A. cGMP-dependent and -independent angiogenesis-related properties of nitric oxide. Life Sci. 2007 Nov 10;81(21-22):1549-54.

[75] Pyriochou A, Beis D, Koika V, Potytarchou C, Papadimitriou E, Zhou Z, et al. Soluble guanylyl cyclase activation promotes angiogenesis. J Pharmacol Exp Ther. 2006 Nov; 319(2):663-71.

[76] Hood J, Granger HJ. Protein kinase G mediates vascular endothelial growth factor-induced Raf-1 activation and proliferation in human endothelial cells. J Biol Chem. 1998 Sep 4;273(36):23504-8.

[77] Parenti A, Morbidelli L, Cui XL, Douglas JG, Hood JD, Granger HJ, et al. Nitric oxide is an upstream signal of vascular endothelial growth factor-induced extracellular sig-

nal-regulated kinase1/2 activation in postcapillary endothelium. J Biol Chem. 1998 Feb 13;273(7):4220-6.

[78] Deguchi A, Thompson WJ, Weinstein IB. Activation of protein kinase G is sufficient to induce apoptosis and inhibit cell migration in colon cancer cells. Cancer Res. 2004 Jun 1;64(11):3966-73.

[79] Zuzga DS, Pelta-Heller J, Li P, Bombonati A, Waldman SA, Pitari GM. Phosphorylation of vasodilator-stimulated phosphoprotein Ser239 suppresses filopodia and invadopodia in colon cancer. Int J Cancer. 2012 Jun 1;130(11):2539-48.

[80] Lincoln TM, Dey N, Sellak H. Invited review: cGMP-dependent protein kinase signaling mechanisms in smooth muscle: from the regulation of tone to gene expression. J Appl Physiol. 2001 Sep;91(3):1421-30.

[81] Francis SH, Busch JL, Corbin JD, Sibley D. cGMP-dependent protein kinases and cGMP phosphodiesterases in nitric oxide and cGMP action. Pharmacol Rev. 2010 Sep;62(3):525-63.

[82] Soh JW, Mao Y, Kim MG, Pamukcu R, Li H, Piazza GA, et al. Cyclic GMP mediates apoptosis induced by sulindac derivatives via activation of c-Jun NH2-terminal kinase 1. Clin Cancer Res. 2000 Oct;6(10):4136-41.

[83] Thompson WJ, Piazza GA, Li H, Liu L, Fetter J, Zhu B, et al. Exisulind induction of apoptosis involves guanosine 3',5'-cyclic monophosphate phosphodiesterase inhibition, protein kinase G activation, and attenuated beta-catenin. Cancer Res. 2000 Jul 1;60(13):3338-42.

[84] Persons DL, Yazlovitskaya EM, Pelling JC. Effect of extracellular signal-regulated kinase on p53 accumulation in response to cisplatin. J Biol Chem. 2000 Nov 17;275(46):35778-85.

[85] Colbran JL, Roach PJ, Fiol CJ, Dixon JE, Andrisani OM, Corbin JD. cAMP-dependent protein kinase, but not the cGMP-dependent enzyme, rapidly phosphorylates delta-CREB, and a synthetic delta-CREB peptide. Biochem Cell Biol. 1992 Oct-Nov; 70(10-11):1277-82.

[86] Idriss SD, Gudi T, Casteel DE, Kharitonov VG, Pilz RB, Boss GR. Nitric oxide regulation of gene transcription via soluble guanylate cyclase and type I cGMP-dependent protein kinase. J Biol Chem. 1999 Apr 2;274(14):9489-93.

[87] Gudi T, Casteel DE, Vinson C, Boss GR, Pilz RB. NO activation of fos promoter elements requires nuclear translocation of G-kinase I and CREB phosphorylation but is independent of MAP kinase activation. Oncogene. 2000 Dec 14;19(54):6324-33.

[88] Gudi T, Huvar I, Meinecke M, Lohmann SM, Boss GR, Pilz RB. Regulation of gene expression by cGMP-dependent protein kinase. Transactivation of the c-fos promoter. J Biol Chem. 1996 Mar 1;271(9):4597-600.

[89] Gudi T, Lohmann SM, Pilz RB. Regulation of gene expression by cyclic GMP-dependent protein kinase requires nuclear translocation of the kinase: identification of a nuclear localization signal. Mol Cell Biol. 1997 Sep;17(9):5244-54.

[90] Chen Y, Zhuang S, Cassenaer S, Casteel DE, Gudi T, Boss GR, et al. Synergism between calcium and cyclic GMP in cyclic AMP response element-dependent transcriptional regulation requires cooperation between CREB and C/EBP-beta. Mol Cell Biol. 2003 Jun;23(12):4066-82.

[91] Deveraux QL, Reed JC. IAP family proteins--suppressors of apoptosis. Genes Dev. 1999 Feb 1;13(3):239-52.

[92] Nishihara H, Hwang M, Kizaka-Kondoh S, Eckmann L, Insel PA. Cyclic AMP promotes cAMP-responsive element-binding protein-dependent induction of cellular inhibitor of apoptosis protein-2 and suppresses apoptosis of colon cancer cells through ERK1/2 and p38 MAPK. J Biol Chem. 2004 Jun 18;279(25):26176-83.

[93] Nishihara H, Kizaka-Kondoh S, Insel PA, Eckmann L. Inhibition of apoptosis in normal and transformed intestinal epithelial cells by cAMP through induction of inhibitor of apoptosis protein (IAP)-2. Proc Natl Acad Sci U S A. 2003 Jul 22;100(15):8921-6.

[94] Sasaki H, Sheng Y, Kotsuji F, Tsang BK. Down-regulation of X-linked inhibitor of apoptosis protein induces apoptosis in chemoresistant human ovarian cancer cells. Cancer Res. 2000 Oct 15;60(20):5659-66.

[95] Fraser M, Leung B, Jahani-Asl A, Yan X, Thompson WE, Tsang BK. Chemoresistance in human ovarian cancer: the role of apoptotic regulators. Reprod Biol Endocrinol. 2003 Oct 7;1:66.

[96] Asselin E, Mills GB, Tsang BK. XIAP regulates Akt activity and caspase-3-dependent cleavage during cisplatin-induced apoptosis in human ovarian epithelial cancer cells. Cancer Res. 2001 Mar 1;61(5):1862-8.

[97] Li J, Feng Q, Kim JM, Schneiderman D, Liston P, Li M, et al. Human ovarian cancer and cisplatin resistance: possible role of inhibitor of apoptosis proteins. Endocrinology. 2001 Jan;142(1):370-80.

[98] Fraser M, Leung BM, Yan X, Dan HC, Cheng JQ, Tsang BK. p53 is a determinant of X-linked inhibitor of apoptosis protein/Akt-mediated chemoresistance in human ovarian cancer cells. Cancer Res. 2003 Nov 1;63(21):7081-8.

[99] Kumar S, Bryant CS, Chamala S, Qazi A, Seward S, Pal J, et al. Ritonavir blocks AKT signaling, activates apoptosis and inhibits migration and invasion in ovarian cancer cells. Mol Cancer. 2009;8:26.

[100] Karam AK, Santiskulvong C, Fekete M, Zabih S, Eng C, Dorigo O. Cisplatin and PI3kinase inhibition decrease invasion and migration of human ovarian carcinoma cells and regulate matrix-metalloproteinase expression. Cytoskeleton (Hoboken). 2010 Aug;67(8):535-44.

[101] Zhou C, Qiu L, Sun Y, Healey S, Wanebo H, Kouttab N, et al. Inhibition of EGFR/PI3K/AKT cell survival pathway promotes TSA's effect on cell death and migration in human ovarian cancer cells. Int J Oncol. 2006 Jul;29(1):269-78.

[102] Peng DJ, Wang J, Zhou JY, Wu GS. Role of the Akt/mTOR survival pathway in cisplatin resistance in ovarian cancer cells. Biochem Biophys Res Commun. 2010 Apr 9;394(3):600-5.

[103] Whitley BR, Beaulieu LM, Carter JC, Church FC. Phosphatidylinositol 3-kinase/Akt regulates the balance between plasminogen activator inhibitor-1 and urokinase to promote migration of SKOV-3 ovarian cancer cells. Gynecol Oncol. 2007 Feb;104(2):470-9.

[104] Park BK, Zeng X, Glazer RI. Akt1 induces extracellular matrix invasion and matrix metalloproteinase-2 activity in mouse mammary epithelial cells. Cancer Res. 2001 Oct 15;61(20):7647-53.

[105] Furuya F, Hanover JA, Cheng SY. Activation of phosphatidylinositol 3-kinase signaling by a mutant thyroid hormone beta receptor. Proc Natl Acad Sci U S A. 2006 Feb 7;103(6):1780-5.

[106] Vasko V, Saji M, Hardy E, Kruhlak M, Larin A, Savchenko V, et al. Akt activation and localisation correlate with tumour invasion and oncogene expression in thyroid cancer. J Med Genet. 2004 Mar;41(3):161-70.

[107] Choi JH, Choi KC, Auersperg N, Leung PC. Gonadotropins activate proteolysis and increase invasion through protein kinase A and phosphatidylinositol 3-kinase pathways in human epithelial ovarian cancer cells. Cancer Res. 2006 Apr 1;66(7):3912-20.

[108] Garcia-Cardena G, Fan R, Shah V, Sorrentino R, Cirino G, Papapetropoulos A, et al. Dynamic activation of endothelial nitric oxide synthase by Hsp90. Nature. 1998 Apr 23;392(6678):821-4.

[109] Takahashi S, Mendelsohn ME. Synergistic activation of endothelial nitric-oxide synthase (eNOS) by HSP90 and Akt: calcium-independent eNOS activation involves formation of an HSP90-Akt-CaM-bound eNOS complex. J Biol Chem. 2003 Aug 15;278(33):30821-7.

[110] Gratton JP, Fontana J, O'Connor DS, Garcia-Cardena G, McCabe TJ, Sessa WC. Reconstitution of an endothelial nitric-oxide synthase (eNOS), hsp90, and caveolin-1 complex in vitro. Evidence that hsp90 facilitates calmodulin stimulated displacement of eNOS from caveolin-1. J Biol Chem. 2000 Jul 21;275(29):22268-72.

[111] Fontana J, Fulton D, Chen Y, Fairchild TA, McCabe TJ, Fujita N, et al. Domain mapping studies reveal that the M domain of hsp90 serves as a molecular scaffold to regulate Akt-dependent phosphorylation of endothelial nitric oxide synthase and NO release. Circ Res. 2002 May 3;90(8):866-73.

[112] Brouet A, Sonveaux P, Dessy C, Moniotte S, Balligand JL, Feron O. Hsp90 and caveolin are key targets for the proangiogenic nitric oxide-mediated effects of statins. Circ Res. 2001 Nov 9;89(10):866-73.

[113] Takahashi S, Mendelsohn ME. Calmodulin-dependent and -independent activation of endothelial nitric-oxide synthase by heat shock protein 90. J Biol Chem. 2003 Mar 14;278(11):9339-44.

Chapter 13

The PI3K/Akt/mTOR Pathway in Ovarian Cancer: Biological Rationale and Therapeutic Opportunities

Alexandra Leary, Edouard Auclin,
Patricia Pautier and Catherine Lhommé

Additional information is available at the end of the chapter

http://dx.doi.org/10.5772/54170

1. Introduction

Ovarian cancer is the most lethal cause of gynecological cancer deaths in the developing world and typically presents at an advanced stage when optimal debulking and platinum based-chemotherapy remain the cornerstone of management. Unfortunately, despite frequent initial responses to chemotherapy, these tumors almost invariably relapse. Thanks to recent large scale molecular profiling studies in ovarian cancer, such as the integrated genomic analyses performed by the Cancer Genome Atlas (TCGA) network, significant headway has been made in our understanding of the molecular pathogenesis of ovarian cancer[1]. However these advances have failed to translate into meaningful clinical benefit for patients. The only approved novel 'targeted' therapy to date in ovarian cancer is the anti-angiogenic antibody, bevacizumab, for which reliable predictive markers still elude us.

With the possible exception of the p53 signaling network, the PI3K/Akt/mTOR cascade is probably the most frequently altered signaling pathway in cancer, including ovarian cancer. First generation inhibitors of mTOR have demonstrated anti-tumor activity and are currently approved for the treatment of renal, pancreatic, breast and some brain cancers. In addition, a huge number of PI3K, Akt and second generation mTOR inhibitors are in early clinical trials.

We propose to provide a brief overview of the PI3K/Akt/mTOR signaling network and discuss the rationale for targeting this pathway in ovarian cancer. Preclinical data and results of recent clinical trials will be presented. In addition, some of the challenges facing the development of these inhibitors in ovarian cancer will be discussed, such as the need for predictive markers and quality tumor samples, drug resistance, managing toxicity, as well as trial design considerations in order to optimize the development of novel therapies against the PI3K pathway in ovarian cancer.

2. The PI3K/Akt/mTOR signaling pathway

The phophatidylinositol 3 Kinase (PI3K) pathway is a complex signaling network coordinating a number of direct upstream inputs from growth factors (EGF, heregulin, TGF, and others), tyrosine kinase receptors (IGF1R, EGFR, HER2…) or other membrane receptors such as Met as well as cross-talk with the Ras-Raf-Mek-Erk pathway via indirect input from Ras (Figure 1). PI3K is composed of a p110 catalytic subunit and a p85 regulatory subunit. The p110 subunit of PI3K phosphorylates phosphatidylinositol-4,5-bisphosphate (PIP2) to the active second messenger, PIP3 which recruits Akt to the plasma membrane, and results in a conformational change and activation of PDK1 and Akt proteins. Akt is a serine threonine kinase that regulates a huge number of downstream targets [2],[3], while the phosphatase and tensin (PTEN) analog protein acts as an endogenous pathway repressor by de-phosphorylating PIP3 back to PIP2. Akt controls critical cellular survival and metabolic processes by influencing some of the following:

1. Via downstream regulation of p53, NFκB (nuclear factor κB) or CREB (cAMP response element-binding protein), Akt promotes the transcription of genes involved in anti-apoptotic and proliferative responses such as XIAP (X-linked inhibitor of apoptosis protein), the apoptosis regulating protein Bcl-2, survivin and others[4].
2. Akt also phosphorylates proteins involved in cell cycle regulation and apoptosis thus promoting cell cycle progression and survival:

a. Phosphorylation of GSK3 inhibits proteosomic degradation of cyclin D1,

b. Phosphorylation of the cyclin-dependent kinase (CDK) inhibitors p21 and p27 commits them to nuclear export and removes their inhibitory effect on cyclin D and cyclin E,

c. Downregulation of the apoptotic effector, caspase 9.

3. In addition downstream signaling via mammalian target of rapamycin (mTOR) activates two key substrates 4EBP1 and p70S6K resulting in increased translation of target genes involved in angiogenesis (VEGF), or cell cycle progression (cyclin D1, c-Myc)[5].

In addition to activation via upstream input, the PI3K pathway can be 'intrinsically' activated due to i) gain of function mutations or amplifications in the p110 subunit of PI3K (*PIK3CA*), ii) mutations in the p85 subunit (*PIK3R*), iii) mutations or amplifications in one of the Akt isoforms (*AKT1, AKT2, AKT3*), or iv) due to loss of its negative regulator, *PTEN* via inactivating mutations, copy number loss or homozygous deletions.

While mTOR is probably the best described direct target of Akt, the mTOR complex is actually composed of two components, the mTORC1-Raptor complex primary coordinator of translational control via 4EBP1 and p70S6K[6]; and the mTORC2-Rictor complex whose function is less well described but likely regulates cell proliferation and survival in part by Akt activation via phosphorylation at Serine 473[7]. Importantly mTORC1 is sensitive to inhibition by rapamycin, while mTORC2 is not. In the presence of selective mTORC1 inhibition, mTORC2 can exert a positive feedback on Akt[8]. As discussed later, this positive feedback loop may have important implications regarding the emergence of resistance to first generation mTOR inhibitors (rapalogs) that exclusively target mTORC1, with no effect on mTORC2.

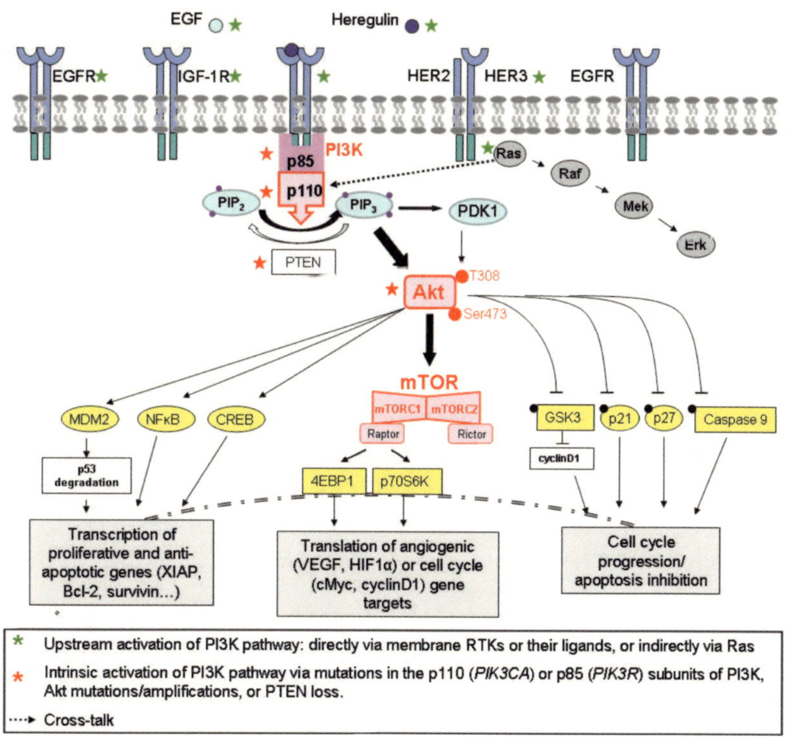

Figure 1. The PI3K/Akt/mTOR signaling pathway. This pathway is up-regulated in a significant proportion of ovarian cancers via either (i) direct upstream stimulation (growth factor receptors and their ligands), (ii) indirect activation via cross-talk with the Ras pathway, or (iii) intrinsically via activating genetic alterations in PI3K or Akt, or via loss of function in the tumor suppressor, PTEN.

3. Relevance of PI3K/Akt/mTOR signaling in ovarian cancer

The PI3K/Akt/mTOR pathway is frequently deregulated in ovarian cancer. Array Comparative Genomic Hybridization (aCGH) studies on 93 ovarian tumors have identified this pathway as the most frequently altered in ovarian cancer [9]. Copy gains in the genes encoding both the p110α (*PIK3CA*) and p110β (*PIK3CB*) subunits of PI3K were associated with a poor prognosis in patients with ovarian cancer. Expression levels of both p110α and pAkt were analyzed in over 500 ovarian cancer tumors and associated with decreased survival. Activation of the pathway as measured by Akt or mTOR phosphorylation levels is almost ubiquitous in ovarian cancer and an independent negative prognostic marker [10-12].

Interestingly, the type of PI3K/Akt/mTOR molecular alteration appears to be histological subtype specific (Table 1). There is mounting evidence that ovarian cancer is a highly heterogeneous disease with marked differences in molecular profile, histology, prognosis and chemosensitivity depending on the subtype [1],[13],[14]. The most common subtype (70%) high grade serous ovarian cancer (HGSOC) is characterized by almost universal p53 mutations (95-97% of cases) and marked genomic instability resulting in frequent somatic copy number alterations (amplifications or deletions)[13]. In HGSOC, oncogenic mutations are rare, but amplifications of the p110 subunit of PI3K (*PIK3CA)* have been described in 20% of cases, amplifications of one of the *AKT* isoforms (*AKT 1, AKT2* or *AKT3*) occur in 15% to 20%, while *PTEN* deletions have been described in 5%[15],[16] (Table 1). Finally *RICTOR* or *RAPTOR* amplifications have also been reported [1]. Rare but potentially relevant mutations in HGSOC include activating *PIK3CA* mutations (3%), or loss of function *PTEN* mutations (1%) [17]. Mutations have also been described in the p85α subunit of PI3K (*PIK3R1*, 4%), resulting in loss of its negative regulation on the p110 subunit and constitutive kinase activity[18]. In summary, 40 to 50% of HGSOC may have constitutive PI3K signaling. In a significant proportion of HGSOC, hyperactive PI3K/Akt/mTOR pathway may also be attributable to upstream deregulations in receptor tyrosine kinases (RTKs) or cross-talk with the Ras/Mek/Mek/Erk pathway. Indeed, amplifications or mutations in RTKs such as *ERBB3, ERBB2, EGFR* or *IGF1R* have been described with frequencies of 1% to 9% [1],[17]. Similarly, the ras pathway is often altered in HGSOC by amplifications in *KRAS* (11%), *MAPK* (20%), loss of the tumor suppressor *NF1* (8%), or less frequent mutations in *KRAS, NRAS*, or *BRAF*.

Whereas individual mutations remain an infrequent event in HGSOC, they are much more prevalent in the rarer subtypes such as low grade serous, mucinous, endometrioid or clear cell ovarian cancer. For example, 20% of endometrioid and 35% of clear cell ovarian tumors display *PIK3CA* mutations[19],[20]. In addition, while *PTEN* loss of function mutations are rare in ovarian cancer in general, they are well documented in up to 20% of endometrioid tumors and *PTEN* deletion occurs in 20% of endometrioid and clear cell ovarian cancers[21]. Low grade mucinous and serous subtypes do not tend to demonstrate intrinsic activation of PI3K effectors, however they frequently exhibit *KRAS* mutations, or amplifications/mutations in *ERBB2[22],[23]*.

Importantly intrinsic activation of the pathway (via *PIK3CA* mutations and *PTEN* loss) has been shown to initiate ovarian tumors in mice and inhibition of PI3K/mTOR in these models delayed tumor growth and prolonged survival, thus providing critical proof of concept for the pathologic relevance of this pathway in OC and its potential as a therapeutic target[24],[25]. Whether amplifications of pathway members actually activate PI3K signaling and confer comparable sensitivity to pathway inhibitors remains to be established. Similarly, while cross-talk with Ras may result in PI3K activation, it is unlikely that this also results in PI3K pathway dependence, however as discussed later, alterations in KRAS may be relevant with regards to predicting benefit from dual PI3K-Ras inhibition.

http://dx.doi.org/10.5772/54170

High grade serous ovarian cancer is exquisitely chemosensitive, with response rates to first-line platinum-based chemotherapy of 75%, but almost invariably relapses with acquired resistance. The rarer subtypes tend to respond poorly to platinum chemotherapy with response rates of only 15% to 30%. Thus both acquired and de novo chemotherapy resistance remains a significant clinical challenge in ovarian cancer. Increased phosphorylation of mTOR has been described in cell lines with acquired cisplatin resistance, and Akt signaling has been implicated in primary platinum resistance[12]. Inhibitors of Akt or mTOR were shown to restore chemo-sensitivity in vitro and in xenograft models [26],[27]. These data suggest a potential role for inhibitors of the PI3K pathway in modulating chemotherapy sensitivity and justify their use in combination with conventional cytotoxics.

Ovarian cancer histological subtype	Intrinsic PI3K pathway activation	PI3K activation via upstream membrane RTKs	PI3K activation via cross-talk with ras
High grade serous (70%)	**Amplifications**: *PIK3CA* (17-20%) AKT1 (3%) AKT2 (6-12%) AKT3 (8%) RICTOR (6%) RAPTOR (4%) **Deletions:** PTEN (7%)	**Amplifications:** *ERBB3* (4%) ERBB2 (3%) IGF1R (4%)	**Amplifications:** *MAPK* (25%) KRAS (11%) **Deletions:** NF1 (8%)
	Mutations: *PIK3CA* (3%) *PIK3R1* (4%) *PTEN* (1%)	**Mutations:** *EGFR* (4-9%) *ERBB2* (1%)	**Mutations:** *NF1* (4%) *KRAS* (1-5%) *NRAS* (1%) *BRAF* (1%)
Clear cell	**Deletions** *PTEN* (20%)	**Amplifications** *ERBB2* (14%)	
	Mutations: *PIK3CA* (33%)		
Endometrioid	**Deletions** *PTEN* (20%)		
	Mutations: *PIK3CA* (20%) *PTEN* (20%)		
Mucinous		**Amplifications:** *ERBB2* (18%)	**Mutations:** *KRAS* (40-60%)
Low grade serous		**Mutations:** *ERBB2* (15%)	**Mutations:** *KRAS* (40%) *BRAF* (1%)

Table 1. Molecular alterations according to ovarian cancer subtype that could contribute to PI3K pâthway activation either directly (deregulated PI3K members) or indirectly via alterations in upstream RTKs or Ras pathway members.

4. Results of clinical trials targeting the PI3K/Akt/mTOR pathway in ovarian cancer

The frequent PI3K/Akt alterations demonstrated in vivo in tumors from patients with ovarian cancer, combined with the evidence for dependence on this oncogenic pathway in preclinical models provide a robust biological rationale for investigating the benefit of targeting PI3K, Akt or mTOR in ovarian cancer. However as detailed throughout this chapter, the intrinsic complexity of this signaling network may limit the anti-tumor potential of inhibiting a single effector along the pathway.

4.1. mTOR inhibitor monotherapy in ovarian cancer (Table 2)

The first inhibitors of the pathway to enter the clinic were rapamycin analogs that bind to the FK506 binding protein-12 of the MTORC1 complex and prevent mTOR activity. Rapamycin was used for years as an immunosuppressant to prevent rejection in solid organ transplants and hematological malignancies; its toxicity profile is therefore well described with main side effects consisting of edema, hypertension, renal toxicity, hematologic toxicity, and hypertriglyceridemia and hypercholesterolemia. In addition, rarer but potentially more concerning side effects included interstitial lung disease, risk of secondary lymphoma, and reactivation of latent infections[28]. Rapamycin analogs with less immunosuppressive properties, such as temsirolimus, everolimus and ridaforolimus have shown activity in a number of tumor types.

A phase II trial of temsirolimus at a flat dose of 25mg IV weekly in patients with ovarian cancer progressing after 1-3 previous regimens met its first stage response and PFS criteria at interim analysis with three responses and seven PFS at 6 months and pursued accrual through the second stage[29]. At final analysis, with 54 evaluable patients, grade 3-4 toxicities were as expected for mTOR inhibitors, mainly gastrointestinal (10%), metabolic (15%), and study drug was discontinued in 6% for interstitial pneumonitis. Unfortunately, objective responses were only seen in 9.3% (5/54) and 6 months PFS was 24% thus the study failed to meet its efficacy endpoint. Exploratory analyses were conducted in order to identify potential predictive markers. Phosphorylated-Akt, p-mTOR, p-p70-S6K, and cyclinD1 were measured in archival tumor samples as surrogates for activation of the PI3K pathway; only cyclinD1 levels were weakly correlated with PFS>6 months (r=0.28). The authors concluded that observed activity was insufficient to justify a phase III trial of temsirolimus in unselected patients with ovarian cancer. As discussed later in the chapter; these negative results may be explained by i) the lack of patient selection, ii) the cytostatic rather than cytotoxic effect of mTOR inhibitors (mTORi) and iii) the fact that these agents may require combinations with chemotherapy or other targeted agents to achieve a robust anti-tumor effect. The trial just fell short of its PFS efficacy endpoint (>24% PFS at 6 months), had the study limited enrollment to clear cell and endometrioid histologies known to show frequent PI3K alterations, the results may have been different.

4.2. mTOR inhibitors in combination with chemotherapy in ovarian cancer (Table 2)

Given the implication of mTOR and Akt in chemo-resistance and the preclinical studies suggesting an additive benefit with chemotherapy, studies have investigated mTORi-cytotoxic combinations. A phase I study of weekly topotecan (1mg/m2 days 1, 8 and 15) and temsirolimus 25mg days 1, 8, 15 and 22 on a 28 day schedule was conducted in 15 patients with gynecological malignancies including 7 patients with ovarian cancer. Dose limiting toxicities were myelosuppression and although efficacy was not a primary objective, 8 of 11 patients had stable disease at first evaluation and one patient with clear cell histology was still progression free at 6 months[30].

A phase Ib dose escalation study of temsirolimus (T) and pegylated liposomal doxorubicin (PLD) in advanced breast and gynaecological malignancies identified T 15mg and PLD 40mg/m2 as the maximum tolerated dose (MTD)[31]. The most frequent grade 3-4 adverse events were fatigue (5%), nausea (16%), mucositis (21%), rash (11%) and hand-foot syndrome (21%). The mean PFS was 4.9 months and the authors concluded that the combination warranted further study.

Two other phase I studies of rapalogs in combination with chemotherapy (temsirolimus plus carboplatin/paclitaxel[32] and everolimus plus weekly paclitaxel[33]) have been conducted with grade 3-4 neutropenia being the major DLT (at 89% and 56%, respectively) as well as fatigue and mucositis. These studies included a small number of patients with advanced ovarian cancer and responses were described (3 of 6 patients with ovarian cancer had a PR to temsirolimus plus carboplatin and paclitaxel). However given the small numbers and the combination with chemotherapy, no robust conclusions may be drawn regarding the added value of the mTOR inhibitor.

These early studies have begun to establish the feasibility and safety of mTORi-cytotoxic combinations, randomized trials will be required to investigate efficacy. In the interim, a number of non-randomized phase I and II studies are ongoing (Table 4). Given the heterogeneity of ovarian cancer, non-randomized phase II studies may require a degree of patient selection by molecular alteration or even histology in order to enrich the trial for potential responders and make the patient population more uniform with regards to natural disease course and chemosensitivity. Indeed studies recruiting patients with both high and low grade tumors with marked differences in tumor growth rates and responsiveness to chemotherapy may mask any benefit from the addition of the mTOR inhibitor. For example, a phase II trial of temsirolimus plus carboplatin and paclitaxel as adjuvant treatment is ongoing for patients with stage III or IV clear cell ovarian cancer (NCT01196429).

4.3. mTOR inhibitors in combination with anti-angiogenics in ovarian cancer (Table 2)

Finally, given the activity of VEGF inhibitors in ovarian cancer and the fact that downstream mTOR targets include angiogenic genes, there is A biological rationale for using mTOR and VEGF inhibitors in combination. A phase II trial of temsirolimus and bevacizumab in ovarian cancer has been conducted[34]. Thirty one (31) patients were evaluable for toxicity and 25 for efficacy. Adverse events included fatigue, mucositis, hypertension and neutropenia. In addition one grade 4 rash and 6% colonic perforations (2/31) were reported. While the confirmed PR rate is only 12% in the first 25 evaluable patients (all in platinum-resistant patients), the 6 months PFS rate of 56% (14/25) met efficacy criteria to justify progression to second stage accrual. Updated results are awaited. It is noteworthy that the study only enrolled patients who had not been exposed to anti-angiogenics; the previously reported RR of 15-21% in early trials of bevacizumab monotherapy among heavily pretreated patients with ovarian cancer raises the possibility that temsirolimus may be adding little anti-tumor effect to bevacizumab alone[35],[36]. A randomized phase II study is ongoing comparing bevacizumab alone to bevacizumab and everolimus in patients with recurrent ovarian cancer (NCT00886691, Table 4). Patients will be stratified according to their platinum-free interval or prior treatment with bevacizumab. This study should provide valuable insight into the potential additive benefit of this combinatorial strategy.

Reference	Phase	Treatment	N, total enrolled	N, ovarian cancer	Selected toxicities	Efficacy
Behbakht et al	II	Temsirolimus, 25mg IV D1, 8, 15, 22 Q28 days	54	54	G3-4 GI (10%), metabolic (15%), pulmonary (6%)	RR=9% 6 month PFS=24%
Temkin et al	I	Temsirolimus IV 25mg D 1, 8, 15, 22 + topotecan 1mg/m2 IV D1, 8, 15 Q28 days	15	7	G3-4 neutropenia and thrombocytopenia	RR=0 One SD for 6 months
Boers-Sonderen et al	Ib	MTD= temsirolimus IV 15mg D1, 8, 15, 22 + PLD IV 40mg/m2 D1 Q28 days	20	NA	G3-4 fatigue (5%), nausea (16%), mucositis (21%), vomiting (16%), rash (11%), hand-foot syndrome (21%)	NA
Kollsmannberger et al	I	MTD= temsirolimus IV 25mg D1 and 8 + carbo AUC5 IV D1 + Pac IV 175mg/m2 D1 Q 21 days	39	6	G3-4 neutropenia (89%), thrombocytopenia (21%), pulmonary (5%)	RR= 50% (3/6) SD=50% (3/6)
Campone et al	I	Everolimus PO 30mg daily + Pac 80mg/m2 D 1, 8, 15 Q 28 days	16	3	G3 neutropenia, anemia, thrombocytopenia, mucositis, fatigue	NA
Morgan et al	II	Temsirolimus IV 25mg D 1, 8, 15, 22 + Bev 10mg/kg D1 and 15 Q 28 days	31	31 evaluable for toxicity and 25 evaluable for efficacy	G3-4 fatigue (13%), mucositis (13%), HTN (6%), neutropenia (10%), rash (3%), colonic perforation (6%)	RR=12% 6month PFS 56%

Abbreviations: N: number of patients; IV: intravenous; D: day; Q: every; G3-4: grade 3-4; RR: response rate; PFS: progression-free survival; SD: stable disease; MTD: maximum tolerated dose; PLD: pegylated liposomal doxorubicin; NA: information not available; carbo: carboplatin; pac: paclitaxel; PO: per os.

Table 2. Completed clinical trials of mTOR inhibitors in ovarian cancer

While the evidence for clinical activity of mTOR inhibitors in ovarian cancer remains quite limited, especially compared to endometrial cancer where efficacy has been more encouraging, a number of phase II trials of mTOR inhibitors alone or in combination with conventional cytotoxics or targeted therapies are currently ongoing. These should help clarify the role mTOR inhibitors may have in the management of patients with ovarian cancer (Table 4).

4.4. Akt inhibitors

Targeting Akt upstream from mTOR may produce a more effective knock-down of signal transduction and a number of Akt inhibitors have therefore been generated. These include ATP-competitive inhibitors, allosteric inhibitors, peptide-based inhibitors and lipid-based inhibitors (reviewed in Stronach et al[37]). Akt inhibitors are still in early stages of clinical development and two compounds have been specifically tested in ovarian cancer (Table 3).

The most mature inhibitor in clinical development is the lipid-based inhibitor, perifosine, it interferes with the cell membrane recruitment of Akt (thus preventing activation). However early data in phase I and II trials in other tumor types were disappointing with frequent gastrointestinal toxicity and a lack of meaningful activity[38]-[41]. Given the suggestion that the narrow therapeutic window of perifosine may limit its clinical usefulness, combination trials with conventional cytotoxics have been conducted in order to improve the therapeutic index. Preclinical studies have shown that perifosine inhibited ovarian cancer cell proliferation, motility and angiogenesis and potentiated paclitaxel sensitivity in vitro and in vivo[42], [43]. On this basis, a phase I trial of perifosine and docetaxel in platinum and taxane resistant ovarian cancer was conducted[42]. Perifosine was given at a loading dose of 100mg every 6 hours for 4 doses followed by a daily dose according to dose level (50, 100 or 150mg daily) in combination with docetaxel 75mg/m2 day 1 every 3 weeks. Twenty one patients were enrolled including 11 at the MTD level of perifosine 150mg. No DLTs were observed, frequent adverse events included nausea, vomiting, anorexia, constipation and fatigue. With regards to efficacy at the MTD (N=11), there was one PR in an endometrioid ovarian cancer with a loss of function *PTEN* mutation (R130Q) and one SD maintained for 4 months in a PI3K mutated clear cell tumor. Two other patients without apparent PI3K alterations achieved SD while two patients with KRAS mutations progressed quickly. The investigators also performed pharmacodynamic studies using reverse phase protein array (RPPA) to detect changes in total and phosphorylated markers in pre-treatment versus day 7 tumor biopsies and functional imaging studies using FDG-PET scans. Bcl2 and ERK2 levels were increased by treatment suggesting that the low response rate may be in part explained by perifosine induced increases in alternate signalling pathways. However FDG-PET responses at one week correlated with inhibition of S6 phosphorylation raising the possibility that FDG-PET may serve as an early surrogate indicator of Akt inhibition.

GSK795 is an oral ATP-competitive pan-Akt inhibitor in early stages of development and a small phase I pharmacodynamic and pharmacokinetic study was conducted in order to characterize the relationship between AKT inhibition by GSK795 and downstream effects in patients with advanced platinum resistant ovarian cancer[44]. Twelve patients were enrolled. The only toxicities were grade 2 anorexia (18%) and vomiting (18%). FDG metabolism decreased in the majority of tumors but there was no dose response relationship. Among 5 patients treated at the higher dose levels, paired pre- and post-treatment tumor biopsies demonstrated downregulation in pAkt and in the tumor proliferative marker, Ki67. Two patients have achieved >6 months PFS with objective tumor regressions of 26% and 11%, respectively.

In addition to the aforementioned inhibitors, Akt isoform specific inhibitors are being developed, however the distinct functions of each of these isoforms and their relevance to different tumor types or individual tumor genetic background is still poorly understood. Studies of AKT isoform knockouts provide some insight into their relative roles: AKT1 loss is associated with impaired fetal development and increased fetal mortality; AKT2 loss leads to diabetes and AKT3 loss results in defective central nervous system development[45].

Reference	Phase	Treatment	N, total enrolled	N, ovarian cancer	Selected toxicities	Efficacy
Fu et al	I	MTD Perifosine orally 150mg/day + docetaxel, 75mg IV D1 Q21 days	21	21	Nausea, vomiting, anorexia, fatigue	At MTD (N=11) PR in 1 PTEN null, SD 3/11.
Gungor et al	I	GSK795 25, 50 or 75mg orqlly/day	12	12	G2 anorexia (18%), vomiting (18%)	16% SD for 6 mo (2/12) with tumor shrinkage of 26% and 11%

Table 3. Completed clinical trials of Akt inhibitors in ovarian cancer

4.5. PI3K inhibitors

The PI3K inhibitors, LY290002 and wortmannin have been used for years as tools in preclinical experiments to demonstrate the biological relevance of PI3K and explore its potential as a therapeutic target in cancer. However, the micromolar IC50 (50% inhibitory concentration) and off-target effects of these agents have limited their clinical applicability. Less toxic PI3K inhibitors are just entering phase II stages of clinical development (reviewed in Kurtz et al[46]). BKM120 is an oral selective PI3K inhibitor with an IC50 for the PI3K kinase of 35nM. A dose escalation phase I trial has shown that the drug is well tolerated at the MTD of 100mg once a day with rash, hyperglycemia, diarrhea and mood alterations in over a third of patients[47]. BKM120 demonstrated dose dependent inhibition of FDG activity and downregulation in p-S6 in skin biopsies. The only response was in a KRAS mutated breast

http://dx.doi.org/10.5772/54170

cancer patient, and 7 patients had stable disease for more than 8 months. Five of these 7 patients had either PTEN loss or PI3K mutation. GDC0941 is an oral selective class I PI3K inhibitor that showed evidence of clinical activity in 3 patients enrolled in a phase I trial, including one ovarian cancer (PTEN negative) patient who remained on study for 5 months with a FDG-PET response, >50% decrease in pS6 staining in paired biopsies, and 80% decrease in CA-125[48]. XL147 is another selective PI3K inhibitor which was well tolerated in a phase I trial with rash as the main DLT. An associated trial of XL147 in combination with carboplatin and paclitaxel demonstrated that the combination was feasible with no evidence of PK interactions or overlapping toxicities and dose expansion cohorts are ongoing in ovarian cancer[49].

5. Challenges of PI3K/Akt/mTOR pathway inhibitors

Despite a strong preclinical rationale, clinical trials of novel agents targeting the PI3K/Akt/mTOR pathway in ovarian cancer have been disappointing. Given the complexity and redundancy of the PI3K signaling network, combined targeting may be required. The fact that all the trials conducted to date enrolled an unselected patient population may have diluted objective activity in a subset. It is therefore crucial that efforts are made to uncover resistance mechanisms, develop rationale combinatorial strategies, identify predictive biomarkers, and explore novel trial designs.

5.1. Resistance

5.1.1. Feedback loops via MTORC2 or IRS1

Compensatory feedback loops may allow escape from blockade of a single effector of the pathway. Early on, paradoxical increases in pAkt were identified in preclinical models and in tumors from patients treated with mTOR inhibitors[8]. As illustrated in Figure 2, rapalogs suppress MTORC1 but do not affect the other subunit of mTOR, MTORC2. MTORC2 is a positive regulator of Akt, and selective inhibition of MTORC1 results in compensatory increase in Akt phosphorylation at Serine 473[50]. Rapalog-induced rebound Akt activation has been proposed as one of the mechanisms accounting for resistance to first generation inhibitors in the clinic. In addition, although the function and downstream effectors of MTORC2 are less well described, it is reasonable to expect that complete abrogation of the whole mTOR complex may be required to achieve a robust anti-tumor effect. As a result, mTORC1/mTORC2 dual inhibitors have been developed such as DS3078a, INK128, AZD8055, OSI027 and AZD2014 (reviewed in [51]).

Another postulated compensatory escape route from mTOR inhibition is via insulin growth factor 1 receptor (IGF1R, see Figure 2)[52]. Insulin receptor substrate-1 is normally under basal negative regulation via phosphorylation by mTOR; mTOR inhibition prevents IRS-1 phosphorylation thus allowing IRS-1 to complex with IGF1R and promote Akt signaling[53] thereby generating another positive feedback loop accounting for resistance.

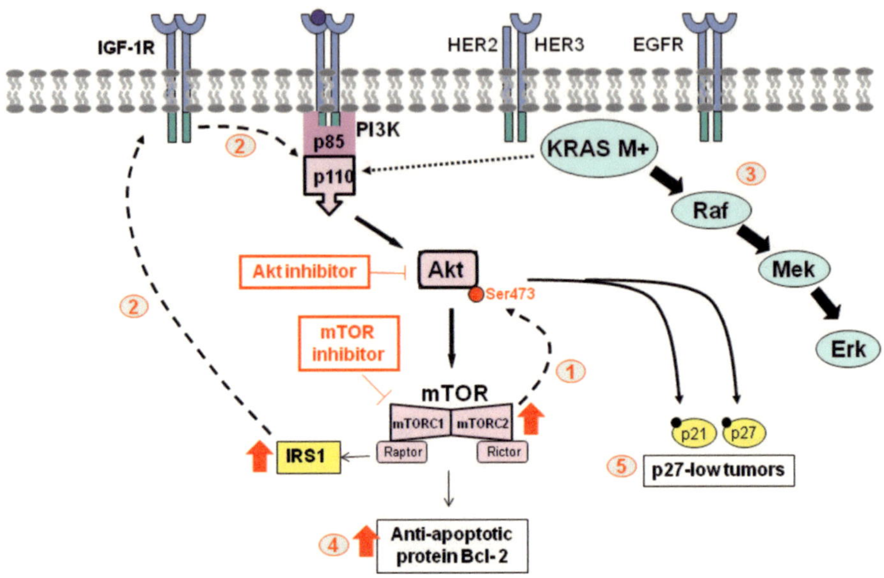

Figure 2. Proposed mechanisms accounting for resistance to inhibitors of the PI3K pathway. (1) Selective blockade of MTORC1 by rapalogs increases MTORC2 and results in positive feedback activation of pAkt. (2) Inhibition of mTOR removes the basal inhibition of IRS1, now free to bind to and activate IGF1R and promote PI£K activation. (3) In the presence of constitutive activation of KRAS, abrogation of the PI3K pathway alone does not inhibit cancer cell growth. (4) A dysfunctional apoptotic pathway (high bcl2, high survivin...) may lead to resistance to the pro-apoptotic effects of PI3K apthway inhibitors. (5) One downstream effect of Akt inhibition is cell cyle arrest via increase in the cdk inhibitors, p21 or p27; p27 low tumors may be resistant to PI3K pathway inhibitor induced cell cycles arrest.

5.1.2. The Ras pathway: KRAS/BRAF mutations and compensatory increases in Erk signaling

Interactions with parallel pathways may also allow escape from PI3K inhibition. Akt has been shown to be phosphorylated via cross-talk with Ras. Thus, in KRAS mutant tumors primarily driven by a constitutively upregulated Ras pathway, PI3k pathway inhibitors alone are unlikely to be effective. This hypothesis is supported by studies demonstrating that KRAS or BRAF mutated tumors are insensitive to mTOR inhibitors. Using a panel of cell lines including ovarian cancer, PI3K mutated tumors were shown to be sensitive, while dual PI3K and KRAS or BRAF mutated tumors were resistant to everolimus[54]. Importantly, they also demonstrated that knock-down of the KRAS mutation in these cells restored everolimus sensitivity in vitro and in vivo. In the presence of KRAS or BRAF mutations, tumors may exhibit 'oncogenic addiction' to an alternate survival pathway, e.g. Ras-Raf-Mek-Erk. This illustrates the fact that sensitivity to PI3K transduction inhibitors may require not only pathway activation but also demonstration of pathway dependence.

In addition to reactivating Akt, rapalogs have been reported to cause treatment induced increases in Mek/Erk signalling. In mice models and human tumors, everolimus increased Erk1/2 activation in post treatment tumor samples, suggesting the existence of crosstalk between the PI3K/mTOR and Mek/Erk signal transduction cascades[55]. Selective targeting of one pathway may simply result in compensatory upregulation in the other, and vice versa.

5.1.3. Dysfunctional apoptotic machinery

Even in tumor types such as renal cell or pancreatic neuroendocrine cancers where mTOR inhibitors have demonstrated sufficient clinical benefit to justify FDA approval, objective tumor responses are sporadic[56]. Some researchers have hypothesized that tumor shrinkage in response to mTOR inhibitors requires a functional apoptotic machinery. Majumder et al demonstrated that rapamycin-resistant SKOV3 ovarian cells have an activated PI3K pathway but upregulated levels of the anti-apoptotic protein, bcl2, and bcl2 knock-down using siRNA restored rapamycin sensitivity[57]. In line with this preclinical data, the Phase I trial of the Akt inhibitor perifosine reported compensatory increases in bcl2 in post treatment tumor biopsies[42].

5.1.4. Cell cycle dependent kinase (cdk) inhibitors

One of the major anti-tumor effects of PI3K blockade is to activate the cdk inhibitors p27 and p21, allow their nuclear translocation where they interact with, and inhibit cdks, thereby promoting cell cycle arrest. p27-null cells are resistant to rapamycin in vitro, some therefore postulate that tumors that have very low levels of p27 may therefore be less responsive to PI3K/Akt inhibition[58].

5.2. Combinatorial strategies

Given the presence of redundant pathways and the adaptive capacity of cancer cells, drug combinations are increasingly being investigated in an effort to abrogate both primary and acquired resistance to PI3K pathway inhibitors. Different approaches include targeting the same pathway at different levels (vertical combinations) or aiming for different pathways (horizontal combinations).

5.2.1. Vertical combinations

With membrane growth factor receptor inhibitors

Activation of the PI3K pathway can be attributable to upstream activation via membrane receptor kinases, and preclinical data suggest that concurrent inhibition of mTOR and EGFR may result in synergistic anti-tumor effect. Studies are investigating the benefit of dual mTOR/EGFR blockade[59]. A completed phase I trial showed that the combination of everolimus, bevacizumab and panitumumab was well tolerated, and three patients with ovarian cancer achieved prolonged disease control for 11 to >40 months[59]. In addition, mTOR inhibition may induce IRS1 expression and promote Akt activation via IGF1R thus attenuating the anti-tumor effects of rapalogs[60]. The addition of IFG1R antibodies to mTOR inhibitors has been shown to improve growth inhibition in vitro[52]. Studies investigating concurrent IGF1R/mTOR targeting have shown that treatment is feasible with an acceptable toxicity profile and encouraging activity in other tumor types[61] and studies using this approach are ongoing in ovarian cancer (Table 4).

Treatment type	Phase	Experimental treatment	Prior treatment	Selection criteria (biomarker vs allcomers)	Secondary endpoints	Clinical trial.gov identifier
PI3K inhibitor	I	BKM120 + Olaparib (PARP inhibitor)	First line platinium-based CT	All comers	MTD for the combination, safety, PK, efficacy. PD markers of PI3K inhibition, determination of BRCA1 IHC, BRCA1 promoter hypermethylation and BRCA1/2 somatic mutation status	NCT01623349
AKT inhibitor	I	GSK2141795	Not specified	All comers	PK and PD by FDG/PET	NCT01266954
	II	MK-2206	Platinum resistant	*P13K* or *AKT* mutation or low PTEN expression	RR, PFS and OS, toxicities of MK-2206, explore the association between select biomarkers and response to MK-2206, to explore the development of feedback loop activation and target inhibition with MK-2206.	NCT01283035
	I	Perifosine + docetaxel	Not specified	All comers	Tumor response	NCT00431054
	I/II	GSK2110183 + carbo+pac	Platinum resistant, "/>2 prior lines of CT	All comers	Phase I : safety and tolerability Phase II : overall RR	NCT01653912
1st generation MTOR inhibitor	I	Sirolimus + ALVAC(2)-NY-ESO-1 vaccine	Not specified	Tumor expression of NY-ESO-1 or LAGE-1	Safety, effectiveness of sirolimus on enhancing vaccine efficacy, antibody titers, NY-ESO-1 specific CD8+ and CD4+ frequency and function, PFS.	NCT01536054
	II	Temsirolimus	Taxane based treatment, <3 prior CT	All comers	PFS, rate and duration of stable diseases, cancer antigen 125 (for ovarian cancer), overall survival, safety and toxicity, quality of life, rate and duration of stable diseases	NCT01460979
	II	Temsirolimus + carbo + pac	Refractory to standard treatment	All comers	MTD, toxicity, RR, PK.	NCT00408655
	I	Everolimus + PLD + carbo	One prior platinum/ taxane-CT	All comers	MTD for the combination, safety/tolerability, anti-tumor activity	NCT01281514
	I	Ridaforolimus + carbo + pac	<4 prior CT lines	All comers	MTD, preliminary efficacity, toxicity	NCT01256268
	II	Adjuvant Temsirolimus + carbo + pac followed by maintenance temsirolimus	First line	Clear cell histology only	PFS at 12 months, median PFS, OS, toxicity and RR. mTOR signaling pathway by IHC.	NCT01196429
1st generation mTOR inhibitor in combination with	II	Everolimus + bevacizumab	Previously treated	All comers	PFS at 6 months, complete response + partial response + stable disease	NCT01031381

Treatment type	Phase	Experimental treatment	Prior treatment	Selection criteria (biomarker vs allcomers)	Secondary endpoints	Clinical trial.gov identifier
antiangiogenic therapy	II	Temsirolimus + bevacizumab	Previously treated	All comers	RR, PFS at 6 months, OS, duration of response, TTP. No specific biomarker objectives specified but blood and tumor collected on all	NCT01010126
	I	Temsirolimus + Cediranib (VEGFR 2 inhibitor)	<2 prior line of CT for recurrent disease	All comers	MTD , response rate, clinical benefit	NCT01065662
	II	Everolimus +/- bevacizumab randomised trial	Platinum-based CT. Stratification according to platinum resistant vs not, measurable disease vs. not and prior bevacizumab vs. not	All comers	PFS, tolerability, OS, RR, CA-125 response.	NCT00886691
mTOR or Akt inhibitor + IGF1R inhibitor	IB	MK-2206 (Akt inhibitor) or ridaforolimus + IGF1R Ab (dalotuzumab), non randomized study	Previously treated. Platinum resistance required for MK-2206 arm	All comers	Number of participants with dose limiting toxicities, number of participants whose best response is a partial response (PR) or complete response (CR)	NCT01243762
mTOR inhibitor in combination with Notch pathway inhibitor	I	Ridaforolimus + MK-0752	<3 prior CT lines	All comers	Number of participants with dose limiting toxicities, AUC for the ridaforolimus + MK-0752 doublet	NCT01295632

Abbreviations: PARP : poly-ADP-ribose polymerase ; CT : chemotherapy ; MTD : maximum tolerated dose, PK : pharmacokinetic ; PD : pharmacodynamic ; BRCA : breast cancer susceptibility gene ; IHC : immunohisotchemistry ; FDG/PET : fluorodeoxyglucose positron emission tomography ; RR : response rate ; PFS : progression-free survival ; OS : overall survival ; carbo : carboplatin ; pac : paclitaxel ; NY-ESO-1 : cancer-testis antigen-1 ; LAGE-1 : cancer-testis antigen-2 ; PLD : pegylated liposomal doxorubicin ; TTP : time to progression ; VEGFR : vascular endothelial growth factor receptor ; IGF1R : insulin-like growth factor receptor ; AUC : area under the curve.

Table 4. Ongoing trials of PI3K pathway inhibitors in ovarian cancer

Combined PI3K-mTOR or Akt-mTOR inhibition

As previously discussed, positive feedback loops generated by selective mTOR inhibition may result in paradoxical activation of Akt via mTORC2 and account for early resistance.

Dual MTORC1 and MTORC2 inhibitors have therefore been developed and shown to result in greater anti-tumor activity than rapalogs in preclinical studies[62]. Another strategy involves co-targeting mTOR as well as upstream PI3K in order to overcome the positive feedback loops via Akt. In addition, simultaneous targeting of several effectors of the PI3K pathway may improve the likelihood of completely shutting down the signaling cascade. A combination of everolimus and the PI3K inhibitor, PI-103 blocked rebound rapalog induced Akt activation and resulted in greater cell cycle arrest than either treatment alone in ovarian cancer cells[63]. NVP-BEZ235 is a novel agent that is both an ATP-competitive PI3K inhibitor and an inhibitor of both mTORC1 and mTORC2. Studies in ovarian cancer cell lines and mouse models have suggested that this drug caused cell cycle arrest and apoptosis, and prolonged survival of mice with established ovarian tumors[64]. A phase I trial of ridaforolimus with the Akt inhibitor MK2206 is ongoing and a dose expansion cohort in ovarian cancer is planned (NCT01295632). Other studies are exploring the benefit of inhibiting further downstream effectors such as p70S6 in combination with everolimus (NCT01115803).

5.2.2. Horizontal combinations

With Mek inhibitors

Given the evidence that oncogenic activation of the ras pathway may be associated with resistance to mTOR inhibitors even in the presence of PI3K oncogenic mutations, targeting both PI3K and Ras pathways simultaneously is worthy of investigation. In a mouse model of ovarian cancer driven by PTEN loss and KRAS mutation, simultaneous blockade of both PI3K and Mek signalling using pharmacological inhibitors resulted in significant tumor regressions and prolonged survival compared to monotherapy[65]. A phase I study comparing the tolerability and efficacy of dual PI3K and Mek targeting to either treatment alone showed that the combination significantly increased the risk of Grade 3-4 toxicity from 18% to 54% (p=0.001), but all patients with alterations in the PI3K pathway and a KRAS or BRAF mutation had tumor regressions with dual targeting[66].

With chemotherapy

One of the earliest explored strategy has been the combination of novel inhibitors with chemotherapy. There has been the theoretical concern that the cytostatic effects of these drugs may in fact antagonize the cell cycle dependent effects of chemotherapy. Preclinical studies in ovarian cancer have indeed suggested that PI3K inhibitor-induced G1 arrest undermined the cytotoxic effects of agents such as cisplatin, paclitaxel, gemcitabine and topotecan that are primarily effective in the S or G2 phase of the cell cycle[67]. However preliminary data from non-randomized studies of mTOR inhibitors in combination with chemotherapy have reported objective response rates comparable to those expected for chemotherapy alone, thus providing indirect evidence for a lack of antagonism. Randomized studies will be required to rule out any antagonism between PI3K inhibitors and conventional cytotoxics.

With anti-angiogenics

Pro-angiogenic factors such as HIF1α and VEGF are downregulated by inhibition of PI3K signaling. This may explain the activity of mTOR inhibitors in HIF1α-driven clear cell renal cancer. Given the putative anti-angiogenic effects of PI3K pathway inhibitors and the known activity of the VEGF antibody, bevacizumab in ovarian cancer, there is a rationale for targeting multiple angiogenic regulators at once in an effort to shut down angiogenesis completely. In fact, clear cell ovarian cancers with their reported angiogenic signature and increased HIF1α signaling[68] may be particularly suited to a therapeutic strategy combining traditional anti-angiogenics with PI3K pathway inhibitors.

5.3. Biomarkers

In light of the heterogeneity of ovarian cancer, predictive as well as pharmacodynamic (demonstrating target downregulation) biomarkers are desperately needed in order to select patients most likely to respond. In addition biomarkers would be useful to identify the subset of patients who may benefit from specific combinations. One question is whether sensitivity can be predicted on the basis of activation status of pathway members.

5.3.1. Constitutive PI3K activity: PIK3CA mutations and PTEN loss of function

The main intrinsic effectors of the pathway that have been studied in preclinical and clinical models have been PTEN loss, and PIK3CA activating mutations. Early studies in cell lines including ovarian cancer demonstrated greater anti-proliferative activity of PI3K pathway inhibitors in PTEN-null or PIK3CA mutated cells[69]-[71], Di Nicolantonio et al, showed in cell lines and in 43 patient tumor samples that PIK3CA mutations sensitized cancer cells to everolimus, but co-existing KRAS or BRAF mutations predicted resistance[54]. More recent clinical and preclinical studies have reported contradictory correlations between PI3K mutations or PTEN loss and response to inhibitors[72],[73]; in particular, a significant number of PI3K mutated tumors fail to respond, while a proportion of tumors lacking PI3K and PTEN alterations respond. This is in contrast to the much stronger association between activating mutations and response to other targeted agents such as EGFR, BRAF or ALK inhibitors. Studies in tumor types with frequent PTEN mutations, such as melanoma have not demonstrated significant responses to mTOR inhibitors suggesting that patient selection on the basis of PTEN loss alone may not identify responders[74]. In a pooled analysis of 3 trials of mTOR inhibitors in endometrial cancers, MacKay et al found no correlation between PIK3CA mutation or PTEN loss and response[75]. However a recent report by Janku and colleagues suggested that PI3K mutations did preferentially identify responders[76]. They conducted mutational analyses on 140 patients with breast and gynecological malignancies (including 60 with ovarian cancer) enrolled in phase I trials of PI3K/Akt/mTOR inhibitors. They demonstrated that the response rate was higher among patients with PIK3CA mutated tumors (RR=30% versus 10%). However these results should be interpreted in light of the fact that all responders were included in a trial of temsirolimus, bevacizumab and liposomal doxorubicin. Given the known activity of bevacizumab and liposomal doxorubicin in ovarian cancer and the fact that half the responding patients had never been previously exposed to liposomal doxorubicin, mutations may simply correlate with prognosis, or with an improved response to treatment in general.

In conclusion, if trials of PI3K/mTOR inhibitors had limited enrolment to PTEN null or PI3K mutated tumors a significant proportion of responding patients would have been missed. In light of the imperfect association between PI3K mutations or PTEN loss and response to PI3K pathway inhibitors, most ongoing trials are enrolling an unselected patient population; unfortunately, most of these studies do not appear to be collecting archival tumor samples for detailed molecular analyses (Table 4).

5.3.2. *pAkt and stathmin*

The level of phosphorylated Akt has been identified as a read-out for activation of the PI3K pathway and thus a potential biomarker for responsiveness to PI3K inhibitors. An in vitro and in silico study using a panel of cell lines and xenograft models treated with PI3K pathway inhibitors showed that pAkt correlated with efficacy, and KRAS or BRAF mutations with resistance; neither PTEN loss nor PIK3CA mutations correlated with response[77]. Udai et al analyzed PI3K signaling output in patient tumor samples by measuring phosphorylation of 3 effectors downstream of PI3K, ie pAkt, p p70S6K and pGSK3beta[78]. No correlation was found between the presence of genomic alterations in PI3K or PTEN and activation of the pathway as measured by phosphorylated downstream targets. In a study of 17 well-characterized ovarian cancer cell lines, the majority failed to respond to Akt inhibitors despite Akt phosphorylation[79]. A high level of pAkt may not only reflect PI3K pathway intrinsic activation, but also result from cross-talk with Ras or other upstream signals.

In addition to being a non-specific measure of PI3K signal transduction, pAkt is a labile phosphorylated tumor marker, its stability is affected by pre-analytical factors such as tissue acquisition, ischemic time and fixation method[80],[81], In an effort to identify more stable biomarkers, Saal et al developed a gene expression signature of PI3K pathway activation and Stathmin, a regulator of microtubule dynamics was an accurate marker of the gene signature. Stathmin can be easily measured by immunohistochemistry and is increasingly being used as a surrogate marker for activation of the PI3K pathway[82].

5.3.3. *KRAS/BRAF*

As previously discussed a number of preclinical studies have demonstrated that KRAS and BRAF mutations confer resistance to inhibitors of the PI3K pathway[54],[77]. Intringingly, in a pooled molecular analysis of patients treated with PI3K/Akt/mTOR inhibitors in phase I trials, Janku et al reported 2 objective responses in patients with co-existing PI3K and KRAS or BRAF mutation[76]. Genomic analyses of tumors and cell lines has established that a subset of ovarian cancers have co-existing Ras and PI3K/Akt amplifications or mutations. This easily identifiable subset may benefit from coordinated inhibition of both pathways, and a trial combining a Mek inhibitor with a PI3K/mTOR inhibitor in ovarian cancer patients harboring KRAS/BRAF and PI3K/Akt genomic alterations is warranted.

6. Practical issues: Samples and trial design

6.1. Access to quality ovarian cancer samples

As the data to date suggest that there is insufficient evidence to select patients for trials of PI3K inhibitors on the basis of specific molecular alterations, it is imperative that future trials enrolling unselected patient populations include parallel biological studies in an effort to uncover candidate biomarkers. Biological assays must be reproducible, robust and require access to high quality tumor samples. As such, pre-analytical variables must be controlled for as much as possible by following standardized sample collection, fixation, processing and storage procedures. When dealing with paraffin-embedded tissue, markers of the PI3K Akt pathway may be particularly susceptible to artefactual loss[80]. In fact, the optimal fixative for in depth genomic analyses is unlikely to be formalin, and may therefore require a shift in routine practice from paraffin to fresh frozen or RNAlater for sample storage.

6.2. Access to post-treatment samples

6.2.1. At relapse

It is likely that clonal evolution and treatment selection pressure will lead to important genomic and/or phenotypic modifications in the tumor in the interval between diagnosis and relapse. An increasing number of phase I and II trials are therefore requesting optional biopsies of metastatic disease and the vast majority of patients are willing to consent this procedure. A study of patients enrolled in phase I trials at our institution revealed that 84% of patients who were proposed optional tumor biopsies consented to the procedure, including sequential pre- and post-treatment biopsies[85]. All procedures were performed using an 18-gauge needle under ultrasound or computed tomography scanning and were associated with low minor complication rates (9/145 tumor biopsies). In 70% of the cases the biopsy met quality criteria for ancillary molecular (RNA and DNA) analyses. Access to samples from relapsed disease is likely to be particularly relevant to high grade ovarian cancer, where the initial disease is exquisitely chemosensitive and repeat profiling of the chemoresistant recurrence may reveal a completely different molecular profile.

6.2.2. Residual disease post-chemotherapy

The molecular characterization of ovarian cancer clones surviving after chemotherapy could identify targets for novel agents designed to eradicate chemoresistant residual disease. As discussed above, the combination of PI3K/Akt/mTOR inhibitors with chemotherapy may not be optimal because of the risk of cumulative toxicities as well as the theoretical risk that these inhibitors may antagonize the cytotoxic effects of chemotherapy. A more attractive approach may be sequential, where primarily chemosensitive ovarian cancer is treated with chemotherapy followed by PI3K inhibitors if indicated by the molecular profile of the residual resistant clones. Although recent trials using such an approach with erlotinib or olaparib after response to platinum based treatment were disappointing, neither trial selected the maintenance treatment on the basis of the profile of residual disease.

6.3. Surrogate tissue

Any effort to sample relapsed disease in ovarian cancer patients invariably faces the challenge of access to tumor. Recurrences tend to be limited to the abdominal cavity with diffuse carcinomatosis which can be difficult to biopsy safely. This is a critical need for more easily accessible surrogate tumor samples which would allow for serial tumor sampling throughout the disease course, to identify both predictive and pharmacodynamic markers. Possibilities include circulating tumor cells, ascites and circulating DNA.

Serial sampling of circulating tumor cells (CTCs) has been shown to provide useful prognostic and/or predictive information in a number of tumor types such as breast and prostate cancer[86],[87]. In the temsirolimus trial, CTCs were detected in 45% of patients before cycle 1 and found to correlate weakly with progressive disease, however no significant change in CTC levels were observed with treatment[29].

Udai et al demonstrated the feasibility of profiling the PI3K pathway from ascites in patients with advanced ovarian cancer: they successfully measured PI3K and PTEN mutations, amplifications and losses as well as PI3K signaling output in ascitic samples by ELISA for phosphorylated proteins[78]. Finally, cancer mutations have been identified by deep sequencing of circulating plasma DNA from patients with advanced ovarian cancer, providing another example of a non-invasive "liquid biopsy"[88].

1) Standardized quality ovarian cancer sample collection protocols at diagnosis and surgery optimized for comprehensive molecular studies.
2) Sequential biopsies for post-treatment/resistant tumor molecular profiling.
3) Studies investigating the feasibility and translational research value of surrogate tissue samples: ascites, circulating tumor cells, circulating DNA

Table 5. Sample-related considerations to enhance the development of PI3K pathway inhibitors in ovarian cancer

6.4. Novel trial designs

Conventional endpoints such as RECIST response may not be appropriate for inhibitors of the PI3K pathway that may result in disease stabilization rather than objective tumor shrinkage. Single arm phase II trials offer little data regarding activity of a novel drug: patient numbers are small, heterogeneous and comparisons with historical controls are intrinsically unreliable. A number of subtle deviations from traditional trial designs could help improve the likelihood that novel PI3K inhibitors make a successful transition from preclinical testing through early and late phase trials. Various strategies are outlined in table 6.

- Randomized placebo controlled phase II trials instead of single arm phase II.
- Randomized discontinuation design: After an initial run-in phase where all patients receive the experimental agent, patients with stable disease are randomized to placebo versus continued drug. This model may be particularly suited to slower growing Type I ovarian cancers where the distinction between treatment induced disease stabilization and natural disease course may be difficult to make.
- When evaluating tumor response on imaging, percentage tumor shrinkage as a continuous variable could be used, rather than categorical RECIST where an arbitrary cut-off of 30% decrease to define response may be more suited to conventional cytotoxics.
- Metabolic response on functional imaging by FDG/PET.
- Using each patient as internal control for evidence of drug activity: the ratio of time to progression (TTP) on experimental drug to TTP on last treatment (TTP_{n+1}/TTP_n), where $TTP_{n+1}/TTP_n \geq 1.3$ would suggest drug activity[89];

Table 6. Suggested modifications to the traditional trial design adapted to testing PI3K pathway inhibitors and other novel therapies

7. Conclusion

The PI3K pathway is emerging as an important and viable therapeutic target. However evidence for efficacy in ovarian cancer remains limited and predictive biomarkers to identify the patients most likely to benefit from this approach are desperately needed. Given the complexicity of the PI3K pathway and its cross-talk with other signaling networks, inhibiting a single member of the pathway may be insufficient to abrogate oncogenic signaling and result in meaningful tumor control. A number of resistance mechanisms to PI3K pathway inhibitors have been identified. Primary resistance may be attributable to co-existing KRAS or BRAF mutations; therefore concurrent PI3K and Mek inhibition in dual PI3K/KRAS mutated ovarian cancer may be worthy of investigation. In addition, treatment induced compensatory increases in alternate pathways (via IGF1R, MTORC2/Akt and others) may allow escape from selective mTOR targeting; response could be improved by appropriately designed combinatorial strategies. This suggests that abrogating adaptive escape pathways will require truly individualized treatment, selected on the basis of on-treatment tumor biopsies to identify the culprit compensatory pathways. A number of trials are ongoing exploring the benefit of combinations, unfortunately few are including correlative biological studies. Finally, for decades, ovarian cancer was treated as a uniform disease, a greater understanding of the biology of epithelial ovarian tumors has encouraged the initiation of a few histology-specific trials. The successful transition of novel PI3K pathway inhibitors from bench to the bedside of patients with ovarian cancer will depend on a greater integration of translation research in trial development. Efforts must be made to include comprehensive molecular profiling both at baseline and sequentially throughout the disease course, and studies investigating the usefulness of novel surrogate tumor markers such as ascites or circulating DNA will likely be essential.

Author details

Alexandra Leary, Edouard Auclin, Patricia Pautier and Catherine Lhommé

*Address all correspondence to: alexandra.leary@igr.fr

Department of Medicine, Gynecological Oncology, Institut Gustave Roussy, Villejuif, France

References

[1] Integrated genomic analyses of ovarian carcinoma. Nature 474:609-15, 2011

[2] Altomare DA, Testa JR: Perturbations of the AKT signaling pathway in human cancer. Oncogene 24:7455-64, 2005

[3] Engelman JA: Targeting PI3K signalling in cancer: opportunities, challenges and limitations. Nat Rev Cancer 9:550-62, 2009

[4] Romashkova JA, Makarov SS: NF-kappaB is a target of AKT in anti-apoptotic PDGF signalling. Nature 401:86-90, 1999

[5] Wullschleger S, Loewith R, Hall MN: TOR signaling in growth and metabolism. Cell 124:471-84, 2006

[6] Montero JC, Chen X, Ocana A, et al: Predominance of mTORC1 over mTORC2 in the regulation of proliferation of ovarian cancer cells: therapeutic implications. Mol Cancer Ther 11:1342-52, 2012

[7] Sarbassov DD, Guertin DA, Ali SM, et al: Phosphorylation and regulation of Akt/PKB by the rictor-mTOR complex. Science 307:1098-101, 2005

[8] Sun SY, Rosenberg LM, Wang X, et al: Activation of Akt and eIF4E survival pathways by rapamycin-mediated mammalian target of rapamycin inhibition. Cancer Res 65:7052-8, 2005

[9] Huang J, Zhang L, Greshock J, et al: Frequent genetic abnormalities of the PI3K/AKT pathway in primary ovarian cancer predict patient outcome. Genes Chromosomes Cancer 50:606-18, 2011

[10] Altomare DA, Wang HQ, Skele KL, et al: AKT and mTOR phosphorylation is frequently detected in ovarian cancer and can be targeted to disrupt ovarian tumor cell growth. Oncogene 23:5853-7, 2004

[11] Kato M, Yamamoto S, Takano M, et al: Aberrant expression of the mammalian target of rapamycin, hypoxia-inducible factor-1alpha, and glucose transporter 1 in the development of ovarian clear-cell adenocarcinoma. Int J Gynecol Pathol 31:254-63, 2012

[12] Mabuchi S, Kawase C, Altomare DA, et al: mTOR is a promising therapeutic target both in cisplatin-sensitive and cisplatin-resistant clear cell carcinoma of the ovary. Clin Cancer Res 15:5404-13, 2009

[13] Kurman RJ, Shih Ie M: Molecular pathogenesis and extraovarian origin of epithelial ovarian cancer--shifting the paradigm. Hum Pathol 42:918-31, 2011

[14] Bowtell DD: The genesis and evolution of high-grade serous ovarian cancer. Nat Rev Cancer 10:803-8, 2010

[15] Bellacosa A, de Feo D, Godwin AK, et al: Molecular alterations of the AKT2 oncogene in ovarian and breast carcinomas. Int J Cancer 64:280-5, 1995

[16] Shayesteh L, Lu Y, Kuo WL, et al: PIK3CA is implicated as an oncogene in ovarian cancer. Nat Genet 21:99-102, 1999

[17] Matulonis UA, Hirsch M, Palescandolo E, et al: High throughput interrogation of somatic mutations in high grade serous cancer of the ovary. PLoS One 6:e24433, 2011

[18] Philp AJ, Campbell IG, Leet C, et al: The phosphatidylinositol 3'-kinase p85alpha gene is an oncogene in human ovarian and colon tumors. Cancer Res 61:7426-9, 2001

[19] Campbell IG, Russell SE, Choong DY, et al: Mutation of the PIK3CA gene in ovarian and breast cancer. Cancer Res 64:7678-81, 2004

[20] Kuo KT, Mao TL, Jones S, et al: Frequent activating mutations of PIK3CA in ovarian clear cell carcinoma. Am J Pathol 174:1597-601, 2009

[21] Obata K, Morland SJ, Watson RH, et al: Frequent PTEN/MMAC mutations in endometrioid but not serous or mucinous epithelial ovarian tumors. Cancer Res 58:2095-7, 1998

[22] Wang SE, Narasanna A, Perez-Torres M, et al: HER2 kinase domain mutation results in constitutive phosphorylation and activation of HER2 and EGFR and resistance to EGFR tyrosine kinase inhibitors. Cancer Cell 10:25-38, 2006

[23] Kelemen LE, Kobel M: Mucinous carcinomas of the ovary and colorectum: different organ, same dilemma. Lancet Oncol 12:1071-80, 2011

[24] Kinross KM, Montgomery KG, Kleinschmidt M, et al: An activating Pik3ca mutation coupled with Pten loss is sufficient to initiate ovarian tumorigenesis in mice. J Clin Invest 122:553-7, 2012

[25] Tanwar PS, Zhang L, Kaneko-Tarui T, et al: Mammalian target of rapamycin is a therapeutic target for murine ovarian endometrioid adenocarcinomas with dysregulated Wnt/beta-catenin and PTEN. PLoS One 6:e20715, 2011

[26] Peng DJ, Wang J, Zhou JY, et al: Role of the Akt/mTOR survival pathway in cisplatin resistance in ovarian cancer cells. Biochem Biophys Res Commun 394:600-5, 2010

[27] Hu L, Hofmann J, Lu Y, et al: Inhibition of phosphatidylinositol 3'-kinase increases efficacy of paclitaxel in in vitro and in vivo ovarian cancer models. Cancer Res 62:1087-92, 2002

[28] Duran I, Siu LL, Oza AM, et al: Characterisation of the lung toxicity of the cell cycle inhibitor temsirolimus. Eur J Cancer 42:1875-80, 2006

[29] Behbakht K, Sill MW, Darcy KM, et al: Phase II trial of the mTOR inhibitor, temsirolimus and evaluation of circulating tumor cells and tumor biomarkers in persistent and recurrent epithelial ovarian and primary peritoneal malignancies: a Gynecologic Oncology Group study. Gynecol Oncol 123:19-26, 2011

[30] Temkin SM, Yamada SD, Fleming GF: A phase I study of weekly temsirolimus and topotecan in the treatment of advanced and/or recurrent gynecologic malignancies. Gynecol Oncol 117:473-6, 2010

[31] Boers-Sonderen M DI, Van Der Graaf WTA, Ottevanger PB, Van Gerpen C.: A phase Ib study of the combination of temsirolimus and pegylated liposomal doxorubcin in advanced or recurrent breast, endometrial and ovarian cancer. J Clin Oncol 30:Abs 5061, 2012

[32] Kollmannsberger C, Hirte H, Siu LL, et al: Temsirolimus in combination with carboplatin and paclitaxel in patients with advanced solid tumors: a NCIC-CTG, phase I, open-label dose-escalation study (IND 179). Ann Oncol 23:238-44, 2012

[33] Campone M, Levy V, Bourbouloux E, et al: Safety and pharmacokinetics of paclitaxel and the oral mTOR inhibitor everolimus in advanced solid tumours. Br J Cancer 100:315-21, 2009

[34] Morgan R OA, Qin R, Laumann KM, Mackay H, Strevel EL, Welch S, Sullivan D, Wenham RM, Chen H, Doyle LA, Gandara DR, Erlichman C: A phase II trial of temsirolimus and bevacizumab in patients with endometrial, ovarian, hepatocellular carcinoma, carcinoid or islet cell cancer: Ovarian cancer subset. J Clin Oncol 29:Abst 5015, 2011

[35] Burger RA, Sill MW, Monk BJ, et al: Phase II trial of bevacizumab in persistent or recurrent epithelial ovarian cancer or primary peritoneal cancer: a Gynecologic Oncology Group Study. J Clin Oncol 25:5165-71, 2007

[36] Cannistra SA, Matulonis UA, Penson RT, et al: Phase II study of bevacizumab in patients with platinum-resistant ovarian cancer or peritoneal serous cancer. J Clin Oncol 25:5180-6, 2007

[37] Stronach EA C-BA, Chen M, Gabra H: Targeting the AKT pathway in ovarian cancer, in al SKe (ed): Emerging therapeutic targets in ovarian cancer, Springer Science, 2011

[38] Crul M, Rosing H, de Klerk GJ, et al: Phase I and pharmacological study of daily oral administration of perifosine (D-21266) in patients with advanced solid tumours. Eur J Cancer 38:1615-21, 2002

[39] Bailey HH, Mahoney MR, Ettinger DS, et al: Phase II study of daily oral perifosine in patients with advanced soft tissue sarcoma. Cancer 107:2462-7, 2006

[40] Knowling M, Blackstein M, Tozer R, et al: A phase II study of perifosine (D-21226) in patients with previously untreated metastatic or locally advanced soft tissue sarcoma: A National Cancer Institute of Canada Clinical Trials Group trial. Invest New Drugs 24:435-9, 2006

[41] Leighl NB, Dent S, Clemons M, et al: A Phase 2 study of perifosine in advanced or metastatic breast cancer. Breast Cancer Res Treat 108:87-92, 2008

[42] Fu S, Hennessy BT, Ng CS, et al: Perifosine plus docetaxel in patients with platinum and taxane resistant or refractory high-grade epithelial ovarian cancer. Gynecol Oncol 126:47-53, 2012

[43] Hennessy BT, Lu Y, Poradosu E, et al: Pharmacodynamic markers of perifosine efficacy. Clin Cancer Res 13:7421-31, 2007

[44] Gungor H SA, Agarwal R, Blagden S, Michael A, Stronach EA, Chen M, PickfordE, Rama NR, Lewis L, Carme SC, Salinas C, Smith DA, Krachey E, Santiago-Walker A, Gunn RN, El-Bajrawy M, Babar SA, Morris R, Gabra H.: Pharmacokinetic/pharmacodynamic analysis of escalating repeat doses of the Akt inhibitor GSK795 in patients with ovarian cancer. J Clin Oncol 29:Abs 5064, 2011

[45] Yang ZZ, Tschopp O, Baudry A, et al: Physiological functions of protein kinase B/Akt. Biochem Soc Trans 32:350-4, 2004

[46] Kurtz JE, Ray-Coquard I: PI3 kinase inhibitors in the clinic: an update. Anticancer Res 32:2463-70, 2012

[47] Bendell JC, Rodon J, Burris HA, et al: Phase I, dose-escalation study of BKM120, an oral pan-Class I PI3K inhibitor, in patients with advanced solid tumors. J Clin Oncol 30:282-90, 2012

[48] Moreno Garcia V BR, Shah KJ, Basu B, Tunariu N, Blanco M, Cassier PA, Pedersen JV, Puglisi M, Sarker, D, Omlin AG, Biondo A, Ware JA, Koeppen H, Levy GG, Mazina KE, De Bone JS: A phase I study evaluating GDC-0941, an oral PI3K inhibitor in patients with advanced solid tumors or multiple myeloma. J Clin Oncol 29:Abstr 3021, 2011

[49] Traynor AM KR, Bailey HH, Attia S, Scheffold C, van Leeuven B, Wu B, Falchook GS, Moulder SL, Xheler J: A phase I safety and pharmacokinetic study of the PI3K inhibitor XL147 in combination with paclitaxel and carboplatin in patients with advanced solid tumors. J Clin Oncol 28:15s (Abs 3078), 2010

[50] Breuleux M, Klopfenstein M, Stephan C, et al: Increased AKT S473 phosphorylation after mTORC1 inhibition is rictor dependent and does not predict tumor cell response to PI3K/mTOR inhibition. Mol Cancer Ther 8:742-53, 2009

[51] Zhang YJ, Duan Y, Zheng XF: Targeting the mTOR kinase domain: the second generation of mTOR inhibitors. Drug Discov Today 16:325-31, 2011

[52] Wan X, Harkavy B, Shen N, et al: Rapamycin induces feedback activation of Akt signaling through an IGF-1R-dependent mechanism. Oncogene 26:1932-40, 2007

[53] Buck E, Eyzaguirre A, Rosenfeld-Franklin M, et al: Feedback mechanisms promote cooperativity for small molecule inhibitors of epidermal and insulin-like growth factor receptors. Cancer Res 68:8322-32, 2008

[54] Di Nicolantonio F, Arena S, Tabernero J, et al: Deregulation of the PI3K and KRAS signaling pathways in human cancer cells determines their response to everolimus. J Clin Invest 120:2858-66, 2010

[55] Carracedo A, Ma L, Teruya-Feldstein J, et al: Inhibition of mTORC1 leads to MAPK pathway activation through a PI3K-dependent feedback loop in human cancer. J Clin Invest 118:3065-74, 2008

[56] Yao JC, Shah MH, Ito T, et al: Everolimus for advanced pancreatic neuroendocrine tumors. N Engl J Med 364:514-23, 2011

[57] Majumder PK, Febbo PG, Bikoff R, et al: mTOR inhibition reverses Akt-dependent prostate intraepithelial neoplasia through regulation of apoptotic and HIF-1-dependent pathways. Nat Med 10:594-601, 2004

[58] Carew JS, Kelly KR, Nawrocki ST: Mechanisms of mTOR inhibitor resistance in cancer therapy. Target Oncol 6:17-27, 2011

[59] Vlahovic G, Meadows KL, Uronis HE, et al: A phase I study of bevacizumab, everolimus and panitumumab in advanced solid tumors. Cancer Chemotherapy and Pharmacology 70:95-102, 2012

[60] O'Reilly KE, Rojo F, She QB, et al: mTOR inhibition induces upstream receptor tyrosine kinase signaling and activates Akt. Cancer Res 66:1500-8, 2006

[61] Quek R, Wang QA, Morgan JA, et al: Combination mTOR and IGF-1R Inhibition: Phase I Trial of Everolimus and Figitumumab in Patients with Advanced Sarcomas and Other Solid Tumors. Clinical Cancer Research 17:871-879, 2011

[62] Janes MR, Limon JJ, So L, et al: Effective and selective targeting of leukemia cells using a TORC1/2 kinase inhibitor. Nat Med 16:205-13, 2010

[63] Mazzoletti M, Bortolin F, Brunelli L, et al: Combination of PI3K/mTOR inhibitors: antitumor activity and molecular correlates. Cancer Res 71:4573-84, 2011

[64] Santiskulvong C, Konecny GE, Fekete M, et al: Dual targeting of phosphoinositide 3-kinase and mammalian target of rapamycin using NVP-BEZ235 as a novel therapeutic approach in human ovarian carcinoma. Clin Cancer Res 17:2373-84, 2011

[65] Kinross KM, Brown DV, Kleinschmidt M, et al: In vivo activity of combined PI3K/mTOR and MEK inhibition in a Kras(G12D);Pten deletion mouse model of ovarian cancer. Mol Cancer Ther 10:1440-9, 2011

[66] Shimizu T, Tolcher AW, Papadopoulos KP, et al: The clinical effect of the dual-targeting strategy involving PI3K/AKT/mTOR and RAS/MEK/ERK pathways in patients with advanced cancer. Clin Cancer Res 18:2316-25, 2012

[67] Fekete M, Santiskulvong C, Eng C, et al: Effect of PI3K/Akt pathway inhibition-mediated G1 arrest on chemosensitization in ovarian cancer cells. Anticancer Res 32:445-52, 2012

[68] Anglesio MS, George J, Kulbe H, et al: IL6-STAT3-HIF signaling and therapeutic response to the angiogenesis inhibitor sunitinib in ovarian clear cell cancer. Clin Cancer Res 17:2538-48, 2011

[69] Neshat MS, Mellinghoff IK, Tran C, et al: Enhanced sensitivity of PTEN-deficient tumors to inhibition of FRAP/mTOR. Proc Natl Acad Sci U S A 98:10314-9, 2001

[70] Noh WC, Mondesire WH, Peng J, et al: Determinants of rapamycin sensitivity in breast cancer cells. Clin Cancer Res 10:1013-23, 2004

[71] Tanaka H, Yoshida M, Tanimura H, et al: The selective class I PI3K inhibitor CH5132799 targets human cancers harboring oncogenic PIK3CA mutations. Clin Cancer Res 17:3272-81, 2011

[72] Weigelt B, Warne PH, Downward J: PIK3CA mutation, but not PTEN loss of function, determines the sensitivity of breast cancer cells to mTOR inhibitory drugs. Oncogene 30:3222-33, 2011

[73] O'Brien C, Wallin JJ, Sampath D, et al: Predictive biomarkers of sensitivity to the phosphatidylinositol 3' kinase inhibitor GDC-0941 in breast cancer preclinical models. Clin Cancer Res 16:3670-83, 2010

[74] Margolin K, Longmate J, Baratta T, et al: CCI-779 in metastatic melanoma: a phase II trial of the California Cancer Consortium. Cancer 104:1045-8, 2005

[75] MacKay H EE, Kamel-Reid S, Clarke B, Walsh W, Karakasis K, Salvesen H, Oza A.: Molecular determinants of outcome with mTOR inhibition in endometrial cancer. J Clin Oncol 30:Abst 5010, 2012

[76] Janku F, Wheler JJ, Westin SN, et al: PI3K/AKT/mTOR inhibitors in patients with breast and gynecologic malignancies harboring PIK3CA mutations. J Clin Oncol 30:777-82, 2012

[77] Dan S, Okamura M, Seki M, et al: Correlating phosphatidylinositol 3-kinase inhibitor efficacy with signaling pathway status: in silico and biological evaluations. Cancer Res 70:4982-94, 2010

[78] Carden CP, Stewart A, Thavasu P, et al: The association of PI3 kinase signaling and chemoresistance in advanced ovarian cancer. Mol Cancer Ther 11:1609-17, 2012

[79] Hanrahan AJ, Schultz N, Westfal ML, et al: Genomic complexity and AKT dependence in serous ovarian cancer. Cancer Discov 2:56-67, 2012

[80] Pinhel IF, Macneill FA, Hills MJ, et al: Extreme loss of immunoreactive p-Akt and p-Erk1/2 during routine fixation of primary breast cancer. Breast Cancer Res 12:R76, 2010

[81] Holzer TR, Fulford AD, Arkins AM, et al: Ischemic time impacts biological integrity of phospho-proteins in PI3K/Akt, Erk/MAPK, and p38 MAPK signaling networks. Anticancer Res 31:2073-81, 2011

[82] Saal LH, Johansson P, Holm K, et al: Poor prognosis in carcinoma is associated with a gene expression signature of aberrant PTEN tumor suppressor pathway activity. Proc Natl Acad Sci U S A 104:7564-9, 2007

[83] Iacovelli R, Palazzo A, Mezi S, et al: Incidence and risk of pulmonary toxicity in patients treated with mTOR inhibitors for malignancy. A meta-analysis of published trials. Acta Oncol, 2012

[84] Lopez-Fauqued M, Gil R, Grueso J, et al: The dual PI3K/mTOR inhibitor PI-103 promotes immunosuppression, in vivo tumor growth and increases survival of sorafenib-treated melanoma cells. Int J Cancer 126:1549-61, 2010

[85] Gomez-Roca CA, Lacroix L, Massard C, et al: Sequential research-related biopsies in phase I trials: acceptance, feasibility and safety. Ann Oncol 23:1301-6, 2012

[86] Cristofanilli M, Budd GT, Ellis MJ, et al: Circulating tumor cells, disease progression, and survival in metastatic breast cancer. N Engl J Med 351:781-91, 2004

[87] Goodman OB, Jr., Fink LM, Symanowski JT, et al: Circulating tumor cells in patients with castration-resistant prostate cancer baseline values and correlation with prognostic factors. Cancer Epidemiol Biomarkers Prev 18:1904-13, 2009

[88] Forshew T, Murtaza M, Parkinson C, et al: Noninvasive identification and monitoring of cancer mutations by targeted deep sequencing of plasma DNA. Sci Transl Med 4:136ra68, 2012

[89] Von Hoff DD, Stephenson JJ, Jr., Rosen P, et al: Pilot study using molecular profiling of patients' tumors to find potential targets and select treatments for their refractory cancers. J Clin Oncol 28:4877-83, 2010

Chapter 14

PARP Inhibitors in Ovarian Cancer

Jeanine Staples and Annekathryn Goodman

Additional information is available at the end of the chapter

http://dx.doi.org/10.5772/52888

1. Introduction

Targeted therapy in cancer has led to intensive searches for the molecular pathways of malignant transformation [1]. In gynecologic malignancies, BRCA 1 and BRCA 2 gene mutations on chromosomes 17 and 13 respectively were identified in the 1990s [2]. Since then, intensive investigation of the pathways for these genes has led to a wealth of information about molecular pathways [3]. The understanding of these molecular pathways has led in turn to the development of novel targeted therapies for women with identified gene mutations [4]. This review reviews the current knowledge of the subset of women with BRCA gene mutations. The characteristics of BRCA deficiency including genetic background and current chemotherapeutic options including mechanisms of resistance are discussed as well. Finally, the data on emerging targeted therapeutic strategies with poly-ADP-ribose-polymerase (PARP) inhibitors and specific PARP clinical trials are reviewed.

2. BRCA genetic background

Hereditary Breast and Ovarian Cancer Syndrome (HBOCS) is characterized by a few distinct features: earlier age of cancer onset, higher incidence of bilateral disease, higher incidence of other cancers, and inheritance in an autosomal dominant pattern [5]. A number of genes, as well as associated syndromes, have been implicated in HBOCS, but none more so than the BRCA genes. Individuals with impaired BRCA protein function have a 50-85% lifetime risk of developing breast cancer and 10-40% lifetime risk of developing ovarian cancer [6]. Although deleterious mutations in either of the 2 BRCA genes significantly increases one's risk for breast and ovarian cancer, mutations in these genes account for only about 5-10% of all breast and ovarian cancer cases [7]. Because of genetic testing, the families of the subset of women with BRCA associated cancers can be tested and early intervention is a possibility [8]. These include tamoxifen therapy, bilateral prophylactic oophorectomy, prophylactic contralateral mastectomy and combinations of these strategies. Such interventions have been shown to offer substantial life expectancy gain for young women with BRCA associated early stage cancer. Currently, treatment of BRCA-associated breast and/or ovarian cancer is no different than that for the general population. Survival data of BRCA positive patients with ovarian cancer suggests that they have prolonged disease free intervals and overall longer survival than their wild-type counterparts [9].

The Breast Cancer Susceptibility genes (BRCA 1 and 2) are considered tumor suppressors, whose job it is to maintain appropriate cell growth, ultimately by upholding genomic stability [10]. No single unified theory exists regarding the action of the BRCA genes. While disruption of either of the BRCA genes demonstrates similar pathophysiological manifestations, they are indeed unique. They lie on 2 separate chromosomes, each have unique primary sequences, and ultimately carry out their responsibilities via discrete (proposed) mechanisms. Furthermore, their unique mechanisms of action give them distinct characteristics that coincide with distinct risks and prognoses with gene disturbance. Both BRCA genes share a relationship with the gene RAD51, which encodes a protein responsible for assisting in repair of DNA double strand breaks via homologous recombination. When there is a double strand break in the genetic sequence, *sequenceX* of a specific chromatid, homologous recombination provides a means for the exchange of the same genetic sequence, *sequenceX*, from the healthy homologous sister chromatid to the damaged one. Rad51 is one of the most important players in HRR. It assists in the search for homology and strand pairing, and its responsibilities are ultimately complemented by the proteins encoded by the 2 BRCA genes [11]. Studies suggest that BRCA2 regulates the intracellular transport and function of RAD51, as well as the enzymatic activity of the RAD51 protein [12]. The relationship between BRCA1 and RAD51 is less clear. There is evidence that BRCA1 physically associates with proteins other than RAD51, creating a complex likely responsible for the creation of resected single-stranded DNA at double strand repair sites [13]. Further data supports BRCA1's role in activation of DNA damage checkpoints. There is also evidence that supports BRCA1's role in altering chromatin structure upon DNA damage to allow easier access for repair.

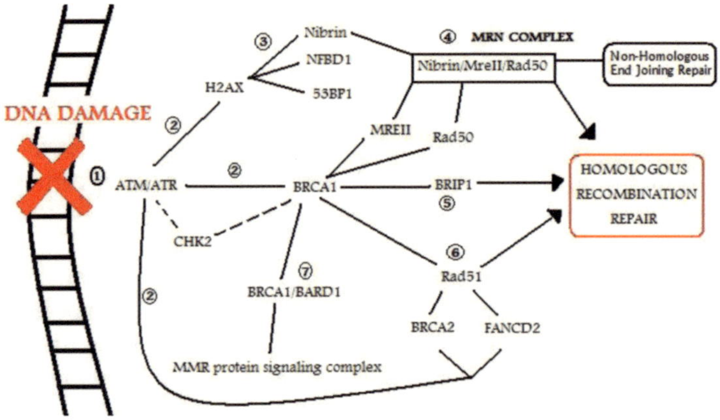

Figure 1. Role of BRCA proteins in Homologous Recombination Repair

(See Figure 1) 1) DNA damage triggers activation of the ataxia-telangiectasia mutated serine-protein kinase as well as the ataxia-telangiectasia and Rad3 related protein kinase [14]. 2) Once activated, these enzymes phosphorylate and activate a number of intracellular items, including the BRCA1 protein, Checkpoint kinase 2 (which also activates BRCA1), BRCA2, the Fanconi anemia protein complex, H2AX histones involved in forming nuclear foci crucial for DNA repair, and a few others [15]. 3) The H2AX histones co-localize and join with other proteins to form nuclear foci at the sites of DNA damage. These other proteins include a tumor binding protein 53BP1, the nuclear factor with BRCT domains protein 1 NFBD1, checkpoint kinase 2, and Nijmegen breakage syndrome 1 protein Nibrin. 4) Nibrin is part of the MRN complex, which also includes Rad50 and MreII. The MRN complex is important in initial processing of double stranded DNA breaks. It directs the cellular process to continue via homologous recombination or non-homologous end joining. BRCA1 plays a part in regulating the MRN complex by inhibiting MreII [16]. This action depresses the NHEJ pathway and stimulates the Rad51 pathway favoring homologous recombination. 5) BRCA1 also activates BRCA1 interacting protein C-terminal helicase 1 (BRIP1), which unwinds DNA strands near sites of damage allowing other repair machinery to access the damaged sites. The gene that encodes BRIP1 may also act as an oncogene in ovarian cancer. 6) Activation of Rad51 allows it to form a complex with BRCA2 and Fanconi anemia complementation group D2 protein, FANCD2 [17]. This complex is a key player in homologous recombination repair as it is involved in searching for homology as well as strand pairing, while causing S-phase and G2 arrest [18]. 7) Certain homologous recombination repair (HRR) promoting activities of BRCA1 are amplified when it forms a complex with BRCA1 associated RING domain protein 1, BARD1 [19]. This complex may also play a role in mismatch repair via downstream action [20].

3. Associated breast and ovarian cancer

Inheritance of a damaging mutation in either BRCA gene can cause disruption of the smoothly regulated replication process of the body's cells, potentially leading to cancer. Though the mechanism is poorly understood, mutations in the BRCA genes show preferential deleterious consequences in breast and ovarian tissues. In the general population, the lifetime prevalence of breast cancer is 12% and ovarian cancer 1.4% [21]. A mutation in the BRCA1 gene puts an individual at a 50-85% lifetime risk of developing breast cancer and a 15-40% risk of developing ovarian cancer. BRCA2 mutation carriers have a 50-85% lifetime risk of developing breast cancer and a 10-20% risk of developing epithelial ovarian cancer. In addition, BRCA mutations are associated with bilateral disease, cancer at a younger age (BRCA1), autosomal dominant inheritance pattern, increased risk of male breast cancer (BRCA2), and increased risk of cancer in other organs [22,23]. Specifically, BRCA positive individuals are at increased risk of epithelial ovarian cancer (EOC), which behaves differently than EOC seen in the general population. Both BRCA1 and 2 carriers have an improved prognosis when compared to their wild-type counterparts. A pooled analysis of 26 observational studies on the survival of women with ovarian cancer, including 1213 EOC cases showed that among patients with invasive EOC, having a BRCA mutation was associated with improved 5-year overall survival, with BRCA2 carriers having the best prognosis [9]. See Table 1.

	BRCA 1 carriers	**BRCA 2 carriers**	**Non-Carriers**
Inheritance	Auto-Dominant	Auto-Dominant	Sporadic
Prevalence of EOC	39%	22%	1.4%
Mean age of onset	54	62	63
Tumor: Stage @ surgery	Advanced	Advanced	Advanced
Histolology	Serous	Serous	Serous
Differentiation	Mod-Poor	Mod-Poor	Mod-poor
Treatment	Surgery + Chemo	Surgery + Chemo	Surgery + Chemo
Recurrence-Free interval	14 months	14 months	7 months
5-year Survival	44%	52%	36%
Other malignancies	Breast, gastric hepatobiliary, renal, testicular, leukemia	Breast (including higher incidence of male breast cancer), prostate, pancreatic	

Table 1. Characteristics of BRCA 1/2 associated Epithelial Ovarian Cancer (EOC) [9,24,25]

BRCA1 associated breast cancers tend to be of the triple-negative type which is significant because it lacks the 3 biomarkers most commonly implicated in breast cancer, the estrogen and progesterone receptors and the human epidermal growth factor receptor 2 (Her2/neu) [26]. The presence of these biomarkers helps in the guidance of treatment options. Estrogen/ progesterone positive breast cancers are typically treated with hormonal therapy (in conjunction with surgery/radiation), and Her2/neu positive breast cancers are treated with an agent that specifically targets the Her2 receptor, such as Herceptin. When these 3 biomarkers are negative in a newly diagnosed breast cancer, the treatment approach becomes more complicated and prognosisis poor. On the other hand, BRCA2 associated breast cancer is typically hormonal in nature [22]. Current evidence suggests no difference in overall prognosis of breast cancers in BRCA carriers compared to sporadic breast cancers, but BRCA deficiency does appear to be predict chemo-sensitivity [27].

4. BRCAness

The term "BRCAness" describes a subset of women with sporadic EOC who display similar phenotypic characteristics to those with a hereditary BRCA mutation [28]. It is widely accepted that a deleterious BRCA mutation adversely affects homologous recombination. While the BRCA genes indeed play a very important role in homologous recombination, they are not the only key players. A defect or hiccup in any of the other genes involved in homologous recombination would in theory, affect this process. This describes the notion of BRCAness: Individuals with structurally healthy BRCA genes that are functionally incapable of carrying out homologous recombination due to a defect elsewhere that hinders the entire process. In fact, about 40-50% of ovarian cancer cases have shown to have some defect in homologous recombination, with a large number of these being associated with BRCA-related defects. See Figure 2.

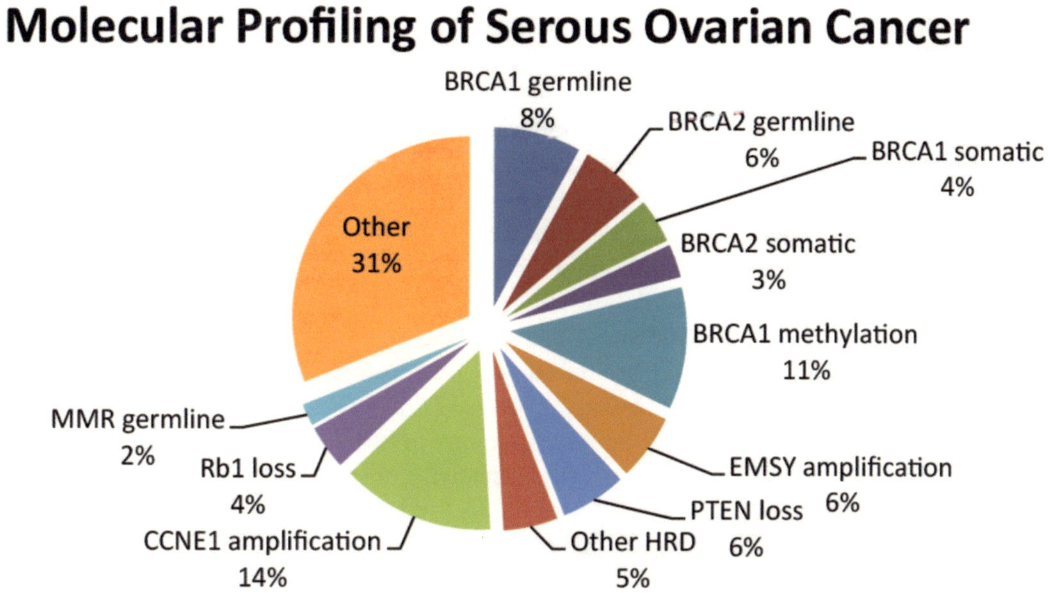

Figure 2. illustrates the molecular profile of serous ovarian cancer. BRCA1 germline, BRCA2 germline, BRCA1 somatic, BRCA2 somatic, BRCA1 hypermethylation, EMSY amplification and PTEN loss have all been shown to lead to impaired homologous recombination, comprising about half of all cases [29]. Sporadic ovarian cancer mutations that affect homologous recombination are clinically significant because they tend to behave like the BRCA cancers. This special sub-group of epithelial ovarian cancer patients show similar therapeutic response and prognosis as their BRCA mutant counterparts which includes improved sensitivity to platinum as well as improved 5 year survival [30]. A few studies have attempted to reveal the mechanism behind BRCAness on a genetic level. There is some data to suggest that transcriptional or post-transcriptional repression of the BRCA1 gene is responsible for such sporadic tumors. For example, hypermethylation of a promotor region upstream from BRCA1 gene that leads to inactivation of BRCA1 protein, causes impaired homologous recombination leading to a sporadic "BRCAness" with an intact yet silenced BRCA1 gene [31].

It should be noted that the specific target of the PARP inhibitor class is not only BRCA mutant cancers; however, it encompasses all that fall under the umbrella of impaired homologous recombination. So in theory, PARP inhibitors should show efficacy in a number of sporadic cancers as well, specifically those that elicit "BRCAness" characteristics [32].

5. Mechanisms of resistance

Currently, there is no difference in management of EOC between BRCA positive patients and BRCA wild type patients. Maximal surgical cytoreduction, with or without neoadjuvant chemotherapy, is the standard initial approach, excluding individuals who are not good surgical candidates or whose disease precludes optimal cytoreduction [34]. The typical chemotherapeutic regimen is a taxane/platinum based combination therapy. The standard post-operative approach would be 6 cycles (21 days each) of IV paclitaxal with carboplatin [35]

The 5-year survival and prognosis for *advanced* stage ovarian cancer, in BRCA or wild-type carriers ranges between 10 and 25 percent. Such poor prognosis is due to an incredibly high recurrence rate of advanced ovarian cancer. The extremely high rate of recurrence is due to the development of drug resistance [36]. Initially, 75% of patients with advanced disease show response to chemotherapy, while the remaining 25% show intrinsic resistance. However, most of the population with initial chemosensitivity will show relapse within 2 years of initial treatment. Patients who have a shorter interval from their last course of chemotherapy to relapse will show decreased response with future courses [37]. For women who relapse within 6 months of treatment completion, there is a less than 10% chance of responding to any future therapies. For women whose disease recurs more than 6 to 12 months after initial therapy, chemotherapy includes platinum-based, multi-agent regimens. These women are considered partially platinum sensitive (relapse within 6-12 months) or platinum sensitive (relapse greater than 12 months after initial treatment). For patients who are platinum resistant (relapse within 6 months) or platinum refractory (no initial response), sequential single agents, such as pegylated liposomal doxorubicin hydrochloride or topotecan are suggested [38]. The slightly superior prognosis of BRCA patients compared to sporadic EOC is likely related to their greater sensitivity to platinum based therapy [33]. However, despite initial chemo-sensitivity of BRCA carriers, they will ultimately develop to platinum resistant recurrent ovarian cancer.

PARP Inhibitors are not unlike the standard therapies for ovarian cancer, in that they too have shown evidence of resistance. Theoretically, their maximum potential is seen in cells with impaired homologous recombination. Researchers have hypothesized that resistance to PARP Inhibitors is through DNA repair mechanisms that actually correct the homologous recombination process. Through compensatory mutations, the initial mutational reading frame is corrected to a reading frame that actually produces a wild type BRCA protein [39]. A restoration in BRCA function would further contribute to platinum resistance and create PARP inhibitor resistance. This will need further investigations.

6. PARP inhibitors

PARP proteins are involved in a number of cellular processes, including DNA replication, transcriptional regulation, and DNA damage repair [40].Of the numerous PARP proteins detected, PARP1 and PARP2, which are associated with DNA stability, have been intensively studied. The PARP enzyme regulates cellular responses to DNA damage, and plays an important role in the repair of single-stranded breaks by excision repair [41]. See Figure 3.

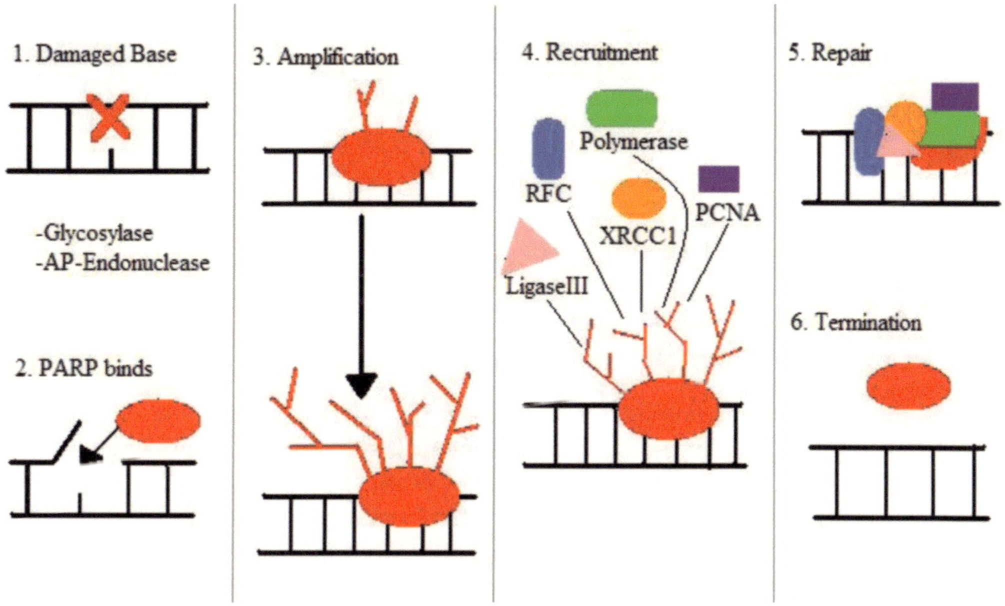

Figure 3. Role of Poly (ADP-ribose) polymerase in Base Excision Repair

The base excision repair (BER) pathway recognizes and removes damaged or inappropriate bases [42]. Damage specific glycosylases recognize the presence of a faulty base and immediately removes it. This leads to the formation of a potentially cytotoxic apurinic or apirimidinic (AP) site. Such sites are then processed by an AP endonuclease, which creates a strand break in the DNA. The enzyme Poly (ADP-ribose) polymerase binds to the strand break and relaxes the chromatin structure to allow for easier access of the BER machinery. Then, PARP transfers ADP-ribose units from NAD+ to nuclear target proteins, histones, and itself. This forms long and branched polymers of poly (ADP-ribose) on the PARP enzyme, that act as a signaling mechanism to recruit the BER machinery, including adaptor factor XECC1, PCNA, RFC, ligase III and DNA polymerase β. The BER complex assembles at the site of damage and facilitates repair in a coordinated fashion. Once complete, the complex disperses [43].

When PARP is inhibited, common single-strand breaks are converted into double-stranded breaks during DNA replication. In normal wild type cells, homologous recombination is the most common mechanism of repair in these double-stranded breaks which provides a safety net in maintaining genomic stability. In the presence of a deleterious BRCA gene, homologous recombination is impaired. These cells and the tumors that they form have increased susceptibility to PARP inhibition, which leads to decreased chromosomal stability and, ultimately, cell death. See Figure 4.

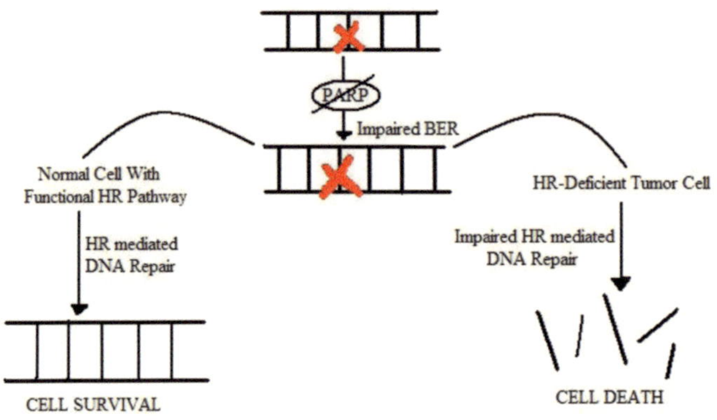

Figure 4. Synthetic Lethality of PARP Inhibition

PARP inhibitors are also hypothesized to increase cytotoxicity of chemotherapeutic agents. Cells treated with chemotherapy, especially platinum based agents, ultimately attain resistance by altering DNA repair processes [44]. It is hypothesized that through PARP inhibition, cells with faulty BRCA function could be prevented from repairing chemotherapy -induced DNA damage [45,46]. Clinical trials have examined PARP inhibitors as single agents in patients with impaired homologous recombination, as well as in combination with chemo-radiation therapy.

7. Clinical trials

Table 2 shows a list of PARP inhibitors that are currently in clinical development [4]. A full list of studies involving all tumor types can be found through the National Institute of Health website, www.clinicaltrials.gov.

Iniparib is one of the first drugs looked at in the PARP inhibitor class. A phase II trial of iniparib in women with advanced ovarian or breast cancer compared the chemotherapeutic regimen carboplatin/gemcitabine with and without iniparib. The iniparib arm showed an improved rate of clinical benefit (56% vs 34%, P=0.01), increased rate of overall response (52% vs 32%, P=0.02), prolonged median progression free survival (5.9 movs 3.6 mo, P=0.01), and increased median overall survival (12.3 mo vs 7.7 mo, P=0.01) [47]. However, a phase III trial of Iniparib for women with triple negative breast cancer proved to be disappointing [48,49]. This trial, which randomized 519 women with triple negative breast cancer to carboplatin with gemcitabine versus carboplatin, gemcitabine plus iniparib demonstrated an increase in progression-free survival among the iniparib arm (5.1 vs 4.1 months, with P=0.027), but did not reach statistical significance. Patients were not stratified based on BRCA status, specific triple negative breast cancer subtype, or level of expression of PARP proteins. More recent studies suggest that Iniparib may not actually inhibit the PARP enzyme in vitro. One in particular compared Iniparib to Olaparib and Veliparib [50]. Olaparib and Veliparib proved to inhibit formation of the poly-ADP-ribose polymer in intact cells, but Iniparib exhibited little or no ability to inhibit poly(ADP-ribose) polymer formation in situ. Other experiments revealed Iniparib's inability to sensitize cells to cisplatin, gemcitabine and paclitaxel [51]. Iniparib's actual role may be modification of cysteine-containing proteins in tumor cells. If this is in fact the case, failure of the Iniparib phase III trial should not be used to guide further decisions about other PARP inhibitors. Keeping that in mind, Iniparib is continuing to be studied in a number of ovarian cancer trials, some showing promise. A phase II trial examining Iniparib in combination with gemcitabine/carboplatin in patients with platinum-resistant recurrent ovarian cancer has to date shown a 25% overall response rate consisting of 8 out of 32 confirmed responses [52]. Progression free survival of 6.4 months (95% CI, 3.0-NE) was demonstrated in an early analysis. The PFS and ORR are significantly improved when compared to a previous study of pegylated liposomal doxorubicin in platinum-resistant recurrent ovarian cancer with an ORR of 11.7% and mean progression free survival of 3.1 months [53]. Once again, these patients were not stratified based on their BRCA carrier status. A similar study looked at iniparib in combination with gemcitabine/carboplatin in patients with platinum-sensitive recurrent ovarian cancer [54]. This study showed an ORR of 65%, consisting of 26 out of 40 patients, as well as a median progression free survival of 9.5 months. Interestingly, there was no indication of a relationship between BRCA status and response.

Agent	Route of Administration	Trial Interests	Side Effects
Iniparib	IV	Ovarian cancer, uterine carcinosarcoma, NSCLC	Fatigue, nausea, diarrhea, dizziness
Olaparib	Oral	Breast and ovarian cancer, the BRCA population, other advanced solid tumors	Nausea, vomiting, fatigue, taste-alteration, anorexia
Veliparib	Oral	TNBC and BRCA deficient breast and ovarian cancer	Myelosuppression, fatigue
Rucaparib	IV	BRCA associated breast cancer, locally advanced or metastatic breast cancer, advanced ovarian cancer	Thrombocytopenia and neutropenia
INO-1001	IV	Melanoma, p53 deficient cancer cells	Myelosuppression, transaminitis
MK-4827	Oral	Advanced solid tumors, ovarian cancer, hematologic malignancies, advanced melanoma, advanced glioblastoma	Fatigue, reversible pneumonitis, myelosuppression, thrombocytopenia
AZD-2461	Oral	Single agent for refractory solid tumors	
CEP-9722	Oral	Single agent for advanced solid tumors	
E7016	Oral	Advanced solid tumors, melanoma, glioblastoma	
BMN-673	Oral	Advanced solid tumors and hematologic malignancies	

Table 2. PARP Inhibitors in Clinical Development

Olaparib, on the other hand, is a considered a bona-fide PARP inhibitor and has shown promising results in phase II trials in the treatment of BRCA-deficient advanced ovarian cancer. A recent study looked at oral Olaparib as a single agent, and its effect on BRCA positive vs. BRCA wild-type patients in women with ovarian and breast cancer [55]. Women with advanced high grade serous and/or undifferentiated ovarian carcinoma or triple-negative breast cancer were enrolled and received olaparib 400 mg twice a day. 91 patients were enrolled in this particular study, 65 with ovarian cancer and 26 with breast cancer. 63 of the 65 ovarian cancer cohorts had target lesions and were evaluable for objective response. Among these 63 patients, 41% of BRCA carriers showed confirmed objective response (7 out of 17 with 95% CI) and a surprising 24% of BRCA wild-type patients showed confirmed objective response (11 of 46 with 95% CI). The 24% response of BRCA wild type patients suggests that Olaparib, if not all PARP inhibitors, may provide significant benefit for all patients with ovarian cancer, and not only those with selective BRCA mutation. As mentioned above, around 40-50% of ovarian cancers, in the absence of a mutation of the BRCA gene, can affect the functional aspect of the BRCA proteins and ultimately homologous recombination. It is for this reason that PARP inhibition likely shows benefit in not just the BRCA mutated population, but a larger population that umbrellas deficient homologous repair. However, for this particular study phase III trials are no longer scheduled to commence because the interim analysis of survival did not show the desired benefit in relation to the benefit in progression free survival. Also, there were no confirmed objective responses reported in the breast cancer patients.

A very similar 2-part study looked at single agent Olaparib, and compared doses (100mg vs. 400mg) in the treatment of advanced breast and ovarian cancer in BRCA deficient individuals [56,57]. Among the 57 ovarian cancer patients, the overall response rate of olaparib 100mg BID was 12.5% with a clinical benefit rate of 16.7%. For the 400mg BID arm, ORR was 33% with a clinical benefit rate of 57.6%. Further stratification showed a response in both platinum-sensitive individuals (38% ORR) and platinum-resistant individuals (30%). Among the 54 breast cancer patients, the overall response of olaparib 100mg BID was 25% with a progression free survival of 3.8months. For the 400mg BID arm, ORR was 42% with PFS of 5.7 months.

Olaparib is also being looked at as maintenance therapy. A phase II trial studied Olaparib as a maintenance therapy in relapsed serous ovarian cancer. The 265 enrolled patients had received at least 2 previous platinum based chemo regimens with eventual relapse [58]. Early analysis has shown a 65% reduced risk of progression in the Olaparib arm, improving progression free survival by 3.6 months (8.4 mo vs. 4.8). Patients were stratified based on BRCA status, age, race, Jewish ethnicity, prior response to platinum regimen and relapse time, and each subgroup showed an improved progression free survival in the Olaparib arm. Overall survival data has not been analyzed.

Another study looking at differences in response to olaparib based on platinum-response status [59]. This trial looked at oral olaparib as a single agent against advanced ovarian cancer in 50 women with BRCA mutations. Results showed a 61.5% response rate in platinum-sensitive patients, a 41.7% response rate in platinum-resistant patients and 15.4% response rate in platinum-refractory patients.

A randomized phase II trial in BRCA deficient advanced ovarian cancer (platinum interval<12 months) enrolled 97 women and looked at olaparib dosing, 200mg vs 400mg, and compared its efficacy to pegylated liposomal doxorubicin [60]. Of the 32 low dose olaparib cohorts (200mg BID), 38 % showed objective response with a median progression free survival of 6.5 months. Of the 32 high dose (400mg BID) cohorts, 59% showed objective response with a median PFS of 8.8 months. These were compared to 33 women who received the standard pegylated liposomal doxorubicin, with an objective response of 38% and median PFS of 7.1 months, results that were not clinically significant. This study, however, does not necessarily rule out Olaparib's action in BRCA deficient patients. Recent studies suggest that women with BRCA associated ovarian cancer may demonstrate increased sensitivity to Doxil than previously reported in unselected cases [61]. One study in particular showed a 57% response rate to PLD among BRCA deficient patients, compared to 20% response rate among those with sporadic EOC. This response was associated with significantly improved progression-free and overall survival. Furthermore, the initial study was actually potentially comparing 2 drugs with particular benefit in BRCA patients and though there is no clinically significant difference among them, they each may show clinical significance when standing alone.

Another PARP inhibitor under investigation is Veliparib. A phase II trial of Veliparib in combination with cyclophosphamide compared to single-agent cyclophosphamide is currently ongoing [62]. This study examines Veliparib's activity against advanced solid tumors and lymphomas. Preliminary results show promising activity in the BRCA subset. Of the 35 patients enrolled, 7 have shown partial response and 6 have stable disease in the veliparib arm. In another study veliparib with or without carboplatin was evaluated in patients with stage III and IV BRCA-associated breast cancer [63]. Of the 22 patients enrolled, only 12 were eligible for evaluation. Complete response was seen in 2 patients and partial response in 6 patients, with a clinical benefit of 75% seen.

A phase I study showed activity of veliparib and temozolomide in combination against metastatic breast cancer [64]. Of the 41 patients enrolled, complete response was seen in 1 patient, partial response in 2, stable disease in 7 and disease progression in 14. BRCA mutation analysis is currently underway. Another study is currently looking at veliparib in combination with doxorubicin and cyclophosphamide for the treatment of breast cancer and other solid tumors [65]. Of the 18 patients enrolled, 14 have breast cancer (including 5 with BRCA mutations), 3 have ovarian cancer, and 1 other solid tumor. There has been objective anti-tumor activity seen in the BRCA mutation carriers. With this particular regimen, dosing was limited by myelosuppresion. Furthermore, although combination therapy has shown to enhance chemotherapeutic effects, myelosuppression appears to be enhanced as well. More than 50 clinical trials examining Veliparib are currently ongoing, looking at gynecologic cancers, solid tumors, lymphomas, brain tumors, GI and prostate cancer. Most of these are currently recruiting, with only a few in Stage II. It will be very exciting to see the end results of these trials, specifically for our purposes, those involving BRCA analysis. Very few updates have been given, as most of these are in the beginning stages.

Agent	Cancer	Summary	Prelim/Conclusions
Iniparib + Carbo/Gem [47]	Metastatic TNBC	Phase 2 -123 enrolled with advanced ovarian or breast cancer, looked at C/G regimen vs. C/G + Iniparib	-clinical benefit rate of 56% in Iniparib arm vs. 34% -Increased ORR (52% vs 32%) -Increased median overall survival (12.3 mo vs 7.7 mo) -Increase in PFS among Iniparib arm (5.1 vs. 4.1mo)
Iniparib + Carbo/Gem [48,49]	Metastatic TNBC	Phase 3 -519 enrolled with TNBC and looked at C/G regimen vs. C/G + Iniparib	-increased median OS (11.8 vs 11.1 mo-did not reach clinical significance *were not stratified on their BRCA status
Iniparib [50]	NA	Study looked at ability of Iniparib to inhibit the PARP enzyme in vitro	-Olaparib and Veliparib proved to inhibit formation of th epoly -ADP-ribose polymer in intact cells, but Iniparib exhibited little or no ability to inhibit PARP in situ.
Iniparib + Carbo/Gem [52]	Platinum resistant recurrent ovarian cancer	48 patients with dx of epithelial ovarian carcinoma, follopian tube cancer, or primary peritoneal carcinoma with platinum-resistant disease	-25% ORR, consisting of 8 out of 32 confirmed responses (compare to ORR of 11.7% w/ PLD) -PFS of 6.4 months (compare to PFS of 3.1 mo w/ PLD)
Iniparib + C/G [54]	Platinum sensitive recurrent ovarian cancer	Single arm study -41 patients with dx of recurrent platinum sensitive ovarian cancer	-ORR 65% (26 out of 40 patients) -9.5mo. median PFS -no indication of relationship between BRCA status and objective response
Olaparib S.A. [55]	Ovarian and breast cancer	91 patients (65 with ovarian ca, 26 with breast ca), stratified based on BRCA status	-41% of BRCA-m ovarian cancer patients showed COR -24% of BRCA-wt ovarian cancer patients showed COR -no COR in breast cancer patients
Olaparib S.A. [59]	Ovarian cancer	50 patients enrolled and stratified based on response to platinum	-61.5% RR in platinum sensitive -41.7% RR in platinum resistant -15.4% RR in platinum refractory
Olaparib S.A. [56]	Advanced breast cancer in BRCA deficient individuals	54 patients with breast cancer	-ORR 42% with 400mgBID, PFS 5.7months -ORR 25% with 100mgBID, PFS 3.8months

Agent	Cancer	Summary	Prelim/Conclusions
Olaparib S.A. [57]	Advanced ovarian cancer in BRCA deficient individuals	57 patients with ovarian cancer	-12.5% ORR of Olaparib 100mg -33% ORR of Olaparib 400mg -Response seen in both platinum sensitive (38%) and platinum resistant (30%) disease -Clinical benefit rate 57.6% w 400mgBID, 16.7% w 100mgBID
Olaparib SA [58]	Relapsed ovarian cancer, platinum-sensitive	265 enrolled with at least 2 previous platinum based chemo regimens	-improved PFS by 3.6mo -65% reduced risk of progression in Olaparib arm -no overall survival benefit
Olaparib SA vs. PLD [60]	BRCA deficient advanced ovarian cancer with platinum interval <12 mo.	97 women enrolled, study compared efficacy/safety of olaparib vs. PLD	-in olaparib low dose group, 38% showed COR, PFS 6.5mo -high dose olaparib group, 59% COR, PFS 8.8mo -PLD group showed 38% COR, PFS 7.1mo
Veliparib with Temozolomide [64]	Metastatic triple negative breast cancer	41 patients	-complete response in 1 patient, partial response in 2 patients, stable disease in 7, progression in 14
Veliparib with Carboplatin [63]	Stage IV breast cancer	22 patients enrolled, 12 eligible for evaluation	-complete response in 2 patients, partial response in 6 patients -clinical benefit of 75% seen
Veliparib with Doxo/ Cyclophosphamide [65]	Breast cancer and other solid tumors	18 patients enrolled, 14 with breast cancer (5 Brca+), 3 with ovarian cancer and 1 other	-objective antitumor activity seen in brca mutation carriers -3/5 BRCA+ TNBC with partial response -stable disease at 12 weeks in 8 breast cancer pt -MTD 100mgBID -dose limited by myelosuppression
Veliparib with Cyclophosphomide [62]	Refractory solid tumors and lymphomas	35 patients	-combination of Cyclophosphamide/ veliparib tolerated well -promising activity in subset of BRCA+ individuals

S.A.- single agent; PFS-progression free survival; ORR-overall response rate; COR-confirmed objective response; BRCA-WT-wild type; BRCA-m-mutant

Table 3. Clinical Trials [47-65]

BMN-673 is the newest PARP inhibitor to be developed and is to date the most potent and selective PARP inhibitor. It has been shown to be up to 700-fold more active in vitro in BRCA deficient cell lines when compared to olaparib [66]. Phase I trials have yet to begin. Rucaparib is another new PARP inhibitor being looked into. It is currently the focus of 3 different clinical trials; examining its activity in combination with several different chemotherapeutic regimens, efficacy in BRCA-associated breast cancer, and treatment of patients with locally advanced or metastatic breast and advanced ovarian cancer [4]. There a few other PARP inhibitors that are currently being evaluated for efficacy and tolerability, and will likely acquire more interest in the near future. Table 3 summarizes the findings of the PARP inhibitors discussed above.

Phase I and II trials demonstrated PARP inhibitor's favorable side effect profile; potentially including fatigue, nausea, vomiting, and mood disturbance. Also, myelosuppression has been noted in higher doses, especially when in combination with chemotherapy. These adverse effects are generally mild, especially in comparison with current chemotherapeutic regimens.

8. Conclusion

PARP inhibitors have been increasingly studied. This new group of drugs has been shown in multiple phase I and II trials to be efficacious with favorable side effect profiles. The preclinical data which suggested the effect of PARP inhibitors in BRCA deficient cells did not take into account the much larger population of tumors deficient in homologous recombination, with physically healthy yet functionally impaired BRCA genes. This new understanding has further raised the bar for the potential of this new class. PARP inhibitors have been shown to increase progression-free-survival and overall response rate in a number of trials. While there have indeed been some setbacks in the development of these new drugs, some of the major concerns have been addressed. Though Iniparib's phase III trial failure was initially viewed as a major disappointment, later studies proved that Iniparib does not have the same efficacy as its counterparts Olaparib/Veliparib, and ultimately may have no role in PARP inhibition of single-strand break repair. Also, the discovery that Olaparib did not show a clinically significant difference when compared to pegylated liposomal doxorubicin, led to the detection of PLD as a particularly potent agent against BRCA deficient cells. So rather than dismissing Olaparib's effect as not clinically significant, this particular study encouraged further investigation of PLD in this special population. Furthermore, the efficacy of PARP inhibition is evident, but the ideal population that could benefit most from this new class has yet to be determined. Future trials involving PARP inhibitors should undergo extremely strict stratification, as it is crucial to reveal precisely which population stands to benefit. Other concerns that need to be further investigated include mechanisms of resistance, use as frontline vs. maintenance vs. recurrent disease therapy, use in mono-therapy vs. combination with chemo or combination with other targeted therapies.

Author details

Jeanine Staples[1] and Annekathryn Goodman[2*]

*Address all correspondence to: agoodman@partners.org

1 Boston University School of Medicine, Boston, USA

2 Harvard Medical School, Massachusetts General Hospital, Department of Obstetrics and Gynecology, Boston, USA

References

[1] Hoeijmakers JH. Genome maintenance mechanisms for preventing cancer. Nature. 2001; 411:366-374

[2] Gayther SA, Warren W, Mazoyer S, Russell PA, Harrington PA, Chiano M, Seal S, Hamoudi R, van Rensburg EJ, Dunning AM, Love R, Evans G, Easton D, Clayton D, Stratton MR, Ponder BA. Germline mutations of the BRCA1 gene in breast and ovarian cancer families provide evidence for a genotype-phenotype correlation. Nat genet, 1995; 11:428-433.

[3] Venkitaraman, Ashok. Functions of BRCA1 and BRCA2 in the biological response to DNA damage. J Cell Sci 2001; 114: 3591-3598.

[4] Underhill C, Toulmonde M, Bonnefoi H. A review of PARP inhibitors: from bench to bedside. Annals Oncology, 2011; 22(2):268-279.

[5] Daly MB, Axilbund JE, Buys S, Crawford B, Farrell CD, Friedman S, Garber JE, Goorha S, Gruber SB, Hampel H, Kaklamani V, Kohlmann W, Kurian A, Litton J,Marcom PK, Nussbaum R, Offit K, Pal T, Pasche B, Pilarski R, Reiser G, Shannon KM, Smith JR, Swisher E, Weitzel JN; National Comprehensive Cancer Network. Genetic/familial high-risk assessment: breast and ovarian. J Natl Compr Canc Netw 2010; 8:562-594.

[6] King MC, Marks JH, Mandell JB. New York Breast Cancer Study Group. Breast and ovarian cancer risks due to inherited mutations in BRCA1 and BRCA2. Science 2003; 302:643.

[7] Breast Cancer Linkage Consortium. Pathology of familial breast cancer: differences between breast cancers in carriers of BRCA1 or BRCA2 mutations and sporadic cases. Lancet 1997; 349:1505-1510.

[8] Schrag D, Kuntz KM, Garber JE, Weeks JC. Life Expectancy Gains From Cancer Prevention Strategies for Women with Breast Cancer and BRCA1 or BRCA2 Mutations. JAMA, 2000; 283(5):617-24.

[9] Bolton KL, Chenevix-Trench G, Goh C, Sadetzki S, Ramus SJ, Karlan BY, Lambrechts D, Despierre E, Barrowdale D, McGuffog L, Healey S, Easton DF,Sinilnikova O, Benítez J, García MJ, Neuhausen S, Gail MH, Hartge P, Peock S, Frost D, Evans DG, Eeles R, Godwin AK, Daly MB, Kwong A, Ma ES, Lázaro C,Blanco I, Montagna M, D'Andrea E, Nicoletto MO, Johnatty SE, Kjær SK, Jensen A, Høgdall E, Goode EL, Fridley BL, Loud JT, Greene MH, Mai PL, Chetrit A,Lubin F, Hirsh-Yechezkel G, Glendon G, Andrulis IL, Toland AE, Senter L, Gore ME, Gourley C, Michie CO, Song H, Tyrer J, Whittemore AS, McGuire V, Sieh W,Kristoffersson U, Olsson H, Borg Å, Levine DA, Steele L, Beattie MS, Chan S, Nussbaum RL, Moysich KB, Gross J, Cass I, Walsh C, Li AJ, Leuchter R, Gordon O, Garcia-Closas M, Gayther SA, Chanock SJ, Antoniou AC, Pharoah PD; EMBRACE; kConFab Investigators; Cancer Genome Atlas Research Network. Association between BRCA1 and BRCA2 mutations and survival in women with invasive epithelial ovarian cancer. JAMA. 2012;307(4):382-390.

[10] Yoshida K, Miki Y. Role of BRCA1 and BRCA2 as regulators of DNA repair, transcription, and cell cycle in response to DNA damage. Cancer science 2004; 95(11): 866-871.

[11] Magwood AC, Mundia MM, Baker MD. High levels of wild-type BRCA2 suppress homologous recombination. J Mol Biol. 2012; 421(1):38-53.

[12] Shin DS, Pellegrini L, Daniels DS, Yelent B, Craig L, Bates D, Yu DS, Shivji MK, Hitomi C, Arvai AS, Volkmann N, Tsuruta H, Blundell TL, Venkitaraman AR,Tainer JA. Full-length archaeal Rad51 structure and mutants: mechanisms for RAD51 assembly and control by BRCA2. The EMBO journal 2003; 22(17):4566-4576.

[13] Somasundaram K. Breast cancer gene 1 (BRCA1): role in cell cycle regulation and DNA repair--perhaps through transcription. Journal of cellular biochemistry 2003;88(6):1084-1091.

[14] Cortez D, Wang Y, Qin J, Elledge SJ. Requirement of ATM-dependent phosphorylation of brca1 in the DNA damage response to double-strand breaks. Science 1999; ; 286(5442):1162-1166.

[15] Zhang J, Willers H, Feng Z, Ghosh JC, Kim S, Weaver DT, Chung JH, Powell SN, Xia F. FChk2 phosphorylation of BRCA1 regulates DNA double-strand break repair. Molecular and cellular biology 2004 Jan; 24(2):708-718.

[16] Zhong Q, Boyer TG, Chen PL, Lee WH. Deficient nonhomologous end-joining activity in cell-free extracts from Brca1-null fibroblasts. Cancer research 2002 Jul 15;62(14): 3966-3970.

[17] Taniguchi T, Garcia-Higuera I, Andreassen PR, Gregory RC, Grompe M, D'Andrea AD. S-phase-specific interaction of the Fanconi anemia protein, FANCD2, with BRCA1 and RAD51. Blood 2002 Oct 1;100(7):2414-2420.

[18] Nakanishi K, Yang YG, Pierce AJ, Taniguchi T, Digweed M, D'Andrea AD, Wang ZQ, Jasin M. Human Fanconi anemia monoubiquitination pathway promotes homol-

ogous DNA repair. Proceedings of the National Academy of Sciences of the United States of America. 2005 Jan 25;102(4):1110-1115 .

[19] Xia Y, Pao GM, Chen HW, Verma IM, Hunter T. Enhancement of BRCA1 E3 ubiquitin ligase activity through direct interaction with the BARD1 protein. The Journal of biological chemistry 2003 Feb 14;278(7):5255-5263.

[20] Chen A, Kleiman FE, Manley JL, Ouchi T, Pan ZQ. Autoubiquitination of the BRCA1*BARD1 RING ubiquitin ligase. The Journal of biological chemistry 2002 Jun 14;277(24):22085-22092.

[21] Stålberg K, Svensson T, Granath F, Kieler H, Tholander B, Lönn S. Evaluation of prevalent and incident ovarian cancer co-morbidity. British Journal Cancer, 2012 May 22;106(11):1860-1865. doi: 10.1038/bjc.2012.164.

[22] Atchley DP, Albarracin CT, Lopez A, Valero V, Amos CI, Gonzalez-Angulo AM, Hortobagyi GN, Arun BK. Clinical and pathological characteristics of patients with BRCA-positive and BRCA-negative breast cancer. J Clin Oncol. 2008; 26:4282–4288

[23] Brekelmans CT, Tilanus-Linthorst MM, Seynaeve C, vd Ouweland A, Menke-Pluymers MB, Bartels CC, Kriege M, van Geel AN, Burger CW, Eggermont AM,Meijers-Heijboer H, Klijn JG. Tumor characteristics, survival and prognostic factors of hereditary breast cancer from BRCA2- BRCA1- and non-BRCA1/2 families as compared to sporadic breast cancer cases. Eur J Cancer. 2007; 43(5):867–876.

[24] Chen S, Iversen ES, Friebel T, Finkelstein D, Weber BL, Eisen A, Peterson LE, Schildkraut JM, Isaacs C, Peshkin BN, Corio C, Leondaridis L, Tomlinson G,Dutson D, Kerber R, Amos CI, Strong LC, Berry DA, Euhus DM, Parmigiani G. Characterization of BRCA1 and BRCA2 mutations in a large United States sample. J Clin Oncol 2006 Feb 20; 24(6):863-871.

[25] Boyd J, Sonoda Y, Federici MG, Bogomolniy F, Rhei E, Maresco DL, Saigo PE, Almadrones LA, Barakat RR, Brown CL, Chi DS, Curtin JP, Poynor EA, Hoskins WJ. Clinicopathologic Features of BRCA-Linked and Sporadic Ovarian Cancer. JAMA 2000 May 3; 283(17):2260-2265.

[26] Bauer KR, Brown M, Cress RD, Parise CA, Caggiano V. Descriptive analysis of estrogen receptor (ER)-negative, progesterone receptor (PR)-negative, and HER2-negative invasive breast cancer, the so-called triple-negative phenotype: a population-based study from the California cancer Registry. Cancer 2007 May 1;109(9):1721-1728.

[27] Narod SA. BRCA mutations in the management of breast cancer: the state of the art. Nat Rev Clin Oncol. 2010 Dec; 7(12):702-707.

[28] Turner N, Tutt A, Ashworth A. Hallmarks of 'BRCAness' in sporadic cancers. Nat Rev Cancer 2004; 4: 814–819.

[29] Levine, D. 2011. The Cancer Genome Atlas, Molecular Profiling of Serous Ovarian Cancer. Data retrieved from cBio Cancer Genomics Portal http://www.cbioportal.org/public-portal/ last accessed August 12, 2012.

[30] Tan DS, Rothermundt C, Thomas K, Bancroft E, Eeles R, Shanley S, Ardern-Jones A, Norman A, Kaye SB, Gore ME. "BRCAness" syndrome in ovarian cancer: a case-control study describing the clinical features and outcome of patients with epithelial ovarian cancer associated with BRCA1 and BRCA2 mutations. J Clin Oncol 2008. Dec 1;26(34):5530-5536.

[31] Russell PA, Pharoah PD, De Foy K, Ramus SJ, Symmonds I, Wilson A, Scott I, Ponder BA, Gayther SA. Frequent loss of BRCA1 mRNA and protein expression in sporadic ovarian cancers. Int J Cancer. 2000; 87:317–321.

[32] McCabe N, Turner NC, Lord CJ, Kluzek K, Bialkowska A, Swift S, Giavara S, O'Connor MJ, Tutt AN, Zdzienicka MZ, Smith GC, Ashworth A. Deficiency in the repair of DNA damage by homologous recombination and sensitivity to poly(ADP-ribose) polymeraseinhibition. Cancer Res 2006; 66: 8109–8115.

[33] Yang D, Khan S, Sun Y, Hess K, Shmulevich I, Sood AK, Zhang W. Association of BRCA1 and BRCA2 mutations with survival, chemotherapy sensitivity, and gene mutator phenotype in patients with ovarian cancer. JAMA. 2011 Oct 12; 306(14): 1557-1565.

[34] Bristow RE, Chi DS. Platinum-based neoadjuvant chemotherapy and interval surgical cytoreduction for advanced ovarian cancer: a meta-analysis. Gynecol Oncol 2006 Dec;103(3):1070-1076.

[35] Bookman MA (2010) the addition of new drugs to standard therapy in the first –line treatment of ovarian cancer Ann Oncol 2010 21 suppl 7: vii211.Cochrane (2000). Chemotherapy for advanced ovarian cancer (2000). Advanced Ovarian Cancer Trialists Group. Cochrane Database Syst Rev 2000 .

[36] Rabik CA, Dolan ME. Molecular mechanisms of resistance and toxicity associated with platinating agents. CancerTreat Rev 2007; 33:9-23.

[37] Vasey PA. Resistance to chemotherapy in advanced ovarian cancer: mechanisms and current strategies. BrJCancer 2003;89 Suppl 3:S23-8.

[38] Chemotherapy for advanced ovarian cancer (2000). Advanced Ovarian Cancer Trialists Group. Cochrane Database Syst Rev. 2000;(2):CD001418.

[39] Hirschhorn R. In vivo reversion to normal of inherited mutations in humans. J Med Genet. 2003 Oct;40(10):721–728

[40] Stewart DJ. Mechanisms of resistance to cisplatin and carboplatin. Crit Rev Oncol Hematol 2007;63:12-31.

[41] Farmer H, McCabe N, Lord CJ, Tutt AN, Johnson DA, Richardson TB, Santarosa M, Dillon KJ, Hickson I, Knights C, Martin NM, Jackson SP, Smith GC,Ashworth A.Targeting the DNA repair defect in BRCA mutant cells as a therapeutic strategy. Nature. 2005 Apr 14;434(7035):917-21.

[42] Heitz F, Harter P, Ewald-Riegler N, Papsdorf M, Kommoss S, du Bois A. Poly(ADP-ribosyl)ation polymerases: mechanism and new target of anticancer therapy. Expert Rev Anticancer Ther. 2010 Jul;10(7):1125-1136.

[43] Ame JC, Splenehauer C, de Murcia G. The PARP superfamily. Bioessays. 2004; 26:882-893.

[44] Fortini P, Dogliotti E. Base damage and single-strand break repair: mechanisms and functional significance of short- and long-patch repair subpathways. DNA Repair 2007 Apr 1;6(4):398-409.

[45] Helleday T, Bryant HE, Schultz N. Poly(ADP-ribose) polymerase (PARP-1) inhomologous recombination and as a target for cancer therapy. Cell Cycle. 2005;4:1176-1178.

[46] Plummer R. Poly(ADP-ribose) polymerase inhibition: a new direction for BRCA and triple-negative breast cancer. Breast Cancer Res. 2011 Aug 16;13(4):218.

[47] Drew Y, Mulligan EA, Vong WT, Thomas HD, Kahn S, Kyle S, Mukhopadhyay A, Los G, Hostomsky Z, Plummer ER, Edmondson RJ, Curtin NJ. Therapeutic potential of poly(ADP-ribose) polymerase inhibitor AG014699 in human cancers with mutated or methylated BRCA1 or BRCA2. J Natl Cancer Inst. 2011 Feb 16;103(4):334-346.

[48] Domagala P, Lubinski J, Domagala W. Iniparib in metastatic triple-negative breast cancer. N Engl J Med. 2011 May 5;364(18):1780-1781.

[49] O'Shaughnessy J, Osborne C, Pippen JE, Yoffe M, Patt D, Rocha C, Koo IC, Sherman BM, Bradley C. Iniparib plus Chemotherapy in Metastatic Triple-Negative Breast Cancer. N Engl J Med 2011 Jan 20;364(3):205-214.

[50] Patel AG, De Lorenzo SB, Flatten KS, Poirier GG, Kaufmann SH. Failure of Iniparib to Inhibit Poly(ADP-Ribose) Polymerase In Vitro. Clin Cancer Res. 2012 Mar 15;18(6): 1655-1662.

[51] Liu X, Shi Y, Maag DX, Palma JP, Patterson MJ, Ellis PA, Surber BW, Ready DB, Soni NB, Ladror US, Xu AJ, Iyer R, Harlan JE, Solomon LR, Donawho CK,Penning TD, Johnson EF, Shoemaker AR. Iniparib nonselectively modifies cysteine-containing proteins in tumor cells and is not a Bona Fide PARP inhibitor. Clin Cancer Res. 2012 Jan 15;18(2):510-523.

[52] Birrer M, Konstantinopoulos P, Penson RT, Roche M, Ambrosio A, Stallings TE, Matulonis U, Bradley CR. A Phase I trial of Iniparib in combination with gemcitabin/ carboplatin in patients with platinum-resistant recurrent ovarian cancer. Presented at 2011 ASCO Annual Meeting. http://www.asco.org/ascov2/Meetings/Abstracts?&vmview=abst_detail_view&confID=102&abstractID=82175 accessed august 12, 2012.

[53] Strauss HG, Hemsen A, Karbe I, Lautenschlager C, Persing M, Thomssen C. Phase II trial of biweekly pegylated liposomal doxorubicin in recurrent platinum-refractory ovarian and peritoneal cancer. Anticancer Drugs. 2008;19:541–545.

[54] Penson R, Whalen C, Lasonde B, Krasner CN, Konstantinopoulos P, Stallings TE, Bradley CR, Birrer MJ, Matulonis U. A Phase II trial of Iniparib in combination with gemcitabin/carboplatin in patients with platinum-sensitive recurrent ovarian cancer. Presented at 2011 ASCO Annual Meeting. http://www.asco.org/ascov2/Meetings/Abstracts?&vmview=abst_detail_view&confID=102&abstractID=82124 accessed August 12, 2012.

[55] Gelmon KA, Tischkowitz M, Mackay H, Swenerton K, Robidoux A, Tonkin K, Hirte H, Huntsman D, Clemons M, Gilks B, Yerushalmi R, Macpherson E,Carmichael J, Oza A. Olaparib in patients with recurrent high-grade serous or poorly differentiated ovarian carcinoma or triple-negative breast cancer: a phase 2, multicentre, open-label, non-randomised study. Lancet Oncol. 2011 Sep; 12 (9): 852-861.

[56] Tutt A, Robson M, Garber JE, Domchek SM, Audeh MW, Weitzel JN, Friedlander M, Arun B, Loman N, Schmutzler RK, Wardley A, Mitchell G, Earl H, Wickens M,Carmichael J.Oral poly(ADP-ribose) polymerase inhibitor olaparib in patients with BRCA1 or BRCA2 mutations and advanced breast cancer: a proof-of-concept trial. Lancet. 2010 Jul 24;376(9737):235-244.

[57] Audeh MW, Carmichael J, Penson RT, Friedlander M, Powell B, Bell-McGuinn KM, Scott C, Weitzel JN, Oaknin A, Loman N, Lu K, Schmutzler RK, Matulonis U,Wickens M, Tutt A. Oral poly(ADP-ribose) polymerase inhibitor olaparib in patients with BRCA1 or BRCA2 mutations and recurrent ovarian cancer: a proof-of-concept trial. Lancet. 2010 Jul 24;376(9737):245-251.

[58] [58]. Ledermann J, Harter P, Gourley C, Friedlander M, Vergote I, Rustin G, Scott C, Meier W, Shapira-Frommer R, Safra T, Matei D, Macpherson E, Watkins C,Carmichael J, Matulonis U. Olaparib maintenance therapy in platinum-sensitive relapsed ovarian cancer. N Engl J Med. 2012 Apr 12;366(15):1382-1392.

[59] Fong PC, Yap TA, Boss DS, Carden CP, Mergui-Roelvink M, Gourley C, De Greve J, Lubinski J, Shanley S, Messiou C, A'Hern R, Tutt A, Ashworth A, Stone J,Carmichael J, Schellens JH, de Bono JS, Kaye SB. Poly(ADP)-ribose polymerase inhibition: frequent durable responses in BRCA carrier ovarian cancer correlating with platinum-free interval. J Clin Oncol. 2010;28:2512-2519.

[60] Kaye SB, Lubinski J, Matulonis U, Ang JE, Gourley C, Karlan BY, Amnon A, Bell-McGuinn KM, Chen LM, Friedlander M, Safra T, Vergote I, Wickens M, Lowe ES,Carmichael J, Kaufman B.Phase II, open-label, randomized, multicenter study comparing the efficacy and safety of olaparib, a poly (ADP-ribose) polymerase inhibitor, and pegylated liposomal doxorubicin in patients with BRCA1 or BRCA2 mutations and recurrent ovarian cancer. J Clin Oncol. 2012 Feb 1;30(4):372-379.

[61] Adams SF, Marsh EB, Elmasri W, Halberstadt S, Vandecker S, Sammel MD, Bradbury AR, Daly M, Karlan B, Rubin SC. A high response rate to liposomal doxorubicin is seen among women with BRCA mutations treated for recurrent epithelial ovarian cancer. Gynecol Oncol. 2011 Dec; 123 (3): 486-491

[62] [62]. Kummar S, Ji J, Morgan R, Lenz HJ, Puhalla SL, Belani CP, Gandara DR, Allen D, Kiesel B, Beumer JH, Newman EM, Rubinstein L, Chen A, Zhang Y, Wang L,Kinders RJ, Parchment RE, Tomaszewski JE, Doroshow JH.A phase I study of veliparib in combination with metronomic cyclophosphamide in adults with refractory solid tumors and lymphomas. Clin Cancer Res. 2012 Mar 15;18(6):1726-1734.

[63] Somlo G, Joseph A. Sparano, Tessa Cigler, et al. ABT-888 (veliparib) in combination with carboplatin in patients with stage IV BRCA-associated breast cancer. A California Cancer Consortium Trial. J Clin Oncol 30, 2012 (suppl; abstr 1010).

[64] Isakoff SJ, B. Overmoyer, N. M. Tung, et al. A phase II trial of the PARP inhibitor veliparib (ABT888) and temozolomide for metastatic breast cancer. J Clin Oncol 28: 15s, 2010 (suppl; abstr 1019)

[65] Tan AR, D. Toppmeyer, M. N. Stein, et al. Phase I trial of veliparib, (ABT-888), a poly(ADP-ribose) polymerase (PARP) inhibitor, in combination with doxorubicin and cyclophosphamide in breast cancer and other solid tumors. J Clin Oncol 29: 2011 (suppl; abstr 3041)

[66] Yugiao Shen, Ying Feng, Bing Wang, et al. Structure and preclinical characterization of BMN 673, a potent and orally active PARP inhibitor as an anticancer agent. Molecular Cancer Therapeutics: Nov 2011; Vol 10, Issue 11, Supplement 1

Section 5

Biomarkers

Chapter 15

The Merit of Alternative Messenger RNA Splicing as a New Mine for the Next Generation Ovarian Cancer Biomarkers

Jean-Philippe Brosseau and Sherif Abou-Elela

Additional information is available at the end of the chapter

http://dx.doi.org/10.5772/53976

1. Introduction

In this review, we discuss the merit of splicing isoforms as a source of biomarkers for ovarian cancer with a special focus on features that distinguish splice variants from global gene expression based markers. Key examples demonstrating the usefulness of alternative splicing (AS) as markers of ovarian cancer are described.

Ovarian cancer is a low incidence cancer with high mortality rate [1]. The asymptomatic nature of this cancer and the late stage diagnosis of most tumors are the reasons for ineffective surgery and chemotherapy [2]. In this sense, intensive research aim at increasing overall patient survival and quality of life by providing biomarkers for 1) early detection and 2) prediction of chemotherapy response and/or suggestion of alternative strategies. CA-125 is a glycoprotein that is usually expressed in a variety of epithelial cells and its serum level rise up in advance ovarian cancer [3]. However, its use as an early detection marker or as a tool to screen the general population has not been approved so far [4,5]. CA-125 level is helpful in treatment-decision making but do not retain the capacity to improve overall survival and quality of life [6,7]. Clearly, there is still great need for biomarkers or combination of biomarkers that could positively identify early ovarian cancer lesions with great certainty or increase patients' survival.

Genome-wide mRNA profiling presents an opportunity to rapidly identify RNA markers. Microarray platform has been applied in numerous occasions to provide gene expression signature correlating prognosis or indicative of chemotherapy response (review in [8]). However, the nature of the platform used to carry the experiments and the analysis methods and sample sets makes inter-laboratory comparison very difficult and finding reliable markers complicated. Indeed, a meta-analysis regrouping 829 samples fails to demonstrate the predictive power of 16 individual gene expression signatures [9]. Consequently, very few microarray markers reached the clinic. In contrast, high-throughput protein signature based on mass spectrometry platform appears to have much more overlap in the peaks found by different experimental studies [10]. However, the pace by which protein biomarkers are translated into clinical setting is relatively slow [11]. Clearly, there is a need for novel methodology to discover ovarian cancer biomarkers that can yield reliable results and produce tests that could be quickly integrated in normal clinical setting. In this chapter, we discuss the potential of splice variant annotations as a tool for the discovery of ovarian cancer markers and discuss the challenges and promises of this hidden mine.

2. Pre-mRNA splicing mechanism and regulation

Transcription of messenger RNA (mRNA) is the first step of converting the DNA code into functional proteins. This process was often seen as a linear cascade of events that include mRNA capping [12], splicing [13], polyadenylation [14], export to the cytoplasm [15] and translation [16] to produce a single protein. However, in reality a single pre-mRNA can produce many mRNAs through the process of AS and this in turn lead to the production of several proteins from a single gene. Splicing is the process by which the protein coding exons (typically hundreds of nucleotides in length) are joined together after the removal of large non-coding introns (typically thousands of nucleotides in length) to form the coding sequence. In some genes, this process leads to one outcome and thus named constitutive (Fig. 1.) but in most cases it leads to more than one outcome and thus called alternative (Fig. 2). Both processes are mediated by the spliceosome, specialized machinery that recognizes consensus RNA sequences [13,17]. The spliceosome component U1snRNP binds the 5′ splice site (5′ss), the splicing Factor 1 (SF1) binds the branch point site (BPS) adenine, U2 auxiliary factor 65 kDa subunit (U2AF65) binds the poly-pyrimidine tract (PPT) and U2 auxiliary factor 35 kDa subunits (U2AF35) binds the 3′ splice site (3′ss) (Fig. 1A). The last two component are further replaced by U2snRNP and following complex base-paring rearrangements and RNA-protein interactions involving hundreds of protein, the spliced mRNA, the intron by-product and the spliceosome component are release [17]. Chemically speaking, the splicing reaction proceeds in two trans-esterification steps (Fig. 1B). The first step involved the attack by the 2′ hydroxyl of the branch point adenine on the phosphate at the 5′ss, releasing at the same time the 3′end of the mRNA. The second step involved the attack by one of the hydroxyl of the terminal phosphate on the phosphate at the 3′ss, liberating the intron in the form of a lariat. This cycle of spliceosome assembly/disassembly is repeated for every intron of a gene on the nascent RNA transcript [18].

When the splice site for some exons become weak or introns with suboptimal sequence exist splicing may become less accurate and may depend on the factors that influence the splicing of competing exons and consequently produce mRNA versions with different exon pairs. AS affected the majority of multi-exons genes and is believed to be the principal driver of proteome diversity [19]. As illustrated in figure 2, two 5′ss can compete for a single 3′ss or inversely, two 3′ss can compete for a single 5′ss. These type of alternative splicing events (ASEs) are referred to alternative 5′ (alt5′, Fig. 2A) and alternative 3′ (alt3′ Fig. 2B), respectively. The most frequent

http://dx.doi.org/10.5772/53976

type of ASE in human is the full skipping of an exon (cassette exon, Fig. 2C). Some exons are also skipped as a bloc (multiple cassette exon, Fig. 2D) or mutually exclusive (Fig. 2E). AS could also be coupled to others regulatory mechanisms such as polyadenylation [14] (Fig. 2F). In this case, the resulting mRNA exhibits a different 3′ untranslated region (UTR), which is further subjected to different regulation by small non-coding RNA (e.g. microRNA). In about 1 out of 3 cases, AS decision introduces a sequence containing premature stop codon [20]. In these cases, the resulting mRNA is flagged to be degraded by the non-sense mediated decay machinery creating an efficient mechanism that control gene expression post-transcriptionally [21] (Fig. 2G). In some cases, ASE occurs outside the coding region and influence regulatory sequence in the UTR [22]. These different forms of splicing isoforms should not be confused with those generated by alternative transcription start site where a single gene might transcribe from different promoters (Fig. 2H). In this case, and unlike alternative splicing, there is little chance that the isoform will have different protein sequence unless a new protein-coding exon is added in frame for translation initiation.

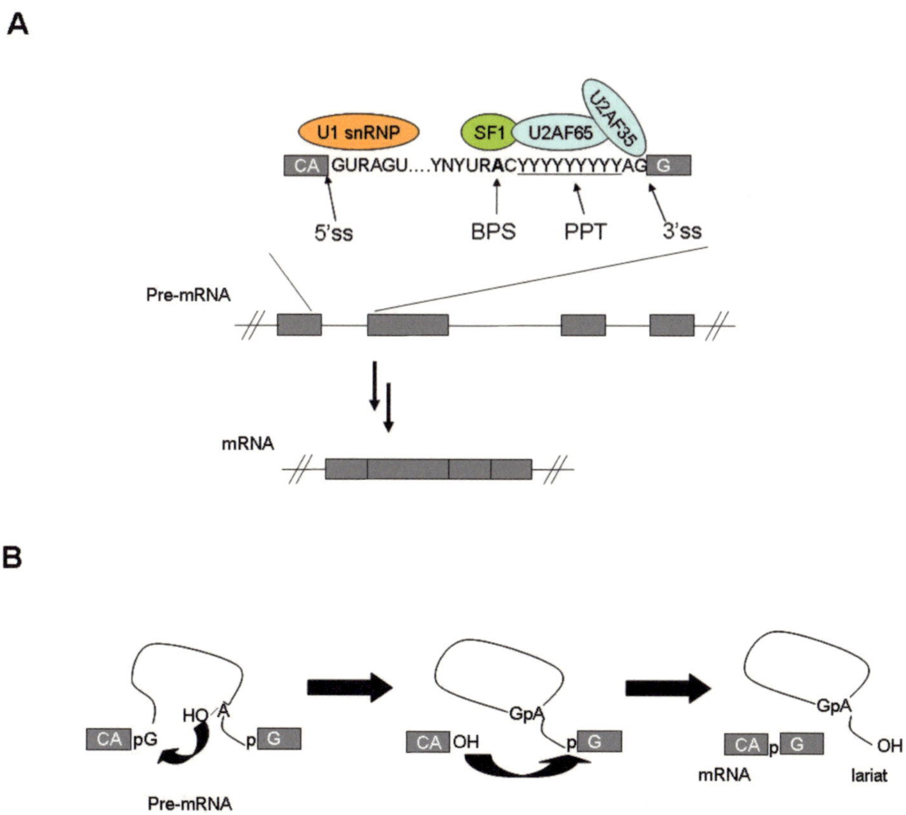

Figure 1. Constitutive splicing. A) Consensus splicing sequences. The 5′ss, BPS, PPT and 3′ss are represented and are binds by U1 snRNP, SF1, U2AF65 and U2AF35, respectively. B) Splicing reaction. The first step involved the attack by the 2′ hydroxyl of the branch point adenine on the phosphate at the 5′ss, releasing at the same time the 3′end of the mRNA. The second step involved the attack by one of the hydroxyl of the terminal phosphate on the phosphate at the 3′ss, liberating the intron in the form of a lariat.

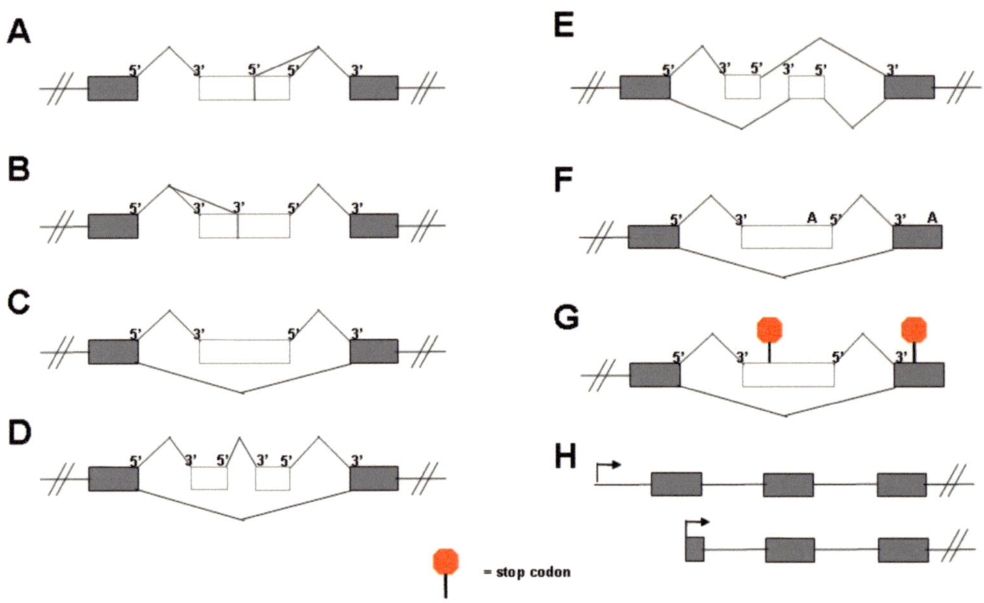

Figure 2. Alternative splicing may take many different forms. A) Alt5′. B) Alt3′. C) Cassette exon. D) Multiple cassette exons. E) Mutually exclusive exons. F) Coupled to alternative polyadenylation. G) Coupled to NMD. H) Alternative transcription initiation. Gray boxes = constitutive exons; white boxes = alternative exons; 5′ = 5′ splice site; 3′ = 3′ splice site; A = polyadenylation site.

ASEs are normally associated with low sequence conservation near the splice site and instead are usually linked to RNA binding motifs that may enhance or repress exon inclusion [23,24]. Motifs that enhance exon inclusion often recruit splicing factors like the SR protein family, which in turn interact with the spliceosome via an arginine serine rich domain to increase weak 5′ss and 3′ss recognition [25] (Fig. 3A). On the other hand, splicing motifs that promotes exon exclusion by binding members of the hnRNP family oligomerized through exon [26], block UsnRNA recruitment [27] or loop out the alternative exon [28] (Fig. 3B to D). Similarly, sequence motifs in intron may bind to SR or hnRNP proteins to influence splicing, but in this case, the SR proteins results in exon exclusion and hnRNP in exon inclusion. This is most likely because hnRNPs define intronic region and SR protein define exons location. Usually, these different enhancers and repressor protein families work together to define the final outcome of any ASEs (Fig. 3E) [29,30]. One of the most conserved intronic motif downstream of alternative exons is the UGCAUG motif [31,32], which bind the tissue-specific splicing factors family RBFOX. In general it is suggested that tissues specific splicing factors favor exon inclusion when bound to introns downstream of alternative exons and exclusion when bound upstream. This rule is beginning to be appreciated for several splicing factor such as Celf [33], epithelial-specific regulatory protein [34], Nova [35] and RBFOX [36] (Fig. 3F).

http://dx.doi.org/10.5772/53976

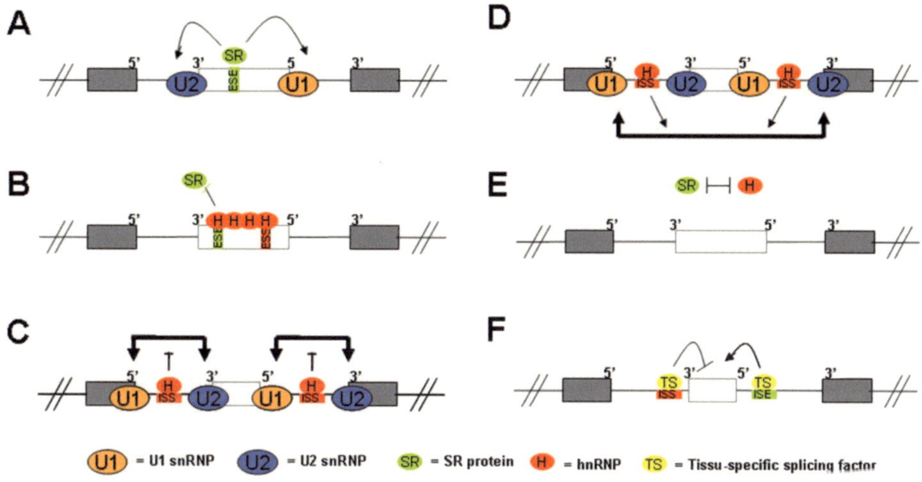

Figure 3. Schematic representation of the different mechanisms regulating alternative splicing. A) SR protein bind to exonic splicing enhancer (ESE) and favor exon inclusion by recruting U1snRNP to 5'ss or U2 snRNP to 3'ss. B) HnRNPs binding to exonic splicing silencer (ESS) and subsequent 3' to 5' oligomerization through exon favor exon exclusion by blocking SR protein access to their exonic splicing enhancer (ESE). C) Intronic splicing enhancer (ISE) binding of hnRNP interferes with intron definition and favor exon definition. D) HnRNP intron looping out. E) SR protein and hnRNPs functional antagonism. F) Tissu-specific splicing factor tend to favor exon inclusion when bound to intronic splicing silencer (ISS) in intron downstream of alternative exon and exclusion when bound upstream. Gray boxes = constitutive exons; white boxes = alternative exons; 5' = 5' splice site; 3' = 3' splice site.

3. The advantage of alternative splicing as a source of ovarian cancer biomarker

Analysis of the ovarian cancer proteome using mass spectrometry is undoubtedly the most direct approach for the identification of biomarkers that could be readily implemented in the clinic. However, the difficulty generating specific antibodies for the large number of potential markers generated via this approach makes marker validation very difficult. In contrast, the validation of nucleic acid markers generated through microarray or deep-sequencing screen is fairly simple and is often achieved by polymerase chain reaction (PCR) [34,37]. Furthermore, the function of these potential markers can easily be verified through the knockdown of gene expression using RNA interference (RNAi) strategies [38]. However, scoring global changes in gene expression as markers for ovarian cancer limits the assay to ~25000 genes in the genome, while it is estimate that the human cells contains at least >100 000 proteins. This limitation is no longer an issue when we consider the expression of specific splice variants, the number of which equal or exceeds the number of cellular proteins [39]. In addition, it is much easier to predict the function of an alternative splice variant than predicting the function of a peptide marker. For examples, while the role of the well established markers CA-125 remain unclear after 25 years of research [40], one could easily predict the function of a marker by the protein domain eliminated or included through AS as is the case of the tyrosine kinase SYK. In this case, exon skipping remove a nuclear localization domain leading to the accumulation of protein in the cytoplasm, elegantly explaining the lost of nuclear function associated with cancer [38]. Predicting the impact of AS is particularly attractive for biomarkers development when the alternative exon encodes a plasma transmembrane domain or an extracellular protease cleavage site [41]. In these cases, one would be able to predict whether the cancer associated marker leads to an increase or decrease in the secretion of membrane anchored protein, an information that is difficult to obtain using global gene expression profiles.

4. The challenges of detecting splicing isoforms

Examples of alternatively spliced genes are steadily accumulating in the literature for more than 20 years and the discovery rate was greatly accelerated by recent technological advances like transcriptome sequencing techniques. Indeed, while early estimation of alternatively spliced genes based on Northern-Blots and endpoint RT-PCR were around 5% of the human genome, transcriptome sequencing revealed ASEs in 95% of the human genes with multiple introns [39]. Different techniques have different capacity to illustrate the number of ASEs (see Table 1) and detecting splice variants remained difficult to detect for many years, which explains the reason they are not regularly considered as a source of biomarkers by most clinicians.

Technique	Throughput	Advantages	Limitations
Northern-Blot	Low	No amplification Several isoforms can be detected in a single sample	Labour-intense Large amount of RNA needed Restricted by gel resolution
Endpoint RT-PCR	Low to medium	Considered as the gold standard for validation Results easy to analyze Throughput is enhanced when coupled to capillary electrophoresis	Labour-intense if polyacrylamide gels are used to separate PCR products Low quantitative range Restricted by gel resolution
Real-time PCR	Low to medium	Provided already validated data Large quantitative range Accurate data in fixed tissues	Custom primer design often needed
Microarray	medium	Some array are commercially available	Complex analysis Results need PCR validation
Next generation Sequencing	Medium to High	Independent of genome annotation (Discovery of novel splicing isoforms)	High cost prevent the use of biological replicates Long multi-step procedure Complex analysis Results need PCR validation

Table 1. Techniques used for the detection of alternative splicing

Back in the 1980's, splicing isoforms were mainly detected by Northern-Blot, which separate transcripts by size [42] and estimate relative mRNA abundance using internal controls. However, this method is difficult to adopt in a clinical setting and require a large amount of RNA (µg), which is difficult to obtain from clinical samples. Later, the discovery of reverse transcription and PCR amplification greatly facilitated the detection of splice variants [43]. Splicing isoform amplification is achived by using PCR primers that are designed to hybridize to constitutive exons flanking the ASE of interest (Fig. 4A). The products are separated in agarose gels or capillary gel electrophoresis [44] and the ratio of the long and short isoform quantified and presented as ψ (percent of splicing index): the molarity of the long over the sum of the long and the short isoforms (Fig. 4A). Even if competitive PCR reaction are limited to a narrow range [43,45], endpoint PCR is still the preferred technique to detect splicing isoforms due to the ease of use and low cost of the experiments.

The gold standard for the mRNA quantification is real-time PCR [46], which unlike standard endpoint PCR, detects the amount of products accumulating after each cycle of amplification and permits accurate comparison of different samples. This type of PCR requires the use of fluorescent probes [47] or dyes [48] that permit detection by specialized sensors. Despite the accuracy of this detection method it is rarely used for the detection of splice variants due to difficulty in achieving isoform specific amplification [43,49]. Primers required for the amplification of the short isoform need to bind to a short unique sequence created by the exon-exon junction, which severely restrict the design (Fig. 4B). However, systematic evaluation of isoform specific design parameters and the availability of new algorithms for primer selection greatly facilitated the detection of ASEs from any species [49]. Indeed, universal PCR conditions and ease of primer design makes real-time PCR reaches the point where it can compete with high-throughput detection methods like microarray in term of ASE coverage [49].

Microarray as a method for genome-wide expression profiling was discovered in 1995 [50], but the use of this method to detect splice variants was reported only in 2003 [51]. It took 8 years to develop methods that could distinguish between the hybridization patterns of two closely related transcripts and develop chips with high enough density to accommodate the thousands of splicing isoforms [51] (Fig. 4C) Early attempts to extract splicing pattern from expression microarrays generated high false positive rate [52]. Therefore, strategies where developed to probe exon-exon junction (junction array) [51]. In this case, alternative exons are defined by very low or very high signals emanating from two consecutive splice junctions [51]. Another popular strategy is to use exonic probe in addition to exon-exon junction probe (exon/junction array) [53]. In every case, the high similarity of exon-exon junction to favor non-specific hybridization and in some analysis procedures the information is restricted to splicing isoform "detection" rather than true quantification [54]. The most successful quantification of splicing isoform by microarray was achieved by relying solely on exonic probe [54-56]. However, the success of this method was limited by its dependence on a small set of pre-selected splice variants [53,57]. To allow the discovery of new splicing isoforms, a fourth strategy that consider all putative exons (tiling array) was developed [58]. However, the high number of probe required for this methods restricted coverage to only a small fraction of the genome. Not surprisingly, these difficulties hampered the application of this method for the study of ovarian cancer splicing isforms. Indeed, to date there is no report of microarray based profiling of ovarian cancer splice variants.

In theory, the most promising approach for the detection of ovarian cancer splicing isoform is the transcriptome sequencing [39]. Next generation sequencing (NGS) technology provide massively parallel sequencing of nucleotidic sequences in miniaturized microsystem. Several platforms are commercially available and their unique technology are discussed elsewhere [59,60]. The specific application of mRNA quantification through sequencing (RNA-seq) was demonstrated for different cancer types (e.g. lung [61] and prostate [62]) but not ovarian cancer thus far. Encouraging development in the refinement of the analytical pipeline to allow accurate quantification of splicing isoforms was recently made [37,63,64]. However, the complexity of the analytical pipeline of sequencing data and the cost of the sequencing read necessary to detect splice variants will reduce the speed by which this technique is applied to the discovery of splicing dependent biomarkers (Fig. 4D). In addition, secondary techniques like PCR will still be needed to confirm and validate the accuracy of the data generated and confirm it in a large number of clinical sample. Indeed, the majority of the AS information in ovarian cancer are derived from PCR-based techniques (see Table 2 and 3).

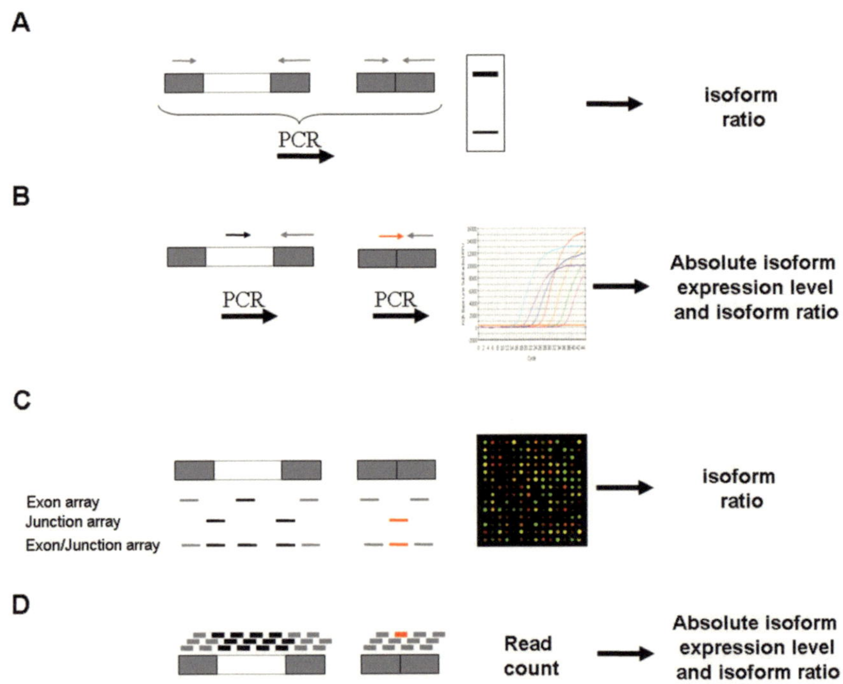

Figure 4. Methodology for splicing isoforms detection. A) Endpoint PCR. B) Real-time PCR. C) Microarray. D) Next Generation Sequencing. Red arrows and lines refer to short isoform specific detection. Gray boxes = constitutive exons; white boxes = alternative exons.

Gene	Technique	Marker type and isoform description	Reference
BRCA1/2	Endpoint RT-PCR	Prognosis Numerous DNA mutation inactivated BRCA1/2 function (deletion of essential domain or protein truncation) through aberrant splicing.	[67]
RUNX1 (AML1)	Real-time RT-PCR	Prognosis AML1b$^{Del179-242}$ expression inversely correlates with overall survival	[69]
KLF6	Real-time RT-PCR	Grade The ratio of total to full length KLF6 expression correlates with ovarian tumor grade	[72]
TP53	Real-time RT-PCR	Chemoresistance p53δ expression is associated to impaired response to first line chemotherapy	[75]
FBLN1	Endpoint RT-PCR	Diagnosis *The ratio of Fibulin C/D increase in ovarian tumors	[77]
SPP1	Real-time RT-PCR	Diagnosis *Osteopontin-c is undetectable in normal ovaries and present in ovarian tumors	[85]

*Potential serum marker

Table 2. Ovarian cancer splicing markers discovered through single gene analysis

Number of ASEs	Technique	Marker type and splicing signature description	Reference
48 ASEs	Endpoint RT-PCR	Diagnosis This signature distinguishes normal ovaries from ovarian tumors regardless of grade, stage or histotype (serous, muscinous, endometriod, mix type)	[44]
288 ASEs	Endpoint RT-PCR	Diagnosis This signature distinguishes normal ovaries from serous high grade ovarian tumors.	[36]
8 ASEs	Real-time RT-PCR	Diagnosis This cancer epithelial signature (CES) distinguishes normal Fallopian tube epithelium tissues from ovarian epithelial cancer cells	[84]
10 ASEs	Real-time RT-PCR	Diagnosis This cancer stromal signature (CSS) distinguishes normal tissues from ovarian tumors independent of the epithelial content of the tissue compared	[84]

Table 3. Ovarian cancer splicing markers derived from high-throughput expression profiling.

5. Example of alternative splicing based ovarian cancer biomarkers

5.1. Gene specific discovery of splicing markers

PCR-based techniques of specific genes associated with ovarian cancer revealed a number of ovarian cancer associated splicing events. The most promising of these potential biomarkers for diagnosis, prognosis, chemoresistance and grade biomarkers are listed in table 2 and are further described in the text below.

BRCA1/2. The ability of DNA mutation in the hereditary gene BRCA1 and BRCA2 (BRCA1/2) to predict the risk of ovarian and breast cancer is known for decades [65,66]. However, in several instance, the clinical relevance of DNA mutation is unknown, making the clinical management difficult to establish properly. Furthermore, the role of these mutations in varying the splicing of BRCA genes was largely ignored despite the fact that any nucleotide changes in the splice site consensus sequences or in any AS regulatory sequence could produce aberrant splicing isoforms. Recently, *in vitro* splicing assay of BRCA1/2 mutation [67], revealed that many cancer associated variants including those with unsuspected synonymous mutations have dramatic effect on splicing. Strikingly, six of the most frequent DNA variants representing 58,5% of BRCA1 families induced aberrant splicing profile [67]. These results, clearly demonstrate the importance of studying cancer associated splicing since it may in many case help explain mutation that cannot be associated with changes in protein sequence. However, the fidelity of splicing signature as a diagnostic marker as compared to DNA sequencing remains to be established.

RUNX1. Runt-related transcription factor 1 is a transcriptional regulator harboring a DNA-binding runt homology domain (RHD). Several layers of regulation (transcription, splicing and translation) fine-tune its tissue-specific expression [68]. RUNX1 is also known as Acute myeloid leukemia (AML) 1 and is often found as oncogenic fusion in leukemia. Nanjundan M and collaborators [69] report the fortuit discovery of a novel isoform that lack exon 6 as compared to isoform AML1b during classical cloning procedure. This novel isoform, subsequently named AML1b$^{Del179-242}$ was found to be the dominant isoform in the majority of the 42 ovarian tumors studied. Functionally speaking, skipping of exon 6 severely abrogated the transactivation potential of the resulting protein and inhibits its tumor suppressive functions. Interestingly, AML1b$^{Del179-242}$ level was either not different from normal cell line (lung cancer) or significantly decreased (breast cancer), suggesting that it may be an ovarian specific marker [69]. Noneoftheless, AML1b$^{Del179-242}$ expression is inversely proportional to the survival rate of patient, suggesting is used as a prognosis marker [69]. As attractive as it sounds, AML1b$^{Del179-242}$ certainly represent an excellent potential target and marker but required further validation in larger cohort and by independent research group.

KLF6. Kruppel-like factor (KLF) 6 is a transcription factor from the well conserved KLF gene family implicated in differentiation, development and cell growth [70,71]. KLF6 is a suspected tumor suppressor gene in several epithelial cancer (see [72] and reference there in). In ovarian cancer, an increase in KLF6 isoforms was noted and correlates with the aggressivity of the tumor in tissues (grade). One of these isoform is produced by the use of the more distal alt5′ ss and produce a protein version lacking the characteristic zinc finger binding domain (KLF6 SV1) and act as a dominant-negative [72]. Although the technical challenges of amplifying specific KLF6 isoforms preclude pinpointing the KLF6 SV1 as the isoform that correlates with grade tumor, a series of *in vitro* and *in vivo* evidence making it likely [72]. It remains to be established whether or not the full length KLF6 over KLF6 SV1 isoform ratio could serve as a prognosis or even early marker.

TP53. The tumor suppressor gene TP53 is mutated in several solid tumors and in almost all of the serous ovarian tumors [73]. Mutations affecting splice site of TP53 are very common [74] and leads to a complex pattern of splicing isoforms that add up to the already complex picture of this gatekeeper. Indeed, the point mutation IVS9-2A>G destroys the splice acceptor and redirect the splicing to include exon 9c. The resulting p53δ protein isoform is truncated in the oligomerization domain and have a new stretch of 27 new residues. In a cohort of 245 ovarian samples, the expression of this isoform is significantly correlated with poor overall survival in multivariate analyses. Moreover, patient having tumor that express p53δ have a higher chance of early relapse after first-line chemotherapy [75]. Since isoform p53δ doesn't correlate with the debulking status, it suggests that expression of p53δ impair platinum-based chemotherapy [75]. In respect to personalized medicine, it would be very interesting to sensitize these tumors by targeting p53δ. Thus, p53δ is not only a potential adverse prognosis marker but could also be a promising target for a subclass of ovarian tumors.

FBLN1. Fibulin (FBLN) 1 is an extracellular matrix (ECM)-associated protein produced by both stromal cells and epithelial cells [76]. Its presence near sites of epithelial cells locally invading stromal boundaries suggests its implication in cell adhesion/motility (see [77] and reference there in). Different C-terminal exons of the FBLN1 gene are alternatively spliced to generate four isoforms. In ovarian tumors, the ratio fibulin 1C / fibulin 1D is significantly increased compared to benign ovarian cystic sample [77]. Interestingly, the isoform ratio between normal and benign cyst is slightly increased in cystic samples (although not significant). It raises the hypothesis that the ratio fibulin 1C / fibulin 1D could potentially serves as an early diagnostic marker. Importantly, the sensitivity and specificity of fibulin splicing isoforms remains to be firmly established using a panel of normal and early lesion tissues and ultimately in patient's serum.

SPP1. Osteopontin is a member of the small integrin-binding ligand, N-linked glycoprotein (SIBLING) family of proteins [78]. It is an important component of the ECM that is secreted by both cancer cells and stromal cells in the tumor microenvironment [79]. Osteopontin interacts with various integrin receptors [80,81] as well as the CD44 receptor [82] to activate the angiogenic switch or enhance cancer cell motility [79]. The level of osteopontin is elevated in patient's plasma when compared to healthy controls by enzyme-linked immuno assay (ELISA) [83]. However, the specificity (80,4%) and sensitivity (80,4%) for the detection of early stage disease are not convincing [83]. These parameters could be increase if one takes advantages of AS. A recent report conducted by real-time PCR indicated that the isoform osteopontin c (excluding exon 4) is absent in normal or benign tissues but always present in ovarian cancer samples. This is supported by our own data from microdissected normal and cancerous ovarian cells indicating that the expression of osteopontin c comes specifically from ovarian epithelial cancer cells [84]. Conditioned medium overexpressing osteopontin c stimulate proliferation of cancer cells more efficiently than either osteopontin a or b, and this effect is revert by specific antibodies against osteopontin c [85]. Based on these data, the biomarker capacity of osteopontin in patient's blood need to be re-established using isoform-specific methodology. As the secretion of osteopontin might be an early event [86-88], it is tempting to speculate that osteopontin c could be an early marker.

5.2. Splicing markers generated through genome-wide expression profiling

The advent of splicing sensitive high-throughput technique opens the doors to monitor a large number of randomly selected ASEs rather than be limited to few candidate genes (see Table 3). The recent use of high-throughput RT-PCR by coupling PCR reaction in 384 wells plate to capillary gel electrophoresis in 96 well Caliper station dramatically increased the number of confirmed ovarian cancer associated splicing events. Initially, exon-exon junctions were systematically analyzed for a set of 600 cancer related genes in four different pools of normal and cancer ovarian samples. The resulting ASEs were subsequently validated using an independent set of 21 normal ovaries and 25 ovarian cancer samples, yielding 48 ASE markers [44]. Later on, a focus on a collection of 2168 highly curated ASEs (RefSeq NCBI build 36) subsequently yield 288 ASEs markers using roughly the same sample set [36]. The relatively high number of ASEs markers found coupled to the fact that several were related to the epithelial-mesenchymal transition raised the possibility that a large fraction of the discovered events might result from difference in the cell type compared (normal ovaries are largely composed of stromal cells where as ovarian tumors have a typical epithelial content around 75% [36]). This question was answered when 9 ovarian tumors were microdissected to isolated the RNA from stromal (tumor microenvironment) and epithelial cancer cells separately. A real-time PCR-based screening strategy coupled to an update version of RefSeq NCBI build 36 (3313 ASEs) yield a low but unambiguous set of cancer-specific splicing isoforms, the cancer epithelial signature (CES) [84]. Surprisingly, the tumor microenvironment appears to contain promising splicing isoforms RNA markers. Indeed, this cancer stromal signature (CSS) might be able to diagnosis early ovarian tumors as it clusters low malignant potential and low-grade tumors within normal ovaries and Fallopian tube samples, although this study was performed on a low number of tissues [84].

The possibility that ovarian tumor microenvironment may be a source of splicing isoforms markers raise interesting questions regarding the studies conducted on whole tumors. First, some of the RNA transcripts detected may actually come from the microenvironment cells. For exemple, fibulin and fibronectin are two ECM components known to be produced and secreted by stromal cells. Pinpointing the cell type that produced those splicing deregulated secreted proteins will certainly help to rationalize the complex autocrine and paracrine pathways implicated in the cell to cell communication that take place into and surrounding the ovarian tumor. Second, AS is a highly tissue-specific process, some of the splicing pattern changes might be the reflection of the different proportion of stromal and epithelial cells of ovarian tumors. Theoretically, those effects would be minimal when ovarian tumors of equivalent epithelial content (typically 50-75%) are compared but maximal when normal ovaries (1% epithelial cells) are used as normal reference. As a consequence, prognosis marker derived from cancer samples comparison should yield more reliable splicing markers than diagnosis marker normalized with normal ovaries.

5.3. Alternative splicing associated protein markers

Interestingly, a number of RNA splicing isoforms markers might be amenable to detection at the protein level using isoform-specific antibodies. Ultimately, these could serve as diagnostic or prognostic tool to either directly detect the presence of cancer cells or indirectly the protein in patient's fluid. Indeed, the product of the genes encoding fibronectin 1, fibulin, osteopontin, galectin 9, platelet derived growth factor A, extracellular sulfatase 2 and slit homolog 2 are all secreted in the extracellular matrix. Even some cytosolic proteins such as utrophin and serine hydroxymethyltransferase 1 were found in patient's serum [89]. Others are cell surface protein (amyloid beta A4 protein, stromal interaction molecule 1, CD97, peptidyl-glycine alpha-amidating monooxygenase and chemokine-like factor) harboring an ASE that encodes for an extracellular domain. More impressively, the exon encoding the transmembrane domain of betacellulin is preferentially excluded in ovarian tumors [44], leading to a secreted version of the protein [90]. Thus in every cases, isoform-specific antibodies could be theoretically raised against the cancer associated isoform to ultimately serve as diagnostic/prognostic tool to either detect cancer cells or detect the protein in patient's fluid.

Inversely, the splicing isoforms of the cell surface receptor Fas and CD44 were mostly studied at the protein level by either immunohistochemistry (IHC) or ELISA. Fas linked extracellular apoptotic signals that converge to the programmed cell death pathway through caspase 8 and 10. Differential usage of exon 6, which encodes the single pass transmembrane domain, results in a soluble version (sFas) and a membrane anchored version (mFas). The level of sFas is increase in ovarian tumor of higher grade compared to low grade [91,92] and correlates with worst prognosis for these patient [91]. Although these studies were performed in small cohort, it elegantly demonstrated that AS can produce isoforms detectable in patient's serum.

The glycoprotein CD44 is a cell surface receptor that binds diverse extracellular matrix ligands such as hyaluronic acid, fibronectin, osteopontin, collagen and laminin [93]. The binding of low molecular weight hyaluronan polymer promotes the motility and invasion properties of CD44 (review in [93]). It is encoded as a 20 exons gene that exhibit extensive AS of the extracellular domain of exons 6 to 15 (also called variable exons 1 to 10). The major isoform present in normal epithelial [94,95] or stromal [96] ovarian cells is the shorter isoform CD44s lacking all variable exons (CD44s for standard isoform). In contrast, a complex pattern of splicing isoforms were detected in cancer tissues, including most of ovarian tumors by mean of RT-PCR [94,97,98] or by IHC using isoform specific antibodies [95,96,99,100]. One of these splicing isoforms, the inclusion of exon v10, appears to correlate with prognosis and is indicative of improved survival in a multivariate analysis of a 142 patient cohort by IHC [96]. However, these findings contrast the initial study of Schroder who found no exon v10 expression although it relies on a smaller cohort [100]. Intriguingly, inclusion of exon v10 in metastatic tumors was correlated with decrease survival [96]. This apparent discrepancy could be rationalized if the exon v10 inclusion is seen as crucial to maintain proper cell adhesion and avoid cell detachment [101]. It remains to be determined if any of the variable exons of CD44 could serve as biomarker at the RNA level.

6. Concluding remarks

AS dramatically increase the diversity of protein expression in human cells and therefore exponentially increase the number of potential disease markers. However, the complexity in detecting AS and the unclear function of the majority of splice variants greatly reduced the rate of AS based ovarian cancer biomarkers. This trend is likely to change in the next few years with the explosion of whole transcriptome sequencing efforts and the inevitable identification of splice variants as byproducts of next generations' expression profiles. The real challenge now is to develop techniques allowing the use of splicing markers in the clinic and prepare pathologists to this new wave. Clearly, a compelling argument is needed to drive this drastic change in clinical practice and it will most likely be driven by the success of AS based screens in rationally predicting secreted protein that may serve as non-invasive ovarian cancer markers.

Author details

Jean-Philippe Brosseau[1,2] and Sherif Abou-Elela[1,3]

*Address all correspondence to: sherif.abou.elela@usherbrooke.ca

1 Laboratoire de Génomique Fonctionnelle de l'Université de Sherbrooke, Canada

2 Département de Biochimie, Faculté de Médecine et des Sciences de la Santé, Université de Sherbrooke, Sherbrooke, Québec, Canada

3 Département de Microbiologie et d'Infectiologie, Faculté de Médecine et des Sciences de la Santé, Université de Sherbrooke, Sherbrooke, Québec, Canada

References

[1] Statistiques canadiennes sur le cancer. Available at: http://www.cancer.ca.

[2] Herbst AL. The epidemiology of ovarian carcinoma and the current status of tumor markers to detect disease. Am J Obstet Gynecol 1994 Apr;170(4):1099-105; discussion 1105-7.

[3] Bast RC,Jr, Klug TL, St John E, Jenison E, Niloff JM, Lazarus H, et al. A radioimmunoassay using a monoclonal antibody to monitor the course of epithelial ovarian cancer. N Engl J Med 1983 Oct 13;309[15]:883-887.

[4] Skates SJ, Jacobs IJ, Knapp RC. Tumor markers in screening for ovarian cancer. In: Bartlett JMS, editor. Ovarian Cancer: Methods and Protocols Totowa, NJ, USA: Humana Press; 2000. p. 61-73.

[5] Muller CY. Doctor, should I get this new ovarian cancer test-OVA1? Obstet Gynecol 2010 Aug;116[2 Pt 1]:246-247.

[6] Bast RC,Jr, Badgwell D, Lu Z, Marquez R, Rosen D, Liu J, et al. New tumor markers: CA125 and beyond. Int J Gynecol Cancer 2005 Nov-Dec;15 Suppl 3:274-281.

[7] Diaz-Padilla I, Razak AR, Minig L, Bernardini MQ, Maria Del Campo J. Prognostic and predictive value of CA-125 in the primary treatment of epithelial ovarian cancer: potentials and pitfalls. Clin Transl Oncol 2012 Jan;14(1):15-20.

[8] Konstantinopoulos PA, Spentzos D, Cannistra SA. Gene-expression profiling in epithelial ovarian cancer. Nat Clin Pract Oncol 2008 Oct;5[10]:577-587.

[9] Fekete T, Raso E, Pete I, Tegze B, Liko I, Munkacsy G, et al. Meta-analysis of gene expression profiles associated with histological classification and survival in 829 ovarian cancer samples. Int J Cancer 2012 Jul 1;131(1):95-105.

[10] Callesen AK, Mogensen O, Jensen AK, Kruse TA, Martinussen T, Jensen ON, et al. Reproducibility of mass spectrometry based protein profiles for diagnosis of ovarian cancer across clinical studies: A systematic review. J Proteomics 2012 Jun 6;75[10]: 2758-2772.

[11] Anderson NL. The clinical plasma proteome: a survey of clinical assays for proteins in plasma and serum. Clin Chem 2010 Feb;56(2):177-185.

[12] Topisirovic I, Svitkin YV, Sonenberg N, Shatkin AJ. Cap and cap-binding proteins in the control of gene expression. Wiley Interdiscip Rev RNA 2011 Mar-Apr;2(2): 277-298.

[13] Will CL, Luhrmann R. Spliceosome structure and function. Cold Spring Harb Perspect Biol 2011 Jul 1;3(7):10.1101/cshperspect.a003707.

[14] Lutz CS. Alternative polyadenylation: a twist on mRNA 3' end formation. ACS Chem Biol 2008 Oct 17;3[10]:609-617.

[15] Oeffinger M, Zenklusen D. To the pore and through the pore: A story of mRNA export kinetics. Biochim Biophys Acta 2012 Jun;1819(6):494-506.

[16] Aitken CE, Lorsch JR. A mechanistic overview of translation initiation in eukaryotes. Nat Struct Mol Biol 2012 Jun 5;19(6):568-576.

[17] Black DL. Mechanisms of alternative pre-messenger RNA splicing. Annu Rev Biochem 2003;72:291-336.

[18] Krummel DA, Nagai K, Oubridge C. Structure of spliceosomal ribonucleoproteins. F1000 Biol Rep 2010 May 24;2:39.

[19] Wang ET, Sandberg R, Luo S, Khrebtukova I, Zhang L, Mayr C, et al. Alternative isoform regulation in human tissue transcriptomes. Nature 2008 Nov 27;456[7221]: 470-476.

[20] Lewis BP, Green RE, Brenner SE. Evidence for the widespread coupling of alternative splicing and nonsense-mediated mRNA decay in humans. Proc Natl Acad Sci U S A 2003 Jan 7;100(1):189-192.

[21] Garneau NL, Wilusz J, Wilusz CJ. The highways and byways of mRNA decay. Nat Rev Mol Cell Biol 2007 Feb;8(2):113-126.

[22] Hughes TA. Regulation of gene expression by alternative untranslated regions. Trends Genet 2006 Mar;22(3):119-122.

[23] Zhang XH, Chasin LA. Computational definition of sequence motifs governing constitutive exon splicing. Genes Dev 2004 Jun 1;18[11]:1241-1250.

[24] Fairbrother WG, Yeh RF, Sharp PA, Burge CB. Predictive identification of exonic splicing enhancers in human genes. Science 2002 Aug 9;297[5583]:1007-1013.

[25] Graveley BR. Sorting out the complexity of SR protein functions. RNA 2000 Sep;6(9): 1197-1211.

[26] Zhu J, Mayeda A, Krainer AR. Exon identity established through differential antagonism between exonic splicing silencer-bound hnRNP A1 and enhancer-bound SR proteins. Mol Cell 2001 Dec;8(6):1351-1361.

[27] Tange TO, Damgaard CK, Guth S, Valcarcel J, Kjems J. The hnRNP A1 protein regulates HIV-1 tat splicing via a novel intron silencer element. EMBO J 2001 Oct 15;20[20]:5748-5758.

[28] Martinez-Contreras R, Fisette JF, Nasim FU, Madden R, Cordeau M, Chabot B. Intronic binding sites for hnRNP A/B and hnRNP F/H proteins stimulate pre-mRNA splicing. PLoS Biol 2006 Feb;4(2):e21.

[29] Mayeda A, Krainer AR. Regulation of alternative pre-mRNA splicing by hnRNP A1 and splicing factor SF2. Cell 1992 Jan 24;68(2):365-375.

[30] Eperon IC, Makarova OV, Mayeda A, Munroe SH, Caceres JF, Hayward DG, et al. Selection of alternative 5' splice sites: role of U1 snRNP and models for the antagonistic effects of SF2/ASF and hnRNP A1. Mol Cell Biol 2000 Nov;20[22]:8303-8318.

[31] Yeo GW, Van Nostrand EL, Liang TY. Discovery and analysis of evolutionarily conserved intronic splicing regulatory elements. PLoS Genet 2007 May 25;3(5):e85.

[32] Voelker RB, Berglund JA. A comprehensive computational characterization of conserved mammalian intronic sequences reveals conserved motifs associated with constitutive and alternative splicing. Genome Res 2007 Jul;17(7):1023-1033.

[33] Kalsotra A, Xiao X, Ward AJ, Castle JC, Johnson JM, Burge CB, et al. A postnatal switch of CELF and MBNL proteins reprograms alternative splicing in the developing heart. Proc Natl Acad Sci U S A 2008 Dec 23;105[51]:20333-20338.

[34] Warzecha CC, Jiang P, Amirikian K, Dittmar KA, Lu H, Shen S, et al. An ESRP-regulated splicing programme is abrogated during the epithelial-mesenchymal transition. EMBO J 2010 Oct 6;29[19]:3286-3300.

[35] Zhang C, Frias MA, Mele A, Ruggiu M, Eom T, Marney CB, et al. Integrative modeling defines the Nova splicing-regulatory network and its combinatorial controls. Science 2010 Jul 23;329[5990]:439-443.

[36] Venables JP, Klinck R, Koh C, Gervais-Bird J, Bramard A, Inkel L, et al. Cancer-associated regulation of alternative splicing. Nat Struct Mol Biol 2009 Jun;16(6):670-676.

[37] Katz Y, Wang ET, Airoldi EM, Burge CB. Analysis and design of RNA sequencing experiments for identifying isoform regulation. Nat Methods 2010 Dec;7[12]: 1009-1015.

[38] Prinos P, Garneau D, Lucier JF, Gendron D, Couture S, Boivin M, et al. Alternative splicing of SYK regulates mitosis and cell survival. Nat Struct Mol Biol 2011 Jun; 18(6):673-679.

[39] Pan Q, Shai O, Lee LJ, Frey BJ, Blencowe BJ. Deep surveying of alternative splicing complexity in the human transcriptome by high-throughput sequencing. Nat Genet 2008 Dec;40[12]:1413-1415.

[40] Bouanene H, Miled A. Tumor Marker CA125: biochemical and molecular properties. Bull Cancer 2009 May;96(5):597-601.

[41] Mittendorf KF, Deatherage CL, Ohi MD, Sanders CR. Tailoring of Membrane Proteins by Alternative Splicing of Pre-mRNA. Biochemistry 2012 Jun 29.

[42] Cheng C, Sharp PA. Regulation of CD44 alternative splicing by SRm160 and its potential role in tumor cell invasion. Mol Cell Biol 2006 Jan;26(1):362-370.

[43] Bracco L, Throo E, Cochet O, Einstein R, Maurier F. Methods and platforms for the quantification of splice variants' expression. Prog Mol Subcell Biol 2006;44:1-25.

[44] Klinck R, Bramard A, Inkel L, Dufresne-Martin G, Gervais-Bird J, Madden R, et al. Multiple alternative splicing markers for ovarian cancer. Cancer Res 2008 Feb 1;68(3): 657-663.

[45] Richards MP, Poch SM. Quantitative analysis of gene expression by reverse transcription polymerase chain reaction and capillary electrophoresis with laser-induced fluorescence detection. Mol Biotechnol 2002 May;21(1):19-37.

[46] Nolan T, Hands RE, Bustin SA. Quantification of mRNA using real-time RT-PCR. Nat Protoc 2006;1(3):1559-1582.

[47] Heid CA, Stevens J, Livak KJ, Williams PM. Real time quantitative PCR. Genome Res 1996 Oct;6[10]:986-994.

[48] Morrison TB, Weis JJ, Wittwer CT. Quantification of low-copy transcripts by continuous SYBR Green I monitoring during amplification. BioTechniques 1998 Jun;24(6): 954-8, 960, 962.

[49] Brosseau JP, Lucier JF, Lapointe E, Durand M, Gendron D, Gervais-Bird J, et al. High-throughput quantification of splicing isoforms. RNA 2010 Feb;16(2):442-449.

[50] Schena M, Shalon D, Davis RW, Brown PO. Quantitative monitoring of gene expression patterns with a complementary DNA microarray. Science 1995 Oct 20;270[5235]: 467-470.

[51] Johnson JM, Castle J, Garrett-Engele P, Kan Z, Loerch PM, Armour CD, et al. Genome-wide survey of human alternative pre-mRNA splicing with exon junction microarrays. Science 2003 Dec 19;302[5653]:2141-2144.

[52] Hu GK, Madore SJ, Moldover B, Jatkoe T, Balaban D, Thomas J, et al. Predicting splice variant from DNA chip expression data. Genome Res 2001 Jul;11(7):1237-1245.

[53] Pan Q, Shai O, Misquitta C, Zhang W, Saltzman AL, Mohammad N, et al. Revealing global regulatory features of mammalian alternative splicing using a quantitative microarray platform. Mol Cell 2004 Dec 22;16(6):929-941.

[54] Cuperlovic-Culf M, Belacel N, Culf AS, Ouellette RJ. Data analysis of alternative splicing microarrays. Drug Discov Today 2006 Nov;11[21-22]:983-990.

[55] Gardina PJ, Clark TA, Shimada B, Staples MK, Yang Q, Veitch J, et al. Alternative splicing and differential gene expression in colon cancer detected by a whole genome exon array. BMC Genomics 2006 Dec 27;7:325.

[56] Clark TA, Schweitzer AC, Chen TX, Staples MK, Lu G, Wang H, et al. Discovery of tissue-specific exons using comprehensive human exon microarrays. Genome Biol 2007;8(4):R64.

[57] Fagnani M, Barash Y, Ip JY, Misquitta C, Pan Q, Saltzman AL, et al. Functional coordination of alternative splicing in the mammalian central nervous system. Genome Biol 2007;8(6):R108.

[58] Bertone P, Stolc V, Royce TE, Rozowsky JS, Urban AE, Zhu X, et al. Global identification of human transcribed sequences with genome tiling arrays. Science 2004 Dec 24;306[5705]:2242-2246.

[59] Metzker ML. Sequencing technologies - the next generation. Nat Rev Genet 2010 Jan; 11(1):31-46.

[60] Pareek CS, Smoczynski R, Tretyn A. Sequencing technologies and genome sequencing. J Appl Genet 2011 Nov;52(4):413-435.

[61] Kalari KR, Rossell D, Necela BM, Asmann YW, Nair A, Baheti S, et al. Deep Sequence Analysis of Non-Small Cell Lung Cancer: Integrated Analysis of Gene Expression,

Alternative Splicing, and Single Nucleotide Variations in Lung Adenocarcinomas with and without Oncogenic KRAS Mutations. Front Oncol 2012;2:12.

[62] Wu Y, Wang X, Wu F, Huang R, Xue F, Liang G, et al. Transcriptome profiling of the cancer, adjacent non-tumor and distant normal tissues from a colorectal cancer patient by deep sequencing. PLoS One 2012;7(8):e41001.

[63] Ameur A, Wetterbom A, Feuk L, Gyllensten U. Global and unbiased detection of splice junctions from RNA-seq data. Genome Biol 2010;11(3):R34.

[64] Anders S, Reyes A, Huber W. Detecting differential usage of exons from RNA-seq data. Genome Res 2012 Jun 21.

[65] Miki Y, Swensen J, Shattuck-Eidens D, Futreal PA, Harshman K, Tavtigian S, et al. A strong candidate for the breast and ovarian cancer susceptibility gene BRCA1. Science 1994 Oct 7;266[5182]:66-71.

[66] Wooster R, Bignell G, Lancaster J, Swift S, Seal S, Mangion J, et al. Identification of the breast cancer susceptibility gene BRCA2. Nature 1995 Dec 21-28;378[6559]: 789-792.

[67] Sanz DJ, Acedo A, Infante M, Duran M, Perez-Cabornero L, Esteban-Cardenosa E, et al. A high proportion of DNA variants of BRCA1 and BRCA2 is associated with aberrant splicing in breast/ovarian cancer patients. Clin Cancer Res 2010 Mar 15;16(6): 1957-1967.

[68] Levanon D, Bernstein Y, Negreanu V, Ghozi MC, Bar-Am I, Aloya R, et al. A large variety of alternatively spliced and differentially expressed mRNAs are encoded by the human acute myeloid leukemia gene AML1. DNA Cell Biol 1996 Mar;15(3): 175-185.

[69] Nanjundan M, Zhang F, Schmandt R, Smith-McCune K, Mills GB. Identification of a novel splice variant of AML1b in ovarian cancer patients conferring loss of wild-type tumor suppressive functions. Oncogene 2007 Apr 19;26[18]:2574-2584.

[70] Bieker JJ. Kruppel-like factors: three fingers in many pies. J Biol Chem 2001 Sep 14;276[37]:34355-34358.

[71] Black AR, Black JD, Azizkhan-Clifford J. Sp1 and kruppel-like factor family of transcription factors in cell growth regulation and cancer. J Cell Physiol 2001 Aug;188(2): 143-160.

[72] DiFeo A, Narla G, Hirshfeld J, Camacho-Vanegas O, Narla J, Rose SL, et al. Roles of KLF6 and KLF6-SV1 in ovarian cancer progression and intraperitoneal dissemination. Clin Cancer Res 2006 Jun 15;12[12]:3730-3739.

[73] Ahmed AA, Etemadmoghadam D, Temple J, Lynch AG, Riad M, Sharma R, et al. Driver mutations in TP53 are ubiquitous in high grade serous carcinoma of the ovary. J Pathol 2010 May;221(1):49-56.

[74] Holmila R, Fouquet C, Cadranel J, Zalcman G, Soussi T. Splice mutations in the p53 gene: case report and review of the literature. Hum Mutat 2003 Jan;21(1):101-102.

[75] Hofstetter G, Berger A, Fiegl H, Slade N, Zoric A, Holzer B, et al. Alternative splicing of p53 and p73: the novel p53 splice variant p53delta is an independent prognostic marker in ovarian cancer. Oncogene 2010 Apr 1;29[13]:1997-2004.

[76] Roger P, Pujol P, Lucas A, Baldet P, Rochefort H. Increased immunostaining of fibulin-1, an estrogen-regulated protein in the stroma of human ovarian epithelial tumors. Am J Pathol 1998 Nov;153(5):1579-1588.

[77] Moll F, Katsaros D, Lazennec G, Hellio N, Roger P, Giacalone PL, et al. Estrogen induction and overexpression of fibulin-1C mRNA in ovarian cancer cells. Oncogene 2002 Feb 7;21(7):1097-1107.

[78] Bellahcene A, Castronovo V, Ogbureke KU, Fisher LW, Fedarko NS. Small integrin-binding ligand N-linked glycoproteins (SIBLINGs): multifunctional proteins in cancer. Nat Rev Cancer 2008 Mar;8(3):212-226.

[79] Ahmed M, Behera R, Chakraborty G, Jain S, Kumar V, Sharma P, et al. Osteopontin: a potentially important therapeutic target in cancer. Expert Opin Ther Targets 2011 Sep;15(9):1113-1126.

[80] Zheng W, Li R, Pan H, He D, Xu R, Guo TB, et al. Role of osteopontin in induction of monocyte chemoattractant protein 1 and macrophage inflammatory protein 1beta through the NF-kappaB and MAPK pathways in rheumatoid arthritis. Arthritis Rheum 2009 Jul;60(7):1957-1965.

[81] Yokosaki Y, Matsuura N, Sasaki T, Murakami I, Schneider H, Higashiyama S, et al. The integrin alpha(9)beta(1) binds to a novel recognition sequence (SVVYGLR) in the thrombin-cleaved amino-terminal fragment of osteopontin. J Biol Chem 1999 Dec 17;274[51]:36328-36334.

[82] Katagiri YU, Sleeman J, Fujii H, Herrlich P, Hotta H, Tanaka K, et al. CD44 variants but not CD44s cooperate with beta1-containing integrins to permit cells to bind to osteopontin independently of arginine-glycine-aspartic acid, thereby stimulating cell motility and chemotaxis. Cancer Res 1999 Jan 1;59(1):219-226.

[83] Kim JH, Skates SJ, Uede T, Wong KK, Schorge JO, Feltmate CM, et al. Osteopontin as a potential diagnostic biomarker for ovarian cancer. JAMA 2002 Apr 3;287[13]: 1671-1679.

[84] Brosseau JP, Lucier JF, Nwilati H, Thibault P, Durand M, Garneau D, et al. Programmed modulation of alternative splicing in the tumor microenvironment. submitted.

[85] Tilli TM, Franco VF, Robbs BK, Wanderley JL, da Silva FR, de Mello KD, et al. Osteopontin-c splicing isoform contributes to ovarian cancer progression. Mol Cancer Res 2011 Mar;9(3):280-293.

[86] Mi Z, Bhattacharya SD, Kim VM, Guo H, Talbot LJ, Kuo PC. Osteopontin promotes CCL5-mesenchymal stromal cell-mediated breast cancer metastasis. Carcinogenesis 2011 Apr;32(4):477-487.

[87] McAllister SS, Gifford AM, Greiner AL, Kelleher SP, Saelzler MP, Ince TA, et al. Systemic endocrine instigation of indolent tumor growth requires osteopontin. Cell 2008 Jun 13;133(6):994-1005.

[88] Pazolli E, Luo X, Brehm S, Carbery K, Chung JJ, Prior JL, et al. Senescent stromal-derived osteopontin promotes preneoplastic cell growth. Cancer Res 2009 Feb 1;69(3): 1230-1239.

[89] Lomnytska M, Dubrovska A, Hellman U, Volodko N, Souchelnytskyi S. Increased expression of cSHMT, Tbx3 and utrophin in plasma of ovarian and breast cancer patients. Int J Cancer 2006 Jan 15;118(2):412-421.

[90] Dunbar AJ, Goddard C. Identification of an alternatively spliced mRNA transcript of human betacellulin lacking the C-loop of the EGF motif and the transmembrane domain. Growth Factors 2000;18(3):169-175.

[91] Konno R, Takano T, Sato S, Yajima A. Serum soluble fas level as a prognostic factor in patients with gynecological malignancies. Clin Cancer Res 2000 Sep;6(9): 3576-3580.

[92] Midis GP, Shen Y, Owen-Schaub LB. Elevated soluble Fas (sFas) levels in nonhematopoietic human malignancy. Cancer Res 1996 Sep 1;56[17]:3870-3874.

[93] Louderbough JM, Schroeder JA. Understanding the dual nature of CD44 in breast cancer progression. Mol Cancer Res 2011 Dec;9[12]:1573-1586.

[94] Cannistra SA, Abu-Jawdeh G, Niloff J, Strobel T, Swanson L, Andersen J, et al. CD44 variant expression is a common feature of epithelial ovarian cancer: lack of association with standard prognostic factors. J Clin Oncol 1995 Aug;13(8):1912-1921.

[95] Darai E, Walker-Combrouze F, Fauconnier A, Madelenat P, Potet F, Scoazec JY. Analysis of CD44 expression in serous and mucinous borderline tumours of the ovary: comparison with cystadenomas and overt carcinomas. Histopathology 1998 Feb; 32(2):151-159.

[96] Rodriguez-Rodriguez L, Sancho-Torres I, Mesonero C, Gibbon DG, Shih WJ, Zotalis G. The CD44 receptor is a molecular predictor of survival in ovarian cancer. Med Oncol 2003;20(3):255-263.

[97] Lee JH, Kang YS, Kim BG, Park SY, Lee ED, Lee KH, et al. Expression of the CD44 adhesion molecule in primary and metastatic gynecologic malignancies and their cell lines. Int J Gynecol Cancer 1995 May;5(3):193-199.

[98] Sanchez Lockhart M, Hajos SE, Basilio FM, Mongini C, Alvarez E. Splice variant expression of CD44 in patients with breast and ovarian cancer. Oncol Rep 2001 Jan-Feb; 8(1):145-151.

[99] Uhl-Steidl M, Muller-Holzner E, Zeimet AG, Adolf GR, Daxenbichler G, Marth C, et al. Prognostic value of CD44 splice variant expression in ovarian cancer. Oncology 1995 Sep-Oct;52(5):400-406.

[100] Schroder W, Rudlowski C, Biesterfeld S, Knobloch C, Hauptmann S, Rath W. Expression of CD44(v5-10) splicing variants in primary ovarian cancer and lymph node metastases. Anticancer Res 1999 Sep-Oct;19(5B):3901-3906.

[101] Chiu RK, Droll A, Dougherty ST, Carpenito C, Cooper DL, Dougherty GJ. Alternatively spliced CD44 isoforms containing exon v10 promote cellular adhesion through the recognition of chondroitin sulfate-modified CD44. Exp Cell Res 1999 Apr 10;248(1):314-321.

Chapter 16

Ovarian Cancer *in vitro* Diagnostics: New Approaches to Earlier Detection

Jorge Tapia, Mercedes de Alvarado,
Benjamín Bustos, Vania Lukoviek and
Gregory E. Rice

Additional information is available at the end of the chapter

http://dx.doi.org/10.5772/53953

1. Introduction

The overall mortality of ovarian cancer has remained unchanged despite new chemotherapeutic agents that have improved 5-year survival rates. In the United States, ovarian cancer is among the most lethal malignant gynaecological pathology. Each year, more than 230,000 new cases of ovarian cancer are diagnosed. More than 90% of these cases occur in women without clearly identifiable risk factors. In the majority of cases, ovarian cancer is first diagnosed as disseminated disease that has a five-year survival rate of less than 30%. Ovarian cancer, thus, remains a significant health care challenge and the most lethal of women's reproductive tract cancers.

Although ovarian cancer is often considered to be a single disease, it is composed of several related but distinct tumour categories, including: surface epithelial tumours, sex-cord stromal tumours, germ cell tumours, and metastatic tumours. The most frequent are the epithelial tumours that are also divided according to their histologic types: serous, mucinous, endometrioid, clear cell, and transitional. Epithelial tumours may be classified into two further groups, according to their clinical behaviour: either low malignant potential (LMP) or high malignant potential (HMP). In addition, HMP epithelial tumours are also divided into type 1 and 2 depending upon whether or not there is a pre-malignant lesion. Considering this new classification, specific mutations have been isolated depending on the type of tumour. Furthermore, the primary origin of serous epithelial ovarian cancer has been questioned. Crum *et al.* (2007), proposed that the majority of ovarian carcinomas originate outside the ovary and are derived from fallopian tube epithelial cells. The identification of cells with a molecular phenotype similar to Type 2 ovarian cancer within the fimbria is consistent with the hypothesis that ovarian cancer may indeed originate from intraepithelial carcinomas of the fallopian tubule.

Despite significant advances in the development of mathematical modelling and validation of *in vitro* diagnostics, to date none have achieved the level of diagnostic performance required for implementation as a screening test for asymptomatic women in the general population. In the absence of a screening test, however, it is important for women presenting to primary care to be diagnosed in the most effective and timely way to ensure that they are directed to the most appropriate clinical treatment available.

Ongoing studies continue to search for the presence of other biomarkers (in addition to CA125 and ultrasound imaging) to detect ovarian cancer in its initial stages. Of recent note has been the identification of tumour-specific exosomes in the blood of women with ovarian cancer. Other novel diagnosis techniques have been described: intra-fallopian tubule sampling, uterine washing sampling and the sampling of cervicovaginal swabs. While these approaches afford some promise of increasing diagnostic performance for asymptomatic populations, they await clinical validation.

2. Reclassification of disease type

According to the classification of the World Health Organisation in 2003, from an histopathological point of view epithelial ovarian tumour are classified in serous (60%), endometrioid (10-20%), clear cell (<10%), transitional (6%), mucinous (5%), and undifferentiated (<1%) [1,2]. Furthermore, ovarian tumours are also classified, according to behaviour, into low malignant potential (LMP) and high malignant potential (HMP) depending on the grade of invasion.[3] High serous malignant tumours are divided into type I and type II [4].

Type I tumours originate from the progressive transformation of low malignant potential ovarian tumours, whose behaviour is considered to be relatively benign. This group include: mucinous carcinoma; endometrioid carcinoma; Brenner tumours; and clear cell carcinoma. Type II tumours, however, do not display a defined pre-malignant lesion, and their behaviour is aggressive, and rapidly progressive, metastising in early stages of diagnosis. Serous carcinomas, sarcocarcinomas and undifferentiated carcinomas belong in this group. Preliminary studies report that epithelial LMP tumours (mucinous, endometrioid, and clear cell carcinoma) could evolve from low to mildle undifferentiated tumours becoming HMP ovarian tumours [5].

The development of a new classification of epithelial ovarian tumours (*i.e.* type 1 and type 2) has led to the identification of specific molecular phenotypes previously unidentified because of the confounding effects of multiple histopathological types of tumours. Type I and type II tumours display different characteristics and activation of molecular pathways. Type I tumours are associated with mutations in the Ras pathway (BRAF, KRAS, ErbB2) while, type II tumours are frequently associated with mutations in the

TP53 pathway, although there is little information relating to other molecular mutations. [6,7]. When stratified by type (*i.e.* high-grade and low-grade serous carcinoma), it became evident that the mutation TP53 is present in almost 100% of type II high-grade serous carcinomas [8]. Taking into account that TP53 mutation is precocious and ubiquitous (at least in advance stages) it remains to be proven whether or not this mutation plays an aetiological role in the development of this phenotype.

Women with mutations in BRCA 1-2 genes have around 30-70% probability of developing ovarian cancer before reaching old age, in most cases, type II HMP tumours.[9] The BRCA 1-2 genes are crucial components in the DNA repair pathway of homologous recombinant required to resolve errors in the double-stranded DNA [10]. It is likely that inherited mutations in BRCA 1-2 genes predispose the epithelial ovarian surface to neoplastic transformation secondary to genetic instability [5]. The loss of function in the BRCA 1-2 genes is often lethal to the cell because of the associated apoptotic response with p53.[11] Since the loss of BRCA gene function is very common in high-grade serous carcinomas, secondary mutations are expected to be present to ensure the survival of the cells involved [3].

There are undoubtedly many mutations involved in the survival and adaptation of epithelial ovarian carcinomas that have yet to be studied. Currently, the processes that occur between an initial carcinoma and its progression to widely disseminated disease remain unknown. It is presumed that there are multiple mutations in the tumourigenesis pathways that allow the tumour to overcome hypoxia, cytokines, the detachment from the basal membrane and the metabolic demands of many rapidly dividing cells. [7]

3. Fallopian tubule involvement in ovarian cancer

Within the advances in histopathological and genetic investigations, recent dogma regarding the origin of serous ovarian cancer involving pre-cancerous lesions from the ovarian surface epithelium or intra–ovarian inclusion cysts has been questioned. In women with BRCA-1 and BRCA-2 germline mutations, tubal intra-epithelial carcinoma in the fimbria has been identified as a very probable precursor of advanced high-grade serous ovarian cancer (particularly in Type 2 ovarian cancer) [12]-[14]. This is also validated by the coexistence of identical TP53 mutations in tubal intra-epithelial carcinoma and in those tumours classified as ovarian in origin [15].

This evidence is consistent with the idea that the fallopian tube (especially its distal portion: the fimbria) is an important site for the initiation of high-grade serous ovarian cancer [16]. Crum et al. (2007), further, proposed that most ovarian carcinomas originate outside the ovary and are derived from fallopian tube epithelial cells. They suggest that fimbrial epithelial cells detach and implant on the deluded, damaged surface of the ovary resulting in the formation of inclusion cysts that subsequently give rise to what until now was known as "ovarian" cancer. The identification of cells with a molecular phenotype similar to Type 2 ovarian cancer within the fimbria is consistent with the hypothesis that ovarian cancer may indeed originate from intraepithelial carcinomas of the fallopian tubule [17].

Even though the genesis of this pathology remains unclear, there are some groups that support the idea of "endosalpingiosis" as the preliminary event. This means that even when the primary tumour seems to originate in the ovary, it is possible that the fallopian tube epithelium provides the originating cell through earlier entrapment in the ovary [16].

These studies potentially have significant impact on clinical practice and raise important questions, including:

- Should the complete removal of the fallopian tube during hysterectomy and/or oophorectomy be a general practice? Bowtell et al. and Dietl et al. consider this approach essential in reducing the risk of high-grade serous cancer [16, 18].
- Is the removal of fallopian tubes a good idea when practicing a prophylactic hysterectomy in women with BRCA mutations? According to Dietl and Wishhusen, a salpingectomy-only for women at increased risk of ovarian cancer would be a proper prophylactic option [18].

Future research should be oriented towards answering these and many other questions related to the development of new surgical and medical techniques in the treatment and prevention of ovarian cancer.

4. Recent advances in the development of IVDs

Early detection and accurate diagnosis of ovarian cancer is a pending issue in gynaecologic oncology. Tools such as physical examination, transvaginal ultrasound and serum markers (*e.g.* Ca125) have limited sensitivity. Moreover, genetic counselling is warranted only in high-risk patients, such as those with a family history of BRCA-1, BRCA-2 or Lynch syndrome [19].

Considering the high mortality of this type of cancer, it is necessary to develop new and more efficient diagnostic strategies. One recent approach to improve diagnostic efficiency has been the development of multivariate index assays (IVDMIA). IVDMIAs were defined by FDA guidelines in 2007 as a tool that: 1. Combines multiple variables using a performance function to obtain a specific result for a specific patient; and 2. Provides a result whose derivation is non-transparent and cannot be independently derived or verified by the end user.[20] The purpose of the multivariate analysis is to integrate different biomarkers into a single test, to optimise the sensitivity and specificity of the diagnostic through non-lineal functions.[21]

To date, such tests are not methods of screening, but diagnostic tools in the evaluation of women with pelvic tumours. They help to determine the likelihood of malignancy and thus the categorisation of urgency at the time of referral to a gynaecological oncologist. [19]

OVA1 (Vermillion, Inc., Austin, TX) is the first ovarian cancer IVDMIA approved by the FDA, and combines five tests: CA125 II, prealbumin, apolipoprotein A-1, β2-microglobulin, and transferrin, obtaining a score of 0-10, in which 10 is the highest risk of malignancy. The cut-off values to define high probability of malignancy in premenopausal women are 5.0 and 4.4 in postmenopausal women. These tests optimise sensitivity compared to physical examination in both nongynecologic oncologists (72% to 92%) as in gynecologic oncologists (78% to 99%), even at 100% stage II in both pre- and postmenopausal women [22]. In addition to its association with physical examination, it has a sensitivity of 96%, while physical examination and CA125 alone have a sensitivity of 75% and 77%, respectively [21].

Even though OVA1 has a high sensitivity, its specificity is low in both nongynecologic oncologists and gynecologic oncologists (being 42% and 26% respectively). Other IVDMIAs have shown greater specificity, for example OvaSure, a 6 IVDMIA analysing protein biomarker, has a sensitivity of 95.3% and a specificity of 99.4% [23], however, OvaSure has yet to be approved by the FDA.

In a recent study, Autelitano et al. analysed a unique multianalyte test that integrates CA125, C-reactive protein, amyloid-A, plasma interleukin-6 and interleukin-8. This test has a high specificity (92.3%) and a moderate sensitivity (76.4%) for the diagnosis of ovarian cancer in symptomatic women. The panel performs significantly better than CA125 alone, as measured by the area under the receiver operator characteristic curve (88.4% and 84.3%, respectively, $p < 0.001$) [24].

The development of IVDMIAs for ovarian cancer based on known candidate biomarkers offers promise for improving diagnostic efficiency of not only adrenal masses but also the earlier detection of ovarian cancer and prognosis.

Optimising preoperative diagnosis and opportune referral to specialists, would not only assist in the development of a specific management strategy for individual patients, but would also allow for more accurate determination of perioperative morbidity and chance of survival. Further studies, however, are needed to validate not only a comparison with classical clinical or serological parameters, but also between different IVDMIAs, to determine which one is the better diagnostic tool.

5. Novel approaches to the diagnosis of ovarian cancer

Ovarian cancer is generally diagnosed in its advanced stages due to the lack of overt symptoms of disease (70% of the cases approximately), resulting in a poor prognosis (rate survival around 30%) [25]. Only a small number of ovarian cancers are detected early and these are the ones that can generally be treated.

The reason ovarian cancer is difficult to diagnose in its initial stage is due to the lack of specific and appropriately sensitive serum biomarkers associated with the unspecific symptoms. The most utilised serum biomarker in the diagnosis of ovarian cancer is CA125, but unfortunately its ability to detect ovarian cancer in a general population is quite low [26, 27].

As a response to this difficult scenario, current investigations include the search for other serum biomarkers that would improve our ability to detect ovarian cancer in its initial stages, possibly in combination with CA125 and ultrasound imaging. The recent identification of tumour-specific nanoparticle (exosomes) in the blood of patients with various diseases/complications, including ovarian cancer, affords an alternative approach to the identification of more effective biomarkers.

Exosomes are small (40-100 nm) membrane vesicles that are released following the exocytotic fusion of multi-vesicular bodies with the cell membrane. They are characterised by: a cup-shaped form; a buoyant density of 1,13-1,19 g / ml [28,29] endosomal origin; and the enrichment of late endosomal membrane markers, including Tsg101, CD63, CD9 and CD81 [30-32]. Exosomes have been identified in plasma under both normal and pathological conditions, and their concentration has been reported to increase in association with disease severity and/or progression. While, the process(es) of exosome formation remains to be fully elucidated, available data support an endosomal origin and formation by the inward budding of multi-vesicular bodies [33].

Tumor cells release exosomes into peripheral circulation [34], indeed the first vesicular structures described in plasma were observed in women with ovarian cancer [35]. In ovarian cancer, the concentration of exosomes (measured as exosomal protein in peripheral blood) increases with disease stage and are associated with tumour-specific microRNA [36]. These results suggest that microRNA profiling of circulating tumor exosomes could potentially be used as surrogate diagnostic markers and may be of utility for screening asymptomatic populations. Recent data further suggests that the release of exosomes from cells may represent a normal mechanism for cell-to-cell communication [37] their role in the pathogenesis of ovarian cancer, however, remain to be established.

Other novel diagnosis techniques have been described: intra-fallopian tubule sampling, the sampling of uterine washings and the sampling of cervicovaginal swabs. While these approaches represent a very promising alternatives for the diagnosis of ovarian cancer, there is a paucity of data and clinical validation to support their implementation as viable alternatives to CA125 and ultrasound imaging.

6. Concluding comments

The alignment of metastatic and molecular phenotypes of ovarian cancer is affording new insights into the aetiology and treatment of this disease cluster.

Recent evidence supports a tubal origin of epithelial ovarian cancer, including the coexistance of similar gene mutations in the tubal intraepithelial carcinoma and those classified as ovarian origin (*e.g.* TP53 gene mutation). On the basis of these data, some have proposed "endosalpingiosis" as the initial event in ovarian cancer, suggesting that the epithelial cells of the tube migrate to the surface of the ovary constituting ovarian cancer genesis. If proven to be correct, new opportunities for the management of ovarian cancer may be realised, particularly for those patients carrying BRCA-1 and -2 mutations that require prophylactic surgery.

Within the field of gynaecologic oncology, an aspect that has been particularly disappointing is the development of early detection tests for ovarian cancer. Classical methods based on physical examination, images and some serum markers such as CA125, have not resulted in significant advances in early detection rates. Tests, such as OvaSure and OVA 1, have integrated various clinical and serum markers for the diagnosis of cancer with different sensitivities and specificities, but are aimed at defining malignancy in patients with ovarian tumours, rather than providing either an earlier diagnosis or a screening test.

A possible answer to the problem is seen with the recognition of specific membrane particles in ovarian tumors (exosomes), as well as other tissue surfaces. These particles are tissue-specific and may allow the identification of specific cell types in preclinical stages of the disease. The potential detection of these specific exosomes in biofluids also offers new perspectives in research on the early detection of ovarian cancer. Such ovarian cancer–specific non-particles may be present in fallopian tubule fluid, uterine washings or even cervicovaginal fluids. Further research is needed in this area to assess the utility of such approaches in order to develop simple and safe methods of detecting ovarian cancer in its early stage.

Acknowledgements

GER wishes to acknowledge and thank the Rotary Club of Williamstown and The RoCan Program for their support of the University of Queensland Centre for Clinical Diagnostic ovarian cancer biomarker discovery program.

Author details

Jorge Tapia[1], Mercedes de Alvarado[2], Benjamín Bustos[2], Vania Lukoviek[2] and Gregory E. Rice[3]

1 Gynaecologic Oncologist, Unniversity of The Andes and Clinica Dávila, Santiago, Chile

2 Department of Obstetrics and Gynaecology, University of the Andes, Santiago, Chile

3 University of Queensland Centre for Clinical Research, Herston, Queensland, Australia

References

[1] Tavassoli FA, Devilee P. Pathology and genetics of tumors of the breast and female genital organs. In: *World Health Organization Classification of Tumors*. Lyon, France: IARC, 2003; 113–145

[2] Lalwani N, Shanbhogue AK, Vikram R, Nagar A, Jagirdar J, Prasad SR. Current update on borderline ovarian neoplasms. *AJR Am J Roentgenol* 2010;194(2):330–336.

[3] Bowtell D. The genesis and evolution of high-grade serous ovarian cáncer. Nat Rev Cancer. 2010 Nov;10(11):803-8. Epub 2010 Oct 14.

[4] Vang, R., Shih Ie, M. & Kurman, R. J. Ovarian low-grade and high-grade serous carcinoma: pathogenesis, clinicopathologic and molecular biologic features, and diagnostic problems. Adv. Anat. Pathol. 16, 267–282 (2009)

[5] Ie-Ming S, Ovarian Tumorigenesis. A Proposed Model Based on Morphological and Molecular Genetic Analysis. Am J Pathol. 2004 May;164(5):1511-8

[6] Daniel W. Et al. National Academy of Clinical Biochemistry Guidelines for the Use of Tumor Markers in Ovarian Cancer. NACB: Practice Guidelines And Recommendations For Use Of Tumor Markers In The Clinic. 2008.

[7] MJJ, Bowtell. The Changing View of High-Grade Serous Ovarian Cancer. Cancer Res. 2012 Jun 1;72(11):2701-4. Epub 2012 May 16

[8] Ahmed AA, Etemadmoghadam D, Temple J, Lynch AG, Riad M, Sharma R, et al. Driver mutations in TP53 are ubiquitous in high grade serous carcinoma of the ovary. J Pathol 2010;221:49–56.

[9] Risch, H. A. et al. Population BRCA1 and BRCA2 mutation frequencies and cancer penetrances: a kin- cohort study in Ontario, Canada. J. Natl Cancer Inst. 98, 1694–1706 (2006).

[10] Venkitaraman, A. R. Linking the cellular functions of *BRCA* genes to cancer pathogenesis and treatment. *Annu. Rev. Pathol.* 4, 461–487 (2009)

[11] Patel, K. J. *et al.* Involvement of *BRCA2* in DNA repair. *Mol. Cell* 1, 347–357 (1998).

[12] Lee, Y. *et al.* A candidate precursor to serous carcinoma that originates in the distal fallopian tube. *J. Pathol.* 211, 26–35 (2007).

[13] Lee, Y. *et al.* Advances in the recognition of tubal intraepithelial carcinoma: applications to cancer screening and the pathogenesis of ovarian cancer. *Adv. Anat. Pathol.* 13, 1–7 (2006).

[14] Folkins, A. K. *et al.* A candidate precursor to pelvic serous cancer (p53 signature) and its prevalence in ovaries and fallopian tubes from women with *BRCA* mutations. *Gynecol. Oncol.* 109, 168–173 (2008).

[15] Kindelberger, D. W. *et al.* Intraepithelial carcinoma of the fimbria and pelvic serous carcinoma: evidence for a causal relationship. *Am. J. Surg. Pathol.* 31, 161–169 (2007).

[16] Bowtell, D. D. L. The genesis and evolution of high-grade serous ovarian cancer. *Nature Rev. Cancer* 10, 803–808 (2010).

[17] Crum, C. P. *et al.* Lessons from *BRCA*: the tubal fimbria emerges as an origin for pelvic serous cancer. *Clin. Med. Res.* 5, 35–44 (2007).

[18] Dietl, J. & Wischhusen, J. The forgotten fallopian tube. 10 Feb 2011 (doi:10.1038/nrc2946-c1).

[19] Goff A. Ovarian Cancer. Screening and Early Detection. Obstet Gynecol Clin N Am 39 (2012) 183-194.

[20] US Department of Health and Human Services. Draft Guidance for Industry, Clinical Laboratories, and Staff: In Vitro Diagnostic Multivariate Index Assays. http://www.fda.gov/downloads/MedicalDevices/ DeviceRegulationandGuidance/ GuidanceDocuments/ ucm071455.pdf. Accessed April 2, 2012.

[21] Zhang Z. An In Vitro Diagnostic Multivariate Index Assay (IVDMIA) for Ovarian Cancer: Harvesting the Power of Multiple Biomarkers. Rev Obstet Gynecol. 2012;5(1):35-41.

[22] Ueland FR, Desimone CP, Seamon LG, et al. Effectiveness of a multivariate index assay in the preoperative assessment of ovarian tumors. Obstet Gynecol. 2011;117:1289-1297.

[23] Visintin I. et al. Diagnostic markers for early detection of ovarian cancer. Clin Cancer Res 2008 14:1065-1072.

[24] Dominic J Autelitano1*, Linda Raineri1, Kate Knight1, Kelly Bannister1 and Gregory E Rice2. Performance of a multianalyte test as an aid for the diagnosis of ovarian cancer in symptomatic women. 2009.

[25] Jemal A, Siegel R, Ward E, Hao Y, Xu J, Murray T, Thun MJ: Cancer statistics, 2008. *CA Cancer J Clin* 2008, 58:71-96.

[26] Bast RC Jr, Badgwell D, Lu Z, Marquez R, Rosen D, Liu J, Baggerly KA, Atkinson EN, Skates S, Zhang Z, *et al.*: New tumor markers: CA125 and beyond. *Int J Gynecol Cancer* 2005, 15(Suppl 3):274-281.

[27] Badgwell D, Bast RC Jr: Early detection of ovarian cancer. *Disease markers* 2007, 23:397-410.

[28] Mignot G, Roux S, Thery C, Segura E, Zitvogel L. Prospects for exosomes in immunotherapy of cancer. Journal of cellular and molecular medicine. 2006;10(2):376-88.

[29] Miranda KC, Bond DT, McKee M, Skog J, Paunescu TG, Da Silva N, et al. Nucleic acids within urinary exosomes/microvesicles are potential biomarkers for renal disease. Kidney international. 2010;78(2):191-9. Epub 2010/04/30.

[30] Thery C, Zitvogel L, Amigorena S: Exosomes: composition, biogenesis and function. *Nature reviews* 2002, 2:569-579.

[31] Andre F, Schartz NE, Movassagh M, Flament C, Pautier P, Morice P, Pomel C, Lhomme C, Escudier B, Le Chevalier T, *et al.*: Malignant effusions and immunogenic tumour-derived exosomes. *Lancet* 2002, 360:295-305.

[32] Taylor DD, Homesley HD, Doellgast GJ: Binding of specific peroxidase- labeled antibody to placental-type phosphatase on tumor-derived membrane fragments. *Cancer Res* 1980, 40:4064-4069.

[33] Mincheva-Nilsson L, Baranov V. The role of placental exosomes in reproduction. Am J Reprod Immunol. 2010;63(6):520-33.

[34] Keller S, Ridinger J, Rupp AK, Janssen JW, Altevogt P. Body fluid derived exosomes as a novel template for clinical diagnostics. Journal of translational medicine. 2011;9:86.

[35] Simons M, Raposo G. Exosomes--vesicular carriers for intercellular communication. Current opinion in cell biology. 2009;21(4):575-81.

[36] Taylor DD, Gercel-Taylor C. MicroRNA signatures of tumor-derived exosomes as diagnostic biomarkers of ovarian cancer. Gynecologic oncology. 2008;110(1):13-21.

[37] Ludwig AK, Giebel B. Exosomes: small vesicles participating in intercellular communication. The international journal of biochemistry & cell biology. 2012;44(1):11-5.

Chapter 17

Disseminated Tumor Cells and Cancer Stem Cells in Ovarian Cancer

Malgorzata Banys, Natalia Krawczyk,
Andreas D. Hartkopf and Tanja Fehm

Additional information is available at the end of the chapter

http://dx.doi.org/10.5772/54391

1. Introduction

Ovarian cancer is currently the fifth most lethal malignancy of women in Europe and the United States [1, 2]. The prognosis of ovarian cancer patients is limited due to lack of specific early symptoms and a high rate of relapse; more than half of all patients will suffer from disease recurrence, resulting in a poor overall survival [3]. Most cases are diagnosed in advanced stages, and although the initial response to chemotherapy is generally good, a significant proportion of patients will suffer from a relapse despite optimal cytoreductive surgery [4]. Since treatment strategies are mainly developed to control locoregional cancer growth, it may be anticipated that more women will die of distant metastatic disease. The identification of novel molecular markers, reflecting current tumor activity, may improve prediction and therapy monitoring and provide valuable insights into process of carcinogenesis. In this regard, oncologic research have increasingly focused on disseminated and circulating tumor cells.

The presence of disseminated tumor cell (DTC) in bone marrow (BM) is a phenomenon observed in almost all solid tumors of epithelial origin. For breast cancer, DTC presence has been demonstrated as a strong independent prognostic factor (level I evidence) [5]. Available data support the notion that hematogenous tumor cell dissemination may be clinically relevant in ovarian cancer as well [6-10]. Detection rates of DTC, as a surrogate parameter for occult hematogenous spread, vary between 30-50% primary ovarian cancer patients.

A provocative hypothesis has been introduced recently with respect to natural history and progression of ovarian cancer. While the 'classical' stochastic model of cancer development holds that any cell may become source of malignant transformation, emerging evidence supports the view that only a minor subpopulation of cancer cells has the potential to initiate cancer growth. These cells, called cancer stem cells (CSC), have the ability to self-renew, propagate tumorigenesis and are usually drug-resistant [11]. Experimental studies on stem cell biology have given new impetus to the cancer stem cell theory. CSC are assumed to play important role in development of various tumor entities, such as breast and gastrointestinal cancer, retinoblastoma and ovarian cancer [12], [13]. Interestingly, ovarian cancer cell lines feature "side population" cells with potential to differentiate into cancers with different histologies, suggesting the pluripotent character of stem cells [14]. Whether DTC in extraperitoneal sites, such as bone marrow, reflect a stem cell-like sub population of tumor cells, remains yet to be cleared.

Of all prognostic factors, monitoring of minimal residual disease is the only one available after the tumor has been removed. Beside monitoring of tumor markers, there is currently a major effort to identify other biological markers which can be assessed with minimally invasive methods and persist beyond surgery. We previously reported on a significant correlation of positive BM status with shortened relapse-free survival in ovarian cancer patients [6]. DTC persistence after completion of platinum-based chemotherapy was also found to be prognostically relevant [15]. Recently, attempts have been made to target DTC by using antibody-based therapy with the trifunctional antibody catumaxomab. Wimberger et al. reported a marked decrease in tumor cells in peripheral blood following intraperitoneal catumaxomab treatment for malignant ascites, indicating a systemic effect of the therapy [16]. However, in comparison with breast cancer, data on DTC detection in gynecological malignancies are so far limited [7], [17], [18], [19], [9].

In this chapter we discuss recent advances in ovarian cancer research with respect to disseminated tumor cells and cancer stem cell hypothesis. Data on prognostic and clinical relevance are presented.

2. Disseminated and circulating tumor cells in ovarian cancer

Detection and characterization of disseminated tumor cells in bone marrow and blood of patients with epithelial carcinomas can be accomplished by various techniques. For the detection of isolated tumor cells, both antibody-based assays and molecular assays have been established [20, 21]. Despite advances in this field, no specific antigen or marker gene has been described for ovarian cancer so far. Therefore, immunocytochemical identification of these cells based on expression of epithelial markers remains the gold standard (Figure 1). Commonly targeted antigens are cytokeratin and EpCAM due to relatively constant and universal expression pattern in cells of epithelial origin [9, 15, 22]. A major difficulty in detecting and characterizing tumor cells is their relatively low frequency. Most protocols include therefore a cell enrichment step (e.g. density gradient centrifugation, immunomagnetic enrichment). These obstacles highlight the need for optimization of the assay (e.g. by minimizing cell loss, preserving cell morphology and producing reliable immunophenotypic and genotypic data) as it is essential for detecting, enumerating and characterizing single tumor cells [21].

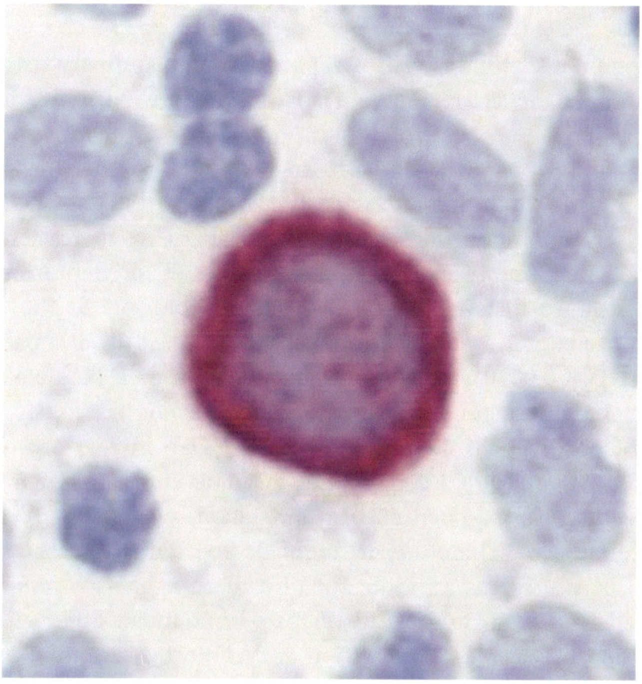

Figure 1. Disseminated tumor cell from ovarian cancer patient with typical cytomorphology and immunophenotype (positive cytokeratin-staining, large nucleus, high nuclear to cytoplasmic ratio, nucleus partially covered by CK-staining, nucleus granular [23].

Detection rates of disseminated tumor cells in ovarian cancer patients stage FIGO I-III reach 20-60% [7, 9, 15, 22]. These results suggest hematogenous spread to be a comparatively frequent phenomenon in ovarian malignancies and indicate the ability of single tumor cells to disseminate to bone marrow in a very early stage of disease. DTC are routinely detected in 13-18% FIGO I ovarian cancer patients [6, 19, 22]. Since bone metastases are relatively rare in ovarian cancer patients, BM seems to serve as a temporary `homing site´ for single tumor cells, from where they are able to migrate and subsequently cause distant metastasis or local recurrence [24]. Assuming that DTC may spread by means of blood stream we cannot exclude that those may also be able to repopulate the peritoneal cavity, an environment which easily supports ovarian cancer growth [11, 25].

Based on numerous studies, no significant relationship has been reported between clinicopathological characteristics of primary tumor and DTC detection. In our latest trial with 414 ovarian cancer patients, DTC status did not correlate with FIGO stage, tumor size, lymph node status, histopathologic grading or resection status [26, 27]. Braun et al., in a cohort of 108 primary ovarian cancer patients, showed no concordance between classical prognostic factors and DTC positivity. The only factor associated with positive DTC status was tumor grading (p = 0.02) [7]. These results could be also confirmed in our earlier study with 112 ovarian cancer patients [6]. Similar findings were obtained by other investigators [8, 9, 15, 19].

2.1. Prognostic relevance of DTC/CTC in ovarian cancer

Detection of disseminated tumor cells in patients with primary ovarian cancer was shown to be of prognostic value (Table 1). However, the currently available data are sparse. In our latest trial bone marrow status of 414 ovarian cancer patients was correlated with clinical follow-up [26]. The presence of DTC predicted a shorter OS ($p < 0.001$) and DFS ($p = 0.035$) compared with BM negative patients [27]; this association was highly significant and confirmed in a multivariable Cox regression analysis. Similar results were found in several smaller studies. Braun et al. demonstrated unfavorable prognosis with regard to distant DFS in BM positive patients at the time of diagnosis [7]. DTC presence remained a strong prognostic factor also in a subset of 64 optimally debulked patients ($p = 0.002$), which highlights the role of DTC detection especially in patients who received successful surgical cytoreduction. We previously reported a significant correlation of positive BM status with reduced DFS in a group of 112 stage FIGO I-III ovarian cancer patients [6]. Interestingly, in some studies, the presence of isolated tumor cells in secondary sites, such as BM and blood, was also associated with higher risk for recurrence [10], [6]. Therefore, it might be speculated that hematogenous tumor cell dissemination may serve as an indicator of a more aggressive phenotype of the primary disease that is likely to cause local relapse. In contrast, other authors reported no significant correlation between DTC detection and clinical outcome in ovarian cancer [19, 28]. This discrepancy might be due to differences in study protocols, e.g. time point of BM sample collection (pre- vs. postoperative aspiration). Hypothetically, a transient increase in cancer cell dissemination from the primary tumor due to intraoperative manipulation could contribute to false-positive results and therefore affect further analysis [29].

2.2. Circulating tumor cells

Bone marrow biopsy represents an invasive procedure not well tolerated by many patients. Therefore, detection of circulating tumor cells (CTC) by simple blood drawing has increasingly become a focus of translational research. Prognostic significance of CTC in peripheral blood has been evaluated in breast cancer both in primary and metastatic disease [33, 34]. Two commercially available kits are currently in use for CTC detection in blood of breast cancer patients: antibody-based CellSearch and RT-PCR-based AdnaTest. Both assays were modified and validated in ovarian cancer patients (Table 1). Recently published trial by Poveda et al. based on a cohort of 216 patients with recurrent ovarian cancer, represents the largest study so far on the impact of CTC presence on survival [10]. Using CellSearch test increased CTC numbers (> 1 cell / 7.5 ml blood) were found in 14% of these patients before the beginning of treatment. Detection of CTC in peripheral blood was associated with significantly impaired prognosis. In the study by Aktas et al., including 86 ovarian cancer patients, a modified AdnaTest kit was used to detect cells expressing EpCAM, MUC-1, HER-2 or CA 125-transcripts [8]. CTC positivity rate of 19% observed in this cohort was associated with significantly shorter survival independent of the time of blood sampling (before surgery or after chemotherapy). Similar results were obtained by Fan et al. in a trial of 66 primary ovarian cancer patients [32]. In contrast, Marth et al. reported a 12% positivity rate irrespective of tumor stage but observed no correlation with clinical outcome [19]. Interestingly, positive finding in the blood was highly associated with DTC detection in bone marrow. Smaller studies showed varying CTC incidence, depending on methodology [35, 36].

Author	N	Method	Median follow-up [months]	Positivity rate	Prognostic significance
Fehm [26]	414	DTC (ICC)	34	27%	OS, DFS [1]
Banys [6]	112	DTC (ICC)	12	25%	DFS
Braun [7]	108	DTC (ICC)	45	30%	DFS
Aktas [8]	95	DTC (ICC)	28	35%	n.s.
Schindlbeck [9]	90	DTC (ICC)	28	23%	DDFS
Marth [19]	73	DTC (immunobeads)	25	21%	n.s.
Wimberger [30]	62	DTC (ICC)	18	54%	DFS [2]
Poveda [10]	216	CTC (ICC: CellSearch) [3]		14% [4]	PFS, OS
Sehouli [17]	167	CTC (ICC)	46		n.s.
Marth [19]	90	CTC (immunomagnetic beads)	25	12%	n.s.
Aktas [8]	86	CTC (Multiplex-RT-PCR: AdnaTest)	28	19%	OS [5]
Heubner [31]	68	Circulating 20S-proteasomes	19	-	OS
Fan [32]	66	CTC (immunofluorescence, cell invasion assay)	18	61%	DFS
Wimberger [30]	62	Circulating nucleosomes, DNA, protease and caspase activity	18	-	DFS, OS

Abbreviations: DFS – disease-free survival, DDFS – distant disease-free survival, DTC – disseminated tumor cells in bone marrow, ICC – immunocytochemistry, n.s. – not significant, PFS – progression-free survival

[1] Determined by multivariate Cox regression analysis

[2] DTC detected after chemotherapy

[3] Relapsed ovarian cancer

[4] Two or more CTC

[5] Both before and after chemotherapy

Table 1. Prognostic relevance of disseminated and circulating tumor cells in ovarian cancer.

2.3. Therapy monitoring

Beyond the prognostic value of DTC/CTC detection, monitoring of minimal residual disease (MRD) during and after treatment offers the opportunity to assess response to therapy and evaluate the residual risk of recurrence. Changes in MRD represent the only clinical parameter available after surgical removal of the primary tumor. While tumor markers are established tools for the evaluation of treatment efficacy in patients with advanced ovarian cancer, CA 125 levels fall during adjuvant chemotherapy and remain often below cut-off values after completion of first line systemic treatment even though significant number of patients will suffer from relapse within five years. Furthermore, the clinical relevance of serial CA125 measurements for early detection and treatment of disease recurrence is currently being controversially discussed [37]. In this regard, the detection of isolated tumor cells in bone marrow or peripheral blood might serve as a parameter for occult tumor load after completion of first line therapy. DTC persistence despite adjuvant treatment is so far an independent prognostic factor in patients with primary breast cancer [38]. Whether persistent DTC influence prognosis in ovarian cancer patients, is currently being investigated. In the study by Wimberger et al. DTC counts before and after the first line systemic treatment were correlated to clinical course of disease in 30 ovarian cancer patients; 54% of these patients presented with DTC after first-line chemotherapy. Marked increase in DTC counts was associated with shortened progression free survival [15].

Evaluation of treatment efficacy in ovarian cancer patients after optimal surgical cytoreduction and completion of first line systemic therapy is based on clinical, radiological and biological (tumor marker CA125) criteria. However, a reliable tool to assess long-term prognosis has so far not been established. Therefore, a solid therapy monitoring tool could help to identify a group of high-risk patients who potentially benefit from additional treatment. New studies are required to evaluate whether persistent DTC indeed predict a worse prognosis and if these cells may be targeted by secondary adjuvant therapy.

3. Cancer stem cell model

An important hypothesis on tumor initiation and progression has attracted much attention in the ovarian cancer research in the past decade. In contrast to stochastic model that postulates every cell as a potential source of malignant transformation, the cancer stem cell model, a theory introduced over a century ago, proposes that tumors are organized in a cellular hierarchy, in which cancer stem cell (CSC) are the only cells with tumorigenic potential. Accordingly, tumors are initiated in cancer stem cells or their immediate progeny through imbalance of self-renewal and apoptosis; these tumors contain a cellular subpopulation that retains key stem cell feature [39]. This small cell group with unlimited proliferative potential is assumed to play a marked role in initiation and development of several tumor entities like retinoblastoma, gastrointestinal cancer as well as breast and ovarian cancer [12]. The cancer stem cell concept has important implications for understanding the process of carcinogenesis as well as for designing new treatment strategies. Due to their long life, CSC are more likely to acquire transforming mutations; further, they seem more resistant to apoptosis and DNA damage and are therefore able to persist beyond therapy. New evidence in support of the cancer stem cell model has arisen due to advances in stem cell biology and the introduction of novel animal models to assess self-renewal and challenge the validity of this concept.

The cancer stem cell hypothesis holds that CSC are responsible for phenomena like drug resistance, tumor dormancy or minimal residual disease and may persist beyond chemotherapy and repopulate the tumor leading to relapse [11]. The stem cell subpopulation, but not the remaining differentiated cancer cells in the tumor, can sustain tumor formation and growth due to their high tumor-initiating potential. So far, such cells have been found in several solid tumors, such as colon [40], breast [41] and ovarian cancer [13, 42, 43]. Indeed, in accordance with recent studies, ovarian cancer cell lines feature 'side population' cells (SP) with potential to differentiate into other morphological entities. Thus, this pluripotent subclone with stem cell-like features is considered a marker of CSC presence [14]. The detection of CSC is based on the presence of extracellular markers assumed to be stem cell-specific; commonly identified markers are CD44, CD133, and CD24, which are found in prostate, breast, pancreas, and ovarian cancer. It remains under discussion whether these parameters are universal markers relevant for CSC derived from all tumor types; for ovarian cancer, multiple markers have been described for the stem cell-like tumor initiating cells.

Owing to aggressive natural course of disease and emergence of multidrug resistance, an essential role of cancer stem cells has been postulated in ovarian cancer [13, 44]. In the study by Szotek et al. SP cells have been encountered in ovarian cancer cell lines as well as in primary ascites cancer cells [13]. In the trial by Hosonuma et al. in 18 of 28 ovarian cancer patients samples side population cells could be detected. SP cells occurred more often in relapsed and metastatic patients and SP positivity predicted significantly reduced overall survival [15]. A high proportion of CD44+ stem cells in ovarian cancer was reported to be an independent predictor of poor progression-free survival [45].

As previously mentioned, CSC are considered responsible for high emergence of drug resistance in the natural history of ovarian cancer, since standard therapies fail to target pluripotent tumor-initiating cells [13]. Latifi et al. could show in their recently published trial, the ability of cisplatin chemotherapy to generate residual tumor cells with mesenchymal stem cell-like characteristics *in vitro* [46]. Accordingly, new therapeutic strategies have to be developed to target these cells by identifying their specific antigens. However, very few tumor characteristics have been described to target the subset of CSC.

Based on an animal model, Bapat et al. reported the isolation and identification of ovarian cancer stem cells [42]. In an *in vitro* model comprised of 19 spontaneously immortalized clones derived from an advanced-stage patient, the authors demonstrated the ability of two clones with stem cell-like characteristics to differentiate to grow as spheroids and form xenografts in an animal model (nude mice). These cells were shown to express CD44, E-cadherin, and the stem cell factors Nestin, Nanong, and Oct-4.

3.1. DTC and cancer stem cell model

A currently discussed theory postulate DTC and CTC, the presumed precursor cells of systemic metastatic disease, to be in fact cancer stem cells. These observations have been so far reported in breast cancer studies. Balic et al. analyzed bone marrow specimens from 50 primary breast cancer patients; 33-100% of DTC of every patient exhibited stem cell-like phenotype: CD44+ / CD24 low/- [47]. This prevalence is estimated for less than 10% in primary tumor suggesting much higher, stem cell like self-renewal and tumorigenic potential in DTC. Aktas et al. detected stem cells markers on CTC in peripheral blood of metastatic breast cancer patients [41]. Moreover, Abraham et al. reported that high proportion of stem cell-like subpopulation in primary breast cancer correlate with a higher prevalence of distant metastases [48]. As breast cancer stem cells have been shown to be generally triple-negative, basal-like CTC, independent of the phenotype of the primary tumor, support the cancer stem cell theory [20, 49, 50]. However, this aspect has not been researched in ovarian cancer so far. Therefore, futher studies have to be performed to evaluate whether isolated tumor cells in extraperitoneal sites, such as blood and bone marrow, may reflect ovarian cancer stem cell population.

4. Conclusions

Despite advances in surgical and systemic therapy, ovarian cancer leads to relapse in 60% of patients within 5 years, resulting in impaired clinical outcome. In the last decades, novel biomarkers have been introduced for better prediction and prognostication [51]. Early hematogenous dissemination of single tumor cells is a general phenomenon observed in most solid tumors of epithelial origin; recent data supports the clinical relevance of disseminated and circulating tumor cells (DTC/CTC) in ovarian cancer. A currently discussed hypothesis postulates isolated tumor cells in secondary sites to be not only the presumed precursors of systemic metastatic disease but in fact pluripotent 'cancer stem cells'. Future research will clarify the implications of these findings for clinical management of ovarian cancer patients. While the published data do not support the use of DTC/CTC detection for early detection or screening purposes, its role as an important prognostic factor has been confirmed in several studies. One of the most promising applications of DTC detection is their use as a therapy monitoring tool. DTC persistence beyond surgery and adjuvant chemotherapy may help to identify patients at risk of developing a relapse.

Author details

Malgorzata Banys[1,2], Natalia Krawczyk[1], Andreas D. Hartkopf[1] and Tanja Fehm[1*]

*Address all correspondence to: tanja.fehm@t-online.de

1 Department of Obstetrics and Gynecology, University of Tuebingen, Tuebingen, Germany

2 Department of Obstetrics and Gynecology, Marienkrankenhaus Hamburg, Hamburg, Germany

References

[1] Ries LAG, Harkins D, Krapcho M, Mariotto A, Miller BA, Feuer EJ, Clegg L, Eisner MP, Horner MJ, Howlader N et al: SEER Cancer Statistics Review, 1975-2003. Bethesda, MD 2006.

[2] Black RJ, Bray F, Ferlay J, Parkin DM: Cancer incidence and mortality in the European Union: cancer registry data and estimates of national incidence for 1990. Eur J Cancer 1997, 33(7):1075-1107.

[3] Tingulstad S, Skjeldestad FE, Halvorsen TB, Hagen B: Survival and prognostic factors in patients with ovarian cancer. Obstet Gynecol 2003, 101(5 Pt 1):885-891.

[4] Cannistra SA: Cancer of the ovary. N Engl J Med 2004, 351(24):2519-2529.

[5] Braun S, Vogl FD, Naume B, Janni W, Osborne MP, Coombes RC, Schlimok G, Diel IJ, Gerber B, Gebauer G et al: A pooled analysis of bone marrow micrometastasis in breast cancer. N Engl J Med 2005, 353(8):793-802.

[6] Banys M, Solomayer EF, Becker S, Krawczyk N, Gardanis K, Staebler A, Neubauer H, Wallwiener D, Fehm T: Disseminated tumor cells in bone marrow may affect prognosis of patients with gynecologic malignancies. Int J Gynecol Cancer 2009, 19(5): 948-952.

[7] Braun S, Schindlbeck C, Hepp F, Janni W, Kentenich C, Riethmuller G, Pantel K: Occult tumor cells in bone marrow of patients with locoregionally restricted ovarian cancer predict early distant metastatic relapse. J Clin Oncol 2001, 19(2):368-375.

[8] Aktas B, Kasimir-Bauer S, Heubner M, Kimmig R, Wimberger P: Molecular profiling and prognostic relevance of circulating tumor cells in the blood of ovarian cancer patients at primary diagnosis and after platinum-based chemotherapy. Int J Gynecol Cancer 2011, 21(5):822-830.

[9] Schindlbeck C, Hantschmann P, Zerzer M, Jahns B, Rjosk D, Janni W, Rack B, Sommer H, Friese K: Prognostic impact of KI67, p53, human epithelial growth factor receptor 2, topoisomerase IIalpha, epidermal growth factor receptor, and nm23 expression of ovarian carcinomas and disseminated tumor cells in the bone marrow. Int J Gynecol Cancer 2007, 17(5):1047-1055.

[10] Poveda A, Kaye SB, McCormack R, Wang S, Parekh T, Ricci D, Lebedinsky CA, Tercero JC, Zintl P, Monk BJ: Circulating tumor cells predict progression free survival and overall survival in patients with relapsed/recurrent advanced ovarian cancer. Gynecol Oncol 2011, 122(3):567-572.

[11] Dyall S, Gayther SA, Dafou D: Cancer stem cells and epithelial ovarian cancer. J Oncol 2010, 2010:105269.

[12] Setoguchi T, Taga T, Kondo T: Cancer stem cells persist in many cancer cell lines. Cell Cycle 2004, 3(4):414-415.

[13] Szotek PP, Pieretti-Vanmarcke R, Masiakos PT, Dinulescu DM, Connolly D, Foster R, Dombkowski D, Preffer F, Maclaughlin DT, Donahoe PK: Ovarian cancer side population defines cells with stem cell-like characteristics and Mullerian Inhibiting Substance responsiveness. Proc Natl Acad Sci U S A 2006, 103(30):11154-11159.

[14] Hosonuma S, Kobayashi Y, Kojo S, Wada H, Seino K, Kiguchi K, Ishizuka B: Clinical significance of side population in ovarian cancer cells. Hum Cell 2011, 24(1):9-12.

[15] Wimberger P, Heubner M, Otterbach F, Fehm T, Kimmig R, Kasimir-Bauer S: Influence of platinum-based chemotherapy on disseminated tumor cells in blood and bone marrow of patients with ovarian cancer. Gynecol Oncol 2007, 107(2):331-338.

[16] Wimberger P, Heubner M, Lindhofer H, Jager M, Kimmig R, Kasimir-Bauer S: Influence of catumaxomab on tumor cells in bone marrow and blood in ovarian cancer. Anticancer Res 2009, 29(5):1787-1791.

[17] Sehouli J, Konsgen D, Nimpsch R, Stengel D, Oskay G, Mustea A, Oertel J, Lichtenegger W: Prognostic significance of epithelial cells in the blood of patients with gynaecological malignancies. Anticancer Res 2003, 23(5b):4133-4140.

[18] Janni W, Hepp F, Strobl B, Rack B, Rjosk D, Kentenich C, Schindlbeck C, Hantschmann P, Pantel K, Sommer H et al: Patterns of disease recurrence influenced by hematogenous tumor cell dissemination in patients with cervical carcinoma of the uterus. Cancer 2003, 97(2):405-411.

[19] Marth C, Kisic J, Kaern J, Trope C, Fodstad O: Circulating tumor cells in the peripheral blood and bone marrow of patients with ovarian carcinoma do not predict prognosis. Cancer 2002, 94(3):707-712.

[20] Fehm T, Hoffmann O, Aktas B, Becker S, Solomayer EF, Wallwiener D, Kimmig R, Kasimir-Bauer S: Detection and characterization of circulating tumor cells in blood of primary breast cancer patients by RT-PCR and comparison to status of bone marrow disseminated cells. Breast Cancer Res 2009, 11(4):R59.

[21] Fehm T, Solomayer EF, Meng S, Tucker T, Lane N, Wang J, Gebauer G: Methods for isolating circulating epithelial cells and criteria for their classification as carcinoma cells. Cytotherapy 2005, 7(2):171-185.

[22] Fehm T, Becker S, Bachmann C, Beck V, Gebauer G, Banys M, Wallwiener D, Solomayer EF: Detection of disseminated tumor cells in patients with gynecological cancers. Gynecol Oncol 2006, 103(3):942-947.

[23] Fehm T, Braun S, Muller V, Janni W, Gebauer G, Marth C, Schindlbeck C, Wallwiener D, Borgen E, Naume B et al: A concept for the standardized detection of disseminated tumor cells in bone marrow from patients with primary breast cancer and its clinical implementation. Cancer 2006, 107(5):885-892.

[24] Pantel K, Brakenhoff RH: Dissecting the metastatic cascade. Nat Rev Cancer 2004, 4(6):448-456.

[25] Lengyel E: Ovarian cancer development and metastasis. Am J Pathol 2010, 177(3): 1053-1064.

[26] Fehm T, Banys M, Marth C, Neubauer H, Hartkopf A, Trope C, Kimmig R, Krawczyk N, Wallwiener D, Wimberger P et al: Detection of disseminated tumor cells in the bone marrow is an independent prognostic factor in primary ovarian cancer patients. in press 2012.

[27] Wimberger P, Banys M, Kasimir-Bauer S, Hartkopf AD, Krawczyk N, Marth C, Kimmig R, Neubauer H, Wallwiener D, Fehm TN: Detection of disseminated tumor cells in bone marrow as an independent prognostic factor in primary ovarian cancer patients (ASCO 2012). J Clin Oncol 2012, 30 (suppl; abstr 5042).

[28] Cain JM, Ellis GK, Collins C, Greer BE, Tamimi HK, Figge DC, Gown AM, Livingston RB: Bone marrow involvement in epithelial ovarian cancer by immunocytochemical assessment. Gynecol Oncol 1990, 38(3):442-445.

[29] Camara O, Kavallaris A, Noschel H, Rengsberger M, Jorke C, Pachmann K: Seeding of epithelial cells into circulation during surgery for breast cancer: the fate of malignant and benign mobilized cells. World J Surg Oncol 2006, 4:67.

[30] Wimberger P, Roth C, Pantel K, Kasimir-Bauer S, Kimmig R, Schwarzenbach H: Impact of platinum-based chemotherapy on circulating nucleic acid levels, protease activities in blood and disseminated tumor cells in bone marrow of ovarian cancer patients. Int J Cancer 2010.

[31] Heubner M, Wimberger P, Dahlmann B, Kasimir-Bauer S, Kimmig R, Peters J, Wohlschlaeger J, Sixt SU: The prognostic impact of circulating proteasome concentrations in patients with epithelial ovarian cancer. Gynecol Oncol 2011, 120(2):233-238.

[32] Fan T, Zhao Q, Chen JJ, Chen WT, Pearl ML: Clinical significance of circulating tumor cells detected by an invasion assay in peripheral blood of patients with ovarian cancer. Gynecol Oncol 2009, 112(1):185-191.

[33] Cristofanilli M, Budd GT, Ellis MJ, Stopeck A, Matera J, Miller MC, Reuben JM, Doyle GV, Allard WJ, Terstappen LW et al: Circulating tumor cells, disease progression, and survival in metastatic breast cancer. N Engl J Med 2004, 351(8):781-791.

[34] Rack BK, Schindlbeck C, Andergassen U, Schneeweiss A, Zwingers T, Lichtenegger W, Beckmann M, Sommer HL, Pantel K, Janni W: Use of circulating tumor cells (CTC) in peripheral blood of breast cancer patients before and after adjuvant chemotherapy to predict risk for relapse: The SUCCESS trial. ASCO Annual Meeting 2010. J Clin Oncol 2010, 28:15s (suppl; abstr 1003).

[35] Ntouroupi TG, Ashraf SQ, McGregor SB, Turney BW, Seppo A, Kim Y, Wang X, Kilpatrick MW, Tsipouras P, Tafas T et al: Detection of circulating tumour cells in peripheral blood with an automated scanning fluorescence microscope. Br J Cancer 2008, 99(5):789-795.

[36] Engel H, Kleespies C, Friedrich J, Breidenbach M, Kallenborn A, Schondorf T, Kolhagen H, Mallmann P: Detection of circulating tumour cells in patients with breast or ovarian cancer by molecular cytogenetics. Br J Cancer 1999, 81(7):1165-1173.

[37] Rustin GJ, van der Burg ME, Griffin CL, Guthrie D, Lamont A, Jayson GC, Kristensen G, Mediola C, Coens C, Qian W et al: Early versus delayed treatment of relapsed ovarian cancer (MRC OV05/EORTC 55955): a randomised trial. Lancet 2010, 376(9747):1155-1163.

[38] Janni W, Rack B, Schindlbeck C, Strobl B, Rjosk D, Braun S, Sommer H, Pantel K, Gerber B, Friese K: The persistence of isolated tumor cells in bone marrow from patients with breast carcinoma predicts an increased risk for recurrence. Cancer 2005, 103(5):884-891.

[39] Wicha MS, Liu S, Dontu G: Cancer stem cells: an old idea--a paradigm shift. Cancer Res 2006, 66(4):1883-1890; discussion 1895-1886.

[40] Ricci-Vitiani L, Lombardi DG, Pilozzi E, Biffoni M, Todaro M, Peschle C, De Maria R: Identification and expansion of human colon-cancer-initiating cells. Nature 2007, 445(7123):111-115.

[41] Aktas B, Tewes M, Fehm T, Hauch S, Kimmig R, Kasimir-Bauer S: Stem cell and epithelial-mesenchymal transition markers are frequently overexpressed in circulating tumor cells of metastatic breast cancer patients. Breast Cancer Res 2009, 11(4):R46.

[42] Bapat SA, Mali AM, Koppikar CB, Kurrey NK: Stem and progenitor-like cells contribute to the aggressive behavior of human epithelial ovarian cancer. Cancer Res 2005, 65(8):3025-3029.

[43] Challen GA, Little MH: A side order of stem cells: the SP phenotype. Stem Cells 2006, 24(1):3-12.

[44] Ponnusamy MP, Batra SK: Ovarian cancer: emerging concept on cancer stem cells. J Ovarian Res 2008, 1(1):4.

[45] Steffensen KD, Alvero AB, Yang Y, Waldstrom M, Hui P, Holmberg JC, Silasi DA, Jakobsen A, Rutherford T, Mor G: Prevalence of epithelial ovarian cancer stem cells correlates with recurrence in early-stage ovarian cancer. J Oncol 2011, 2011:620523.

[46] Latifi A, Abubaker K, Castrechini N, Ward AC, Liongue C, Dobill F, Kumar J, Thompson EW, Quinn MA, Findlay JK et al: Cisplatin treatment of primary and metastatic epithelial ovarian carcinomas generates residual cells with mesenchymal stem cell-like profile. J Cell Biochem 2011.

[47] Balic M, Lin H, Young L, Hawes D, Giuliano A, McNamara G, Datar RH, Cote RJ: Most early disseminated cancer cells detected in bone marrow of breast cancer patients have a putative breast cancer stem cell phenotype. Clin Cancer Res 2006, 12(19):5615-5621.

[48] Abraham BK, Fritz P, McClellan M, Hauptvogel P, Athelogou M, Brauch H: Prevalence of CD44+/CD24-/low cells in breast cancer may not be associated with clinical outcome but may favor distant metastasis. Clin Cancer Res 2005, 11(3):1154-1159.

[49] Dontu G, Al-Hajj M, Abdallah WM, Clarke MF, Wicha MS: Stem cells in normal breast development and breast cancer. Cell Prolif 2003, 36 Suppl 1:59-72.

[50] Asselin-Labat ML, Shackleton M, Stingl J, Vaillant F, Forrest NC, Eaves CJ, Visvader JE, Lindeman GJ: Steroid hormone receptor status of mouse mammary stem cells. J Natl Cancer Inst 2006, 98(14):1011-1014.

[51] Banys M, Krawczyk N, Fehm T: New Tumor Biomarkers in Ovarian Cancer and Its Prognostic and Clinical Relevance. In: Ovarian Cancer - Basic Science Perspective. Edited by Farghaly SA: InTech; 2012.